Elastography of the Liver and Beyond

Mirella Fraquelli

Editor

Elastography of the Liver and Beyond

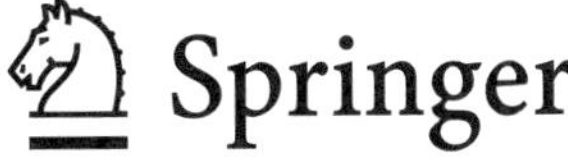 Springer

Editor
Mirella Fraquelli
Gastroenterology and Endoscopy Unit
Fondazione IRCCS Ca' Granda Ospedale Maggiore Policlinico
Milan
Italy

ISBN 978-3-030-74134-1   ISBN 978-3-030-74132-7   (eBook)
https://doi.org/10.1007/978-3-030-74132-7

This Springer imprint is published by the registered company Springer Nature Switzerland AG
The registered company address is: Gewerbestrasse 11, 6330 Cham, Switzerland

Foreword

In the era of precision medicine, accurate staging of a disease stands out as a must whenever a trustable prognostication is needed and prioritization to costly therapies is to be decided based on sophisticated cost efficacy analyses. In the liver domain, the histopathological examination of the liver tissue via a percutaneous liver biopsy has long been the pillar of the process of clinical staging, though its employment has been limited by cost, sampling error, and poor agreement among pathologists and complications. There is no question that, in patients with more than one risk factor, the liver biopsy is a priority as it stands as the sole approach able to define the contribution of each underlying comorbidity to the whole picture of the disease, thereby providing a guide to select the proper therapeutic approach in many circumstances. Though in other contexts involving a majority of patients with chronic viral hepatitis and non-alcoholic fatty liver, disease staging with the canonical histopathological approach has come of age, being replaced either by cheap scores for disease severity stratification that are based on simple demographic and clinical parameters or by user friendly imaging techniques which assess liver stiffness. These noninvasive tests have gained popularity as they have successfully been applied to identify and stage liver disease across multiple etiologies and proved useful to identify subclinical hepatic injury not accompanied by symptoms and/or abnormalities of serum liver chemistries, stage severity of overt chronic liver disease, and confirm resolution of an acute liver injury. On the assumption that they could fill the diagnostic gap of the classical serum chemistries, a majority of these assays were initially conceived as markers of hepatic fibrosis, the relevant determinant of prognosis of most chronic liver disorders. Lately, the same noninvasive assays were more appropriately converted into tests of disease severity, as it became clear that these tests are also altered in the presence of necro-inflammation and degeneration of liver cell and biliary injury. This book is devoted to elastography to assess liver stiffness, a technique which should be commended by all hepatologists for having revolutionized the approach to liver disease staging and management of most patients with chronic liver disorders. At the onset, the prototype FibroScan made the process of disease severity stratification simple and user friendly as it was required for prioritizing patients with viral hepatitis to treatment with exceedingly expensive antiviral regimens. In the last decade, elastography has evolved different technical modalities in the context of ultrasound and magnetic resonance imaging that have been applied to cost effectively manage patients with non-alcoholic fatty liver with respect to patient stratification for surveillance versus therapeutic interventions. Not surprisingly, the restless revolution started with elastography has overcome the boundaries of liver disease, ultimately engaging the spleen for the noninvasive evaluation of portal hypertension and the gastrointestinal tract where in cooperation with endoscopy, elastography has proven useful to investigate pancreas, colon strictures, and inflammatory bowel diseases.

Milan, Italy   Massimo Colombo

Preface

Over the last two decades, the application of sono-elastographic techniques, conceived to assess tissue stiffness, has experienced a dramatic boost in the field of hepatology and gastroenterology.

Liver stiffness measured by Vibration-Controlled Transient Elastography (VCTE), also commonly known as transient elastography (TE or Fibroscan®), has been widely validated as an accurate tool for the indirect staging of liver fibrosis. More recently, liver stiffness has been demonstrated to be a valid prognostic marker of disease severity in patients with chronic liver diseases (CLDs), as it is able to predict such clinically relevant outcomes as survival, OLT, decompensation, and development of liver cancer.

The book is not just a simple overview of the main practical applications of sono-elastography to date as far as hepatological and gastroenterological diseases are concerned, but it is also specifically intended to illustrate, with a clear critical methodological approach, the correct indication for the use of these diagnostic techniques in specific clinical settings. We have taken into account the existing diagnostic pathways, the actual diagnostic accuracy of elastographic techniques and their impact on clinical practice in terms of improvement of clinically relevant outcomes and cost-saving clinical management.

In the first part dedicated to the correct methodology to assess diagnostic accuracy of noninvasive techniques, we have discussed the architecture of diagnostic research and emphasized the correct study design for each phase of a diagnostic study development.

In the second part of this book, we have focused on clarifying the definition of normal value for liver stiffness and the role of VTCE in dealing with patients with liver diseases of different etiology by measuring liver stiffness towards the assessment of liver fibrosis and as a prognostic marker for the development of CLD-related complications.

We have provided a critical comparison of the different existing elastographic techniques, i.e., VTCE vs. ARFI technologies as implemented on standard ultrasound machines.

In the third part of the book, the spotlight is on the role of liver and spleen stiffness measurement in advanced liver diseases as predictors of portal hypertension and as a prognostic marker of clinically relevant outcomes.

The fourth part is devoted to the role of elastography in some fields of gastroenterology, such as the study of the pancreas (for instance, in chronic pancreatitis and alcoholic abuse), the intestine (in patients with chronic inflammatory bowel diseases), and of hematological and vascular diseases.

At last, the book offers a series of case studies on specific practical issues with critical discussion to improve the appropriate use of these technologies.

We remain available to comments and suggestions on how to add to the comprehensiveness of the present endeavors.

Milan, Italy   Mirella Fraquelli

Contents

Part I

Introduction to Elastography

Elastographic Measures: A Methodological Approach

1

Agostino Colli, Mirella Fraquelli, and Giovanni Casazza

At the end of the twentieth century, such techniques as ultrasonography, computerized tomography and magnetic resonance imaging were developed and made available to hepatologists enabling them to watch their patients' liver morphology and to detect even small focal lesions in the parenchyma. The viscoelastic properties of the liver were still assessed by palpation: a hard liver was associated with severe fibrosis [1]. Palpation, the use of the tactile sense to determine the characteristics of an organ, is one of the four cardinal principles of physical examination and relies on both qualitative and subjective estimations. So, a system for the quantitative assessment of tissue stiffness was needed. Furthermore, the diagnosis and staging of chronic hepatitis and, more generally, chronic liver diseases were mainly based on histological scores requiring liver biopsy, which is an invasive procedure. Thus, a non-invasive test was needed.

Over the recent years, a new method for measuring the shear velocity in soft tissues through transient elastography was developed [2]. TE consists in a pulsed excitation driven by a piston vibrating perpendicularly to the surface of a half-space viscoelastic medium. The axial component of the displacements induced by the transient shear wave is estimated with an ultrasonic transducer placed on the opposite side of the medium allowing the estimates of both shear elasticity and shear viscosity [2, 3]. Further progressive improvements have led to the development of an easy-to-use device that allowed the measurement of liver stiffness [3, 4]. The

A. Colli (✉)
Department of Transfusion Medicine and Haematology, Fondazione IRCCS Ca' Granda Ospedale Maggiore Policlinico, Milan, Italy

M. Fraquelli
Gastroenterology and Endoscopy Unit, Fondazione IRCCS Ca' Granda Ospedale Maggiore Policlinico, Milan, Italy

G. Casazza
Department of Biomedical and Clinical Sciences "L. Sacco", Università degli Studi di Milano, Milan, Italy

© Springer Nature Switzerland AG 2021
M. Fraquelli (ed.), *Elastography of the Liver and Beyond*,
https://doi.org/10.1007/978-3-030-74132-7_1

"

next steps have been to evaluate this system for the diagnosis and staging of chronic liver diseases: hepatic fibrosis was recognized as the main factor for the prognosis of chronic liver diseases [5, 6], and many studies have aimed to evaluate the accuracy of transient elastography in diagnosing liver fibrosis [7, 8]. TE has proved to be an accurate tool to evaluate liver fibrosis in different chronic liver diseases, with accuracy estimates quite similar to those of the reference standard, i.e. liver histology. The staging of liver disease through elastography seems even more accurate than through histology as shown by a large-cohort prognostic study [9].

This is the story of a real success of a diagnostic test from the bench to the bedside: a new tool that allows both a quantitative assessment of liver stiffness overcoming old-fashioned palpation and an accurate estimate of liver disease severity.

In this chapter, we aimed to summarize the different phases of the development of a new diagnostic test, from bench to the bedside, outlining and discussing the proper approaches to the different questions and the methodological problems [10].

1.1   Phase 0

This is the preclinical phase with the in-laboratory assessment of the properties of the new diagnostic tool, not yet on patients but rather on phantoms, animals or a small number of healthy participants. The aim is to assess:

1. *Validity*: the extent to which a test measures what it is intended to measure.
2. *Reliability*: the consistency of any variation of the test measurements with the true variations, usually subdivided in:
    (a) *Repeatability*: the ability to reproduce the same results in identical settings (same device, same operator) when testing the same patient.
    (b) *Reproducibility*: the ability to obtain the same results when testing the same patient under changing conditions (different operators or different devices).

The new technique, TE, measures liver elasticity using a shear elasticity probe over a short time (less than 100 ms) reducing boundary and movement artefacts [1, 2, 11]; its reliability, as to repeatability and reproducibility, was assessed in chronic liver disease (CLD) patients [10, 11], and the overall inter-observer and intra-observer agreement intraclass correlation coefficients were 0.98 [12].

It is interesting to note that manual palpation with judgement of normal/hard consistency shows low reproducibility (Cohen's $k = 0.4$) which is usual for most physical signs [13].

The answer to these preliminary questions about validity, reliability and reproducibility is the first step and is necessary for furthering the evaluation of a test. The diagnostic accuracy of a test can be estimated only if its reproducibility has been considered acceptable. Moreover, the modalities of test performance, which ensure the best validity and reproducibility, are defined and described in this phase [4, 12].

1.2 Phase 1

This phase focuses on the definition of the range of the new test results in healthy people and the influence of sex, age, BMI and other anthropometric characteristics (narrow intercostal spaces or overweight). The elastographic measures of the liver are expressed as a continuous variable in the International System of Units (SI) of pressure kiloPascal (kPa); the distribution of its values is asymmetric, and the reference values fall between the 2.5th and 97.5th percentile of the distribution for healthy individuals. This is the simplest way to establish a "normal" value: ignoring the distribution shape and simply referring to the highest and lowest values as "abnormal" [14]. However, the implicit assumption that all the diseases they represent should have exactly the same frequency, i.e. around 5%, is clearly a clinical nonsense: it would mean that 5% healthy people should, by definition, have "abnormal" values and should be tested further to assess whether they are true "false-positive" or not. On the contrary, the aim of this phase should be to estimate the clinical reference interval assessing the distribution with a sample, in general, or a healthy population large enough to show that the observed "false-positive" proportion is less than a pre-specified value. This early phase may be initially skipped, and the pertinent studies not published. The distribution of the test results and evaluation of the influence of patient characteristics on these results can be assessed in the next phase, which compares healthy controls to patients affected by the disease under investigation.

There are some examples of Phase 1 studies assessing liver stiffness in healthy volunteers, blood donors and general population [15–17]. They have shown that the distribution of reference values was very similar in all three groups and that the liver stiffness values were not influenced by age and were positively related to male sex, increased BMI, fatty liver and metabolic syndrome variables [15].

1.3 Phase 2

The studies in this phase aim to assess the diagnostic accuracy of the index test (Fig. 1.1). Diagnostic accuracy is a measurement of the agreement between the index test and the reference standard in discriminating diseased from non-diseased study participants. Accuracy can be evaluated as a whole, i.e. the proportion of correct results of the index test against those of the reference standard; however, it is more informative to assess how many participants with and without the target disease are correctly defined by the test with two other estimates, which are sensitivity and specificity. Sensitivity is the measure of concordance between the index test and the reference standard for diseased participants, i.e. the proportion of diseased participants detected by the index test. Specificity is the measure of the concordance for

> **Index test:** a diagnostic test under assessment
>
> **Target disease:** the pathological condition that the index test aims to identify
>
> **Reference standard:** a test or procedure taken to best identify a patient's true state (diseased or non-diseased).
>
> **Diagnostic accuracy:** the proportion of correct results of the index test.
>
> **The 2-by-2 table:**
>
> | Index test | | Diseased | Non-diseased |
> |---|---|---|---|
> | | **Positive** | true positive | false positive |
> | | **Negative** | false negative | true negative |
>
> **Sensitivity:** the proportion of true positive results (proportion of positive test results among the study participants with the target disease)
> **Specificity:** the proportion of true negative results (proportion of negative test results among the study participants without the target disease)
>
> **Positive likelihood ratio:**
> the ratio of the probability of a positive test result among the participants with the target disease to the probability of a positive test result among the participants without the target disease
>
> **Negative likelihood ratio:**
> the ratio of the probability of a negative test result among the participants with the target disease to the probability of a negative test result among the participants without the target disease

Fig. 1.1 Glossary and definitions of diagnostic studies

non-diseased participants, i.e. the proportion of non-diseased participants correctly identified by the index test.

In this phase, a logical sequence of diagnostic studies can be recognized. They start from preliminary questions allowing the correct design of further studies, hopefully having a progressive increase in the strength of evidence in favour of the index test, in order to obtain an actual definition and assessment of the test's diagnostic accuracy.

The first question is whether the test results obtained in affected patients differ from those in healthy individuals. It relates not only to the distribution of test results among diseased and healthy participants but also to the degree of their overlap. The lower the degree of overlap, the more accurate the test is considered to be. The inter-individual true variability within well-designed, well-conducted Phase 0 studies can provide an explanation about the variability of test results in Phase 2 studies. The usual design format of such Phase 2 studies is one in which affected and healthy participants are sampled and the obtained test value is measured once (case-control design) (Fig. 1.2). These studies are relatively simple and can readily advise on whether a more in-depth assessment of the test accuracy should or should not be performed.

A further preliminary question is whether the results of the index test obtained in patients with the target disease are different from those obtained in patients in whom the target disease could have been suspected but is not present. The study design format is again case-control; nevertheless, "controls" are no more healthy individuals, but participants with some clinical suspicion of the target disease and a negative result of the reference standard test. They are compared to "cases", i.e. participants with a positive reference standard test.

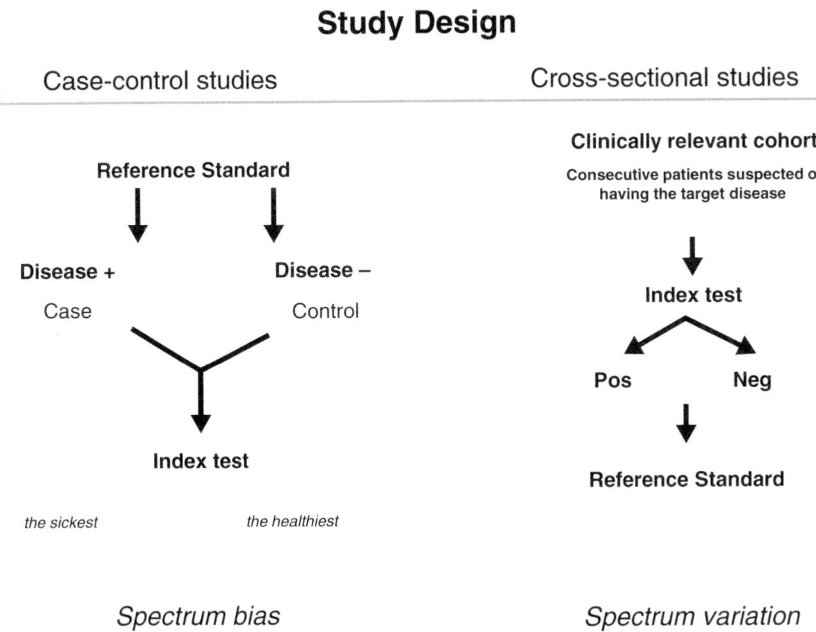

Fig. 1.2 Design of diagnostic accuracy studies: case-control and cross-sectional design formats

Another preliminary question regards the results of the index test in patients with different stages of the target disease. A case-control study can answer this question selecting groups of patients with a known stage of the disease.

A further step aims to explore whether the abnormal results to the index test are specifically associated with the target disease. Other diseases might produce the same results as the target disease or patients affected by the target disease and by another concomitant disease might present different results than patients affected only by the target disease. Again, case-control studies can answer these questions: two pertinent groups of participants are selected and compared.

Case-control studies will establish whether the index test can discriminate between the affected and non-affected patients, but such studies are not yet intended to estimate true sensitivity and specificity in a clinical context. In fact, the estimates can be flawed as a consequence of the inclusion of participants on the basis of the results of the reference standard test. In case-control studies, the participants have to undergo the reference standard before the index test: people known to be affected by the target disease ("cases") and people who are not affected ("controls"; i.e. healthy people or people with other diseases than the target condition) are selected according to the results of the reference standard. Thus, a spectrum bias is potentially introduced with a consequent overestimation of the index test's accuracy. In fact, the participants do not represent the actual spectrum of the severity of the target disease as well as alternative conditions, particularly if the sickest of the sick ones are compared to the healthiest of the healthy people (Fig. 1.2).

Concerning elastography and liver fibrosis, there are some examples of studies answering these preliminary questions. High values of liver stiffness, comparable to those obtained in patients with severe liver fibrosis, have been shown in such conditions as cholestasis or heart failure with increased hepatic venous pressure [18, 19]. Other studies have shown that, in patients with acute hepatitis or a flare of chronic hepatitis, liver stiffness values paralleled those of alanine aminotransferase (ALT), thus showing that the results of the index test are influenced by the presence of acute hepatitis with inflammation and necrosis (concurrent disease) on chronic hepatitis with fibrosis (the target disease) [20, 21].

Cross-sectional studies on consecutive series of participants are not flawed by spectrum bias (Fig. 1.2). Among the enrolled participants, there should only be participants with symptoms suggesting the target disease, but no patients with full-blown severe manifestations of the target disease and no healthy controls. This is the proper Phase 2A study design format, which addresses the question whether the index test is able to detect the target condition among patients suspected of having the target disease, and to assess the index test accuracy (sensitivity and specificity).

The accuracy of the index test is a measure of the concordance of its results with those obtained by the reference standard (Fig. 1.1). A "reference standard" is a test or procedure considered as best identifying the true state (diseased or non-diseased); actually no test is perfectly accurate (a.k.a. "gold standard"), but the test with the relatively best and accepted accuracy can be used as reference. In order to define this concordance, two measures are needed: sensitivity and specificity. Sensitivity is the proportion of true-positive patients, i.e. those with the target disease and positive results of the index test, among the patients with the target disease. Specificity is the proportion of true-negative patients, i.e. those without the target disease and with negative results of the index test, among the patients without the target disease. The two-by-two table provided facilitates the presentation and classification of the index results: two columns, diseased and non-diseased patients, and two rows, positive and negative index test. Sensitivity and specificity are two properties of the index tests and they cannot be separately estimated and evaluated. Likelihood ratios allow the simultaneous consideration of sensitivity and specificity and can be interpreted as the relative risk of being positive (or negative) to the index test for diseased compared to non-diseased patients. The likelihood ratio of the index test can inform on how much the probability of having the target disease varies after the test (post-test probability) if the results of the index test are positive or negative. The higher the value of the positive likelihood ratio (LR+), the higher the probability of having the target disease; the lower the negative likelihood ratio (LR−), the lower this probability.

Many diagnostic tests, and elastography is one of these, produce an explicit continuous measure, which is dichotomized at some threshold value to call the result positive or negative. Identifying the optimal threshold value to use in practice is usually of crucial clinical importance. Youden's J index (J = sensitivity + specificity − 1) can help in defining the cut-off value associated with highest accuracy; nevertheless, the optimal cut-off value is not always the one that ensures best accuracy. In fact, this index assumes that sensitivity and specificity are of equal importance, and this assumption is not true in most clinical contexts. If the test is intended to exclude the presence of a condition, for instance, severe hepatic fibrosis by elastography, a false-negative result could be more relevant than a false-positive one. An alternative and more clinically oriented approach would be to consider the downstream effects of testing in terms of false-negative and false-positive results: such an approach would identify those patients with the minimum degree of "abnormality" requiring treatment [17].

Dichotomizing test results implies that some information is lost. In fact, two individuals close to, but on opposite sides of, the cut-off point are characterized as being quite different rather than very similar [22]. Anyway, grouping simplifies the statistical analysis and leads to the easy interpretation and presentation of results. Considering the role of the index test, two cut-off values can be chosen: one to exclude the presence of the target disease and one to confirm its presence. This choice produces a grey zone of indeterminate results for which further testing is needed: the more patients are in this zone, the less useful the test is.

Cut-off values are defined in cross-sectional Phase 2 studies, including consecutive participants with symptoms or signs suggesting the target disease. When these threshold values are derived from the obtained data, the accuracy of the index test is overestimated and validation studies are needed [23].

Sometimes, the results of the index test cannot be classified as either positive or negative. The test is unable to produce assessable results in all patients and some results are inadequate or indeterminate. This technical failure is not rare for elastographic measurements in that obesity, ascites and hepatic steatosis may impair the validity and reliability of the results. About 10% of patients cannot be assessed by transient elastography [4, 12, 17], and this proportion is even higher for spleen stiffness measurement [24] or ultrasound surveillance of hepatocellular carcinoma in patients with cirrhosis [25]. Simply excluding from analysis these non-assessable results overestimates the test accuracy: there is no consensus on how to handle this circumstance. Applying an intention-to-diagnose approach can provide a more realistic picture of the clinical potential of diagnostic tests [26]. According to this approach, also known as worst-case scenario [27], non-assessable results are classified as false-positive if they had a negative reference standard, or false-negative with a positive reference standard.

The accuracy of the index test, once assessed, can be compared to that of other tests (Phase 2B). The question is which of two or more tests is more or most accurate? The answer is possible with two different study design formats. The first format is the cross-sectional study including consecutive participants who are likely to harbour the target disease and who undergo the index test as well as the reference standard. Thus, a direct comparison of sensitivity and specificity between the different index tests is possible. An example is the direct comparison of different elastography techniques [28]: 349 participants with liver disease underwent supersonic shear imaging, acoustic radiation force impulse (ARFI) and TE as index tests and liver biopsy as the reference standard. The second study design format is the randomized clinical trial (RCT): consecutive participants suspected of having the target disease are randomized to the different index tests. This study design format allows for only indirect comparison of sensitivity and specificity between the two different index tests in two groups made comparable by randomization [29]. This design is rarely used and should be selected when participants cannot undergo both tests because of their risk of harm or costs or both.

The further phase (Phase 2C) studies explore the possible consequences of the introduction of the index test into clinical practice. The diagnostic strategy incorporating the index test is compared with the current standard evaluation. These studies are conducted on participants in whom it is clinically sensible to suspect the target disease in order to assess any immediate downstream consequence of testing and offering treatment, based on that testing [30]. These studies are designed to compare the new diagnostic-therapeutic strategy that incorporates the index test, against the current best diagnostic strategy for managing these patients. The studies should mainly address safety aspects by enabling the capturing of possible harms as a consequence of introducing the index test. Harms from diagnosis can result from misclassification with two opposite types of error (false-negative or false-positive). The risk is not only to overlook the target disease but also to overdiagnose it. On considering the prognosis of an untreated disease and the effectiveness and possible harm of available treatments, one has to define what types of error to avoid. The objective is to minimize the penalty of being wrong. Sometimes, it is better to minimize the number of false-negative results and, other times, that of false-positive results. A direct, or even indirect, comparison between sensitivity and specificity of the index test with existing tests makes it possible to hypothesize the role of the index test in a new strategy to diagnose the target disease: as a replacement for the existing test, as an add-on test after the existing test or as a triage test before the existing test [31]. In general, a more accurate (higher sensitivity and higher specificity) or safer test can replace the existing ones. On the other hand, tests with remarkably high sensitivity can rule the target disease out and could be proposed as triage tests before any further harmful or costly testing, whereas tests with remarkably high specificity can be purposed as add-on tests. Thus, the operative characteristics of the new test and its risk of harm and/or costs suggest a possible role for the test. It is in this role that the new diagnostic test should properly be evaluated in Phase 2C and subsequent Phase 3 randomized clinical trials (RCTs), which assess the downstream effects of the new strategy.

1.4   Phase 3

Phase 3 studies aim to assess the benefits and harms of a diagnostic test. No diagnostic test can, by itself, ever be of benefit for a patient. However, through a diagnostic test, we can reach a decision about which treatment to offer patients. Therefore, the question posed in Phase 3 RCTs deals not only with the test accuracy but also with the benefits and harms of any treatment decided on the basis of the test results. The appropriate study design format is, again, an RCT or, more appropriately, an RCT on diagnostic plus therapeutic strategies. The most important methodological issues are allocation sequence generation, allocation concealment, blinding, follow-up, reporting of all outcomes and transparency regarding conflicts of interest that are central in a therapeutic RCT. They should also be considered for the diagnostic-therapeutic RCT to secure internal and external validity. Furthermore, the "critical comparison" between the new diagnostic-therapeutic strategy and the current strategy should be identified. If the index test is intended to improve the sensitivity of the diagnostic strategy, the benefits and harms of the treatment in the additional positive patients should be assessed. Provided that previous trials have shown the efficacy of the treatment among patients detected by the current standard test, the benefits and harms of the treatment in the additional patients detected by the index tests may not be the same, and this needs to be evaluated. If the new test is intended to improve the specificity of the diagnostic strategy, then the possible benefit of fewer false-positive results has to be assessed. Furthermore, an improvement in specificity usually entails impairment in sensitivity and vice versa. A more sensitive test is expected to be less specific, and the consequences of this possible trade-off should be carefully explored. The downstream effects of the additional false-negative or false-positive results have to be accurately assessed.

Diagnostic test-therapeutic trials are appropriate to solve the problem of the target diseases for which there is no reference standard or the one available is imperfect. In this case, the index test results classified as false may actually be true ones. In fact, a result of the index test named false-positive might be a true-positive and a false-negative of the imperfect (less sensitive) reference test. On the contrary, a false-negative result of the index test might be a true-negative as a consequence of a more specific index test. RCTs that compare the downstream effects of the application of the index test versus the test regarded as the current reference test are able to estimate which test is more effective and thus indirectly more accurate.

1.5 Phase 4

Phase 4 studies are conducted after the index test has been introduced into clinical practice to reassess the benefits and harms of the index-test treatment versus the reference-test treatment strategies. They are designed as large RCTs or cohort studies of patients tested with the index test; they play a role in redefining the accuracy of the index test. This may be required in case of an imperfect reference standard in order to verify discordant results. Through planning the adequate follow-up of the patients with different results for the index test and the reference standard test (i.e. classified as false-positive or false-negative), these longitudinal studies would allow detecting the actual appearance of the target disease or its complications.

As an example, a large-cohort study compared the accuracy of liver stiffness measurement and liver biopsy in predicting overall survival or complications and decompensation of liver cirrhosis in participants with discordant results of the two tests [9]. This longitudinal observation allows to answer the question: in case of disagreement between the index test and the reference standard test, which are the right results?

1.6 Conclusions

Looking back at the history of liver elastography, we have described the five-phase development of a new diagnostic test from the definition of its properties and operative characteristics up to the demonstration of its value to clinical practice. The early phases are necessary for the correct design of the later phases, hopefully progressively increasing the strength of evidence in favour of the index test. However, even if logically consecutive, the progression of diagnostic research may be non-linear. An earlier phase may be initially skipped, or its answer be provided by later-phase studies.

This categorization carries the advantage of being more comparable to the phases of therapeutic research (e.g. as for drugs or medical devices). It is essential that the diagnostic accuracy assessment should not be perceived as the final objective of diagnostic research, but only as a necessary step in the introduction of a test to clinical practice. In fact, for most tests, the clinical consequences of their application to clinical practice are not sufficiently obvious from the definition of their sensitivity and specificity. To address this question, we require diagnostic-treatment RCTs, even if very few trials have been conducted to date. When two or more diagnostic-treatment RCTs have been completed, their systematic reviews, possibly with meta-analyses, are warranted and should be conducted before such new tests are introduced into clinical practice. Then, large-cohort surveillance studies would enable the determination of the actual effects. These final studies are very important because they represent a unique opportunity to assess the real effect of the test on the clinical practice and because such studies can reliably measure a test's benefits as well as identify rare instances of harm that may not be captured through RCTs.

References

1. Zoli M, Magalotti D, Grimaldi M, Gueli C, Marchesini G, Pisi E. Physical examination of the liver: is it still worth it? Am J Gastroenterol. 1995;90:1428–32.
2. Catheline S, Wu F, Fink M. A solution to diffraction biases in sonoelasticity: the acoustic impulse technique. J Acoust Soc Am. 1999;105:2941–50.
3. Sandrin L, Tanter M, Gennisson JL, Catheline S, Fink M. Shear elasticity probe for soft tissues with 1-D transient elastography. IEEE Trans Ultrason Ferroelectr Freq Control. 2002;49:436–46.

4. Sandrin L, Fourquet B, Hasquenoph JM, Yon S, Fournier C, Mal F, et al. Transient elastography: a new non-invasive method for assessment of hepatic fibrosis. Ultrasound Med Biol. 2003;29:1705–13.
5. Bedossa P, Poynard T. An algorithm for the grading of activity in chronic hepatitis C. The METAVIR Cooperative Study Group. Hepatology. 1996;24(2):289–93.
6. Poynard T, Bedossa P, Opolon P. Natural history of liver fibrosis progression in patients with chronic hepatitis C. the OBSVIRC, METAVIR, CLINIVIR, and DOSVIRC groups. Lancet. 1997;349(9055):825–32. https://doi.org/10.1016/s0140-6736(96)07642-8.
7. Friedrich-Rust M, Ong MF, Martens S, Sarrazin C, Bojunga J, Zeuzem S, Herrmann E. Performance of transient elastography for the staging of liver fibrosis: a meta-analysis. Gastroenterology. 2008;134(4):960–74.
8. Tsochatzis EA, Gurusamy KS, Ntaoula S, Cholongitas E, Davidson BR, Burroughs AK. Elastography for the diagnosis of severity of fibrosis in chronic liver disease: a meta-analysis of diagnostic accuracy. J Hepatol. 2011;54(4):650–9.
9. Vergniol J, Foucher J, Terrebonne E, Bernard PH, le Bail B, Merrouche W, et al. Non-invasive tests for fibrosis and liver stiffness predict 5-year outcomes of patients with chronic hepatitis C. Gastroenterology. 2011;140:1970–9.
10. Colli A, Fraquelli M, Casazza G, Conte D, Nikolova D, Duca P, Thorlund K, Gluud C. The architecture of diagnostic research: from bench to bedside. Research guidelines using liver stiffness as an example. Hepatology. 2014;60:408–18.
11. Sandrin L, Tanter M, Gennisson JL, Catheline S, Fink M. Shear elasticity probe for soft tissues with 1D transient elastography. IEEE Trans Ultrason Ferroelec Freq Control. 2002;49:436–46.
12. Fraquelli M, Rigamonti C, Casazza G, Conte D, Donato MF, Ronchi G, Colombo M. Reproducibility of transient elastography in the evaluation of liver fibrosis in patients with chronic liver disease. Gut. 2007;56:968–73.
13. Mc Gee SR. Evidence-based physical diagnosis. Philadelphia: W.B. Saunders Co; 2001. p. 38.
14. Sackett DL, Haynes RB. The architecture of diagnostic research. In: Knottnerus JA, editor. The evidence base of clinical diagnosis. London: BMJ Books; 2002. p. 19–38.
15. Roulot D, Czernichow S, Le Clesiau H, Costes JL, Vergnaud AC, Beaugrand M. Liver stiffness values in apparently healthy subjects: influence of gender and metabolic syndrome. J Hepatol. 2008;48:606–13.
16. Colombo S, Belloli L, Zaccanelli M, Badia E, Jamoletti C, Buonocore M, et al. Normal liver stiffness and its determinants in healthy blood donors. Dig Liver Dis. 2011;43:231–6.
17. Colli A, Fraquelli M, Prati D, Riva A, Berzuini A, Conte D, Aghemo A, Colombo M, Casazza G. Deciding on interferon-free treatment for chronic hepatitis c: updating liver stiffness cut-off values to maximize benefit. PLoS One. 2016;11(10):e0164452. https://doi.org/10.1371/journal.pone.0164452.
18. Millonig G, Reimann FM, Friedrich S, Fonouni H, Mehrabi A, Büchler MW, et al. Extrahepatic cholestasis increases liver stiffness (FibroScan) irrespective of fibrosis. Hepatology. 2008;48:1718–23.
19. Colli A, Pozzoni P, Berzuini A, Gerosa A, Canovi C, Molteni EE, et al. Decompensated chronic heart failure: increased liver stiffness measured by means of transient elastography. Radiology. 2010;257:872–8.
20. Sagir A, Erhardt A, Schmitt M, Haussinger D. Transient elastography is unreliable for detection of cirrhosis in patients with acute liver damage. Hepatology. 2008;47:592–5.
21. Arena U, Vizzutti F, Corti G, et al. Acute viral hepatitis increases liver stiffness values measured by transient elastography. Hepatology. 2008;47:380–4.
22. Altman DG, Royston P. The cost of dichotomising continuous variables. BMJ. 2006;332:1080.
23. Leeflang MM, Moons KG, Reitsma JB, Zwinderman AH. Bias in sensitivity and specificity caused by data-driven selection of optimal cut-off values: mechanisms, magnitude, and solutions. Clin Chem. 2008;54:729–37.
24. Colecchia A, Montrone L, Scaioli E, Bacchi-Reggiani ML, Colli A, Casazza G, Schiumerini R, Turco L, Di Biase AR, Mazzella G, Marzi L, Arena U, Pinzani M, Festi D. Measurement

of spleen stiffness to evaluate portal hypertension and the presence of esophageal varices in patients with hcv-related cirrhosis. Gastroenterology. 2012;143(3):646–54.

25. Simmons O, Fetzer DT, Yokoo T, et al. Predictors of adequate ultrasound quality for hepatocellular carcinoma surveillance in patients with cirrhosis. Aliment Pharmacol Ther. 2017;45(1):169–77.

26. Schuetz GM, Schlattmann P, Dewey M. Use of 3x2 tables with an intention to diagnose approach to assess clinical performance of diagnostic tests: meta-analytical evaluation of coronary CT angiography studies. BMJ (Clinical Research Ed). 2012;345:e6717.

27. Cohen JF, Korevaar DA, Altman DG, Bruns DE, Gatsonis CA, Hooft L, et al. STARD 2015 guidelines for reporting diagnostic accuracy studies: explanation and elaboration. BMJ Open. 2016;6:e012799.

28. Cassinotto C, Lapuyade B, Hiriat JB, et al. Non-invasive assessment of liver fibrosis with impulse elastography: comparison of supersonic shear imaging with ARFI and FibroScan®. J Hepatol. 2014;61(3):550–7.

29. Ezoe Y, Muto M, Uedo N, Doyama H, Yao K, Oda I, et al. Magnifying narrowband imaging is more accurate than conventional white-light imaging in diagnosis of gastric mucosal cancer. Gastroenterology. 2011;141(6):2017–25.

30. Ferrante di Ruffano L, Hyde CJ, McCaffery KJ, Bossuyt PM, Deeks JJ. Assessing the value of diagnostic tests: a framework for designing and evaluating trials. BMJ. 2012;344:e686.

31. Bossuyt PM, Irwig L, Craig J, Glasziou P. Comparative accuracy: assessing new tests against existing diagnostic pathways. BMJ. 2006;332:1089–92.

Liver Stiffness: Thresholds of Health

Daniele Prati, Alessandra Berzuini, Fateh Bazerbachi, and Luca Valenti

2.1 Preamble: The Concept of Normality in Medicine

All organisms extend along a line. At one end is Basedow's disease, which implies the generous, mad consumption of vital force at a precipitous pace, the pounding of an uncurbed heart. At the other end are the organisms depressed through organic avarice, destined to die of a disease that would appear to be exhaustion but which is, on the contrary, sloth. The golden mean between the two diseases is found in the center and is improperly defined as health, which is only a way station … This is the way it's been made, with goiter at one end and edema at the other, and there's no help for it. In the middle are those who have either incipient goiter or incipient edema, and along the entire line, in all mankind, absolute health is missing [1]

As underlined by Agostino Colli and colleagues in Chap. 1, studies on normal (or healthy) individuals are an essential component in the architecture of diagnostic research [2]. Unfortunately, deciding what is normal in medicine is not so straightforward. The above quotation has been taken from *Zeno's Conscience*, a novel by Italo Svevo published in 1923 [1]. Taking thyroid disease as an example, the author describes the difficulties of defining normality and abnormality when the aim is to identify human diseases. It is not surprising that the main character of the

D. Prati (✉) · A. Berzuini
Department of Transfusion Medicine and Haematology, Fondazione IRCCS Ca' Granda Ospedale Maggiore Policlinico, Milan, Italy
e-mail: daniele.prati@policlinico.mi.it

F. Bazerbachi
Division of Gastroenterology, Massachusetts General Hospital and Harvard Medical School, Boston, MA, USA

L. Valenti
Department of Transfusion Medicine and Haematology, Fondazione IRCCS Ca' Granda Ospedale Maggiore Policlinico, Milan, Italy

Department of Pathophysiology and Transplantation, University of Milano, Milan, Italy

© Springer Nature Switzerland AG 2021
M. Fraquelli (ed.), *Elastography of the Liver and Beyond*,
https://doi.org/10.1007/978-3-030-74132-7_2

novel is a neurotic man, who is writing his confessions at the behest of his psychiatrist: the issue of how to define normality in medicine has been scientifically addressed mainly in the field of neurosciences [3]. However, in any clinical context, the concept of "normality" constitutes the central nucleus on which ideas, theories, diagnoses, and clinical decisions are based. The term "normality" was commonly used in medicine well before it came to its methodological systematization: it was considered equivalent to the idea of health, where "abnormality" was synonymous with disease. These definitions are still valid, even if the concept of biological normality has been completed and enriched following the increasing use of mathematics in the medical field. For continuous variables, the "normal" (or "Gaussian") distribution model was initially developed when it was observed for the first time that measurement errors tend to be distributed in a characteristic and symmetrical way ("bell curve"). Later, it was extended to the classification of the values of a variable, observed in different individuals within a particular population. This required some simplification: actually, it was soon realized that a perfect Gaussian distribution is rarely observed in nature. However, the model was very successful, and the concept of "statistical normality," supported by the probabilistic theory, is still the fundamental basis to describe the biological phenomena. For most clinical or laboratory continuous variables, those values that are distributed in a range that includes 95% of the cases defined as "healthy" are considered normal. To indicate an upper reference limit, the sum of the mean value plus two standard deviations is generally used, which includes by definition 95% of cases in a Gaussian distribution. Alternatively, to overcome the problems encountered when the distribution is not perfectly normal, for example, when it is bimodal, the 95th percentile can be used [4, 5].

This probabilistic approach for the definition of normal values, although easy to apply and well standardized on a methodological level, presents some conceptual weaknesses. First, it assumes rather artificially that the possibility of subclinical disease is constant (5%) for all pathologies and for all clinical markers. An important consequence for this simplification is that a healthy person who undergoes multiple independent diagnostic tests (independent in the sense that they are probing totally different organs or functions) has a likelihood of testing normal that will be inversely related to the number of tests. For a single diagnostic test, the possibility is 95% or 0.95. For two tests, it will be $0.95 \times 0.95 = 0.90$. So, the likelihood of any individual being called normal is 0.95 raised to the power of the number of independent diagnostic tests performed. Thus, a healthy subject who undergoes 30 tests has only 0.95^{30}, or about 1 chance in 5, of being called normal at the end of the workup. An additional limitation of the Gaussian theory is that the normal distribution tends by definition to infinity, and therefore the model implicitly accepts the existence of individuals with levels of the marker so high or so low that cannot exist in nature [4, 5]. Another main problem, however, is how to define and select the "normal" ("healthy") population to be used in the creation of reference standards. This requires the identification and exclusion of "abnormal" ("sick") individuals according to a process which, as we will see in detail in the case of liver disease diagnostics, is often complicated and imprecise [6].

In recent decades, the concept of normality has undergone new changes. Increasingly, different reference standards are created (by age group, gender, race, etc.), in an attempt to individualize the interpretation of laboratory results. Furthermore, the development of theories related to clinical epidemiology has provided more solid bases for describing and interpreting biological variables. Bayesian analysis, based on concepts such as sensitivity, specificity, and predictive value, has provided very valuable tools for the evaluation of diagnostic tests. Nevertheless, it is important to remember that each of these approaches is based on the concept of the reference population.

2.2   Healthy Ranges in Liver Disease Diagnostics

In the case of tests for liver disease, the definition of a healthy range can be particularly problematic. First, it is very difficult to identify and exclude subjects with liver disease from the reference population, as the reference standard remains liver biopsy, which is not applicable for ethical reasons in those without any sign or symptom of liver disease. In addition, it is now agreed that populations composed of apparently healthy individuals (the so-called reference populations, for example, blood donors, or subjects recruited from the general population) include substantial proportions of individuals with subclinical liver disease (20–35% depending on the prevalence of risk factors for liver disease in the population), mostly related to hepatic steatosis ("fatty liver disease"). This issue was clearly demonstrated almost 20 years ago, in a study aimed at redefining the healthy thresholds for alanine aminotransferase (ALT) levels. The exclusion of subjects at risk for liver disease (i.e., overweight, with high serum lipids or glucose levels) from the reference sample caused a left shift of the ALT value distribution and a significant reduction of the 95th percentile, chosen as the upper reference limit [7]. In keeping with these results, Takyar et al. [8] have recently reviewed the records of 3160 subjects who participated as healthy volunteers in 149 clinical trials (1–29 trials per subject). They found that 1732 of these subjects (55%) were overweight and 1382 (44%) had abnormal liver biochemistry. This underscores the importance of an a priori definition of the criteria to select the appropriate reference population when the aim is to set the healthy ranges for any laboratory or instrumental test to detect the presence of liver disease. As already described in detail elsewhere [7], individuals to be included in the reference population for liver disease diagnostics should meet some clinical and laboratory criteria, including the absence of specific sign and symptoms for liver disease, negative serology for hepatitis B and C, normal body mass index (BMI) and/or waist circumference, as well as normal parameters of lipid and carbohydrate metabolism. These criteria ensure that only subjects at low risk for viral hepatitis and metabolic-associated fatty liver disease (MAFLD) are included.

2.3   Definition of Healthy Ranges for Liver Stiffness

The measurement of liver stiffness (LS) by transient elastography (TE) was introduced in the early 2000s. Since then, several studies have confirmed its role in the identification of different stages of liver fibrosis compared with the reference standard of liver histology. In particular, the diagnostic performance of TE has been evaluated in cohorts of patients with hepatitis B and C, as well as in other forms of liver disease, including MAFLD [9]. These studies allowed the identification of diagnostic thresholds to rule in or rule out significant fibrosis and cirrhosis in specific clinical contexts, as thoroughly discussed in the following chapters of this book.

In normal-weight individuals, TE has good inter- and intra-observer concordance [9, 10]. In a study including 200 patients with different liver diseases, reproducibility between two operators had intraclass correlation coefficients (ICCs) of 0.98 for inter- and intra-observer agreement, while lower concordance was observed in the presence of mild fibrosis, steatosis, or an increased body mass index (BMI >25 kg/ m^2) [10].

A total failure rate of 3.1% was reported in a series of 13,369 transient elastography examinations [11]. In addition, results were deemed unreliable in an additional 16%. Factors associated with unreliable results included BMI >30 kg/m², age >52 years, female sex, operator inexperience, and type 2 diabetes mellitus.

It is agreed that fluid and parietal adipose tissues attenuate shear wave propagation, which can result in invalid examinations in patients with anatomic distortions, ascites, and elevated central venous pressures or in those who are obese [11, 12]. In particular, the risk of overestimating LS values may emanate from a non-fasting state, excess of alcohol intake, physical exercise, acute hepatitis, inflammatory flares, congestive heart failure, hepatic parenchymal infiltration, cholestasis, and portal vein thrombosis [11–16]. Thus, TE should be performed in fasting patients (for at least 2 h), and results interpreted in light of potential confounders [9]. In addition, even hepatic steatosis may decrease the accuracy of transient elastography [17]. In a study of 253 patients with nonalcoholic fatty liver disease (NAFLD), the stage of fibrosis was often overestimated in patients with severe steatosis [18]. However, these results were not confirmed in other studies [19]. In addition, in healthy individuals, undernutrition and leanness, manifested by lower BMI, seem to increase LS values in a similar way as obesity does, providing a U-shaped distribution. This finding, initially described by Das and colleagues in Indian subjects [20], has been confirmed in a series of more than 1500 Italian blood donors (Berzuini A, unpublished data, 2020). Thus, special probes for overweight patients (XL probe) and children (S probe) have been developed to account for the thickness of the thoracic wall and depth of the liver. These probes may improve accuracy in assessing the degree of liver fibrosis in subjects at extremes of body weight [9, 16].

The description of how LS measurement performs among healthy individuals is of great importance as it establishes whether, and to what extent, the results among diseased and healthy participants overlap. In this regard, the lower the degree of overlap, the more accurate is considered the test [2]. Furthermore, studies on normal individuals provide a necessary background to set healthy thresholds for LS to be used in screening and epidemiological studies. Most data on LS from normal individuals have been obtained by transient elastography, and, for the sake of simplicity, the discussion will be limited to this technique.

The main studies so far conducted in healthy subjects are summarized in Table 2.1. They were highly heterogeneous in terms of studies design, not only for the choice of the population base (i.e., blood or living organ donors, general population, etc.) and the number and ethnic background of participants but also for the selection criteria used to define a healthy status [20–32].

In particular, some studies included subjects with normal liver biochemical tests, no history of chronic liver disease, and/or absence of hepatic steatosis on ultrasound. Others also included individuals with hepatic steatosis. Few studies have considered the effects of factors and comorbidities potentially influencing the risk for subclinical liver disease in apparently normal individuals.

The average values of LS roughly ranged between 4 and 5.5 kPa, and upper thresholds (mostly calculated as 95th percentile of the distribution or as mean value plus two times the standard deviation) between 6 and 8.5 kPa. Most studies agreed that LS measurement is related to sex (values were higher in males than in females) and with factors associated with the metabolic syndrome [20–32]. Recently, Bazerbachi et al. [33] conducted an individual participant data meta-analysis from published studies evaluating LS by TE among healthy individuals and in those at risk for liver disease. Twenty-six cohorts, which included 16,082 individuals, were ultimately selected. Statistically significant modifiers of stiffness included diabetes, dyslipidemia, waist circumference, aspartate aminotransferase (AST), and systolic blood pressure. The mean stiffness in the subgroup of 3882 healthy nonobese individuals (BMI, <30 kg/m^2) was 4.68 kPa (CI, 4.64–4.73). The same database of healthy individuals was used to generate a threshold to rule out fibrosis in individuals at risk. Outliers were removed using a method based on nonlinear regression with a 1% false discovery rate [34]. In order to favor sensitivity, even at the price of a slightly lower specificity, the 90th percentile of the LS measurement (instead of the 95th percentile) was chosen as the upper reference limit. Thus, the healthy threshold was set at 6.47 kPa for males and 6.01 kPa for females (Bazerbachi F, unpublished data, 2020). However, the choice of TE thresholds in a context of a population with a low pretest probability of substantial liver diseases should be modulated in relation to the clinical question. On the one hand, following a screening strategy, the choice of a low threshold would be important to maximize test sensitivity in order to reduce the rate of FN results and avoid underdiagnosis. On the other hand, to limit the number of false-positive cases and unnecessary investigations, it may be proposed to employ an higher cutoff, for example, the upper limit the 95th percentile of the distribution observed in healthy blood donors (i.e., 7.8 kPa for males, 7.4 kPa for females) [22]. However, as this approach by itself would miss a substantial proportion of individuals with significant/severe liver fibrosis, it should be applied together with concurrent clinical evaluation of medical history, risk factors, and other biomarkers of liver disease.

Table 2.1 Studies on the LSM measurement by TE in healthy subjects

Author	Country	N. of subjects	Age, years Mean ± SD or median (range)	Reference population(s)	LS measurement distribution Mean ± SD or median (range)	Healthy thresholds 95th percentile or mean + 2SD	Other findings/observations
Prati et al. [21] Colli et al. [22]	Italy	1001 (59% males)	39.9 ± 10.1	Blood donors at low risk for liver disease	4.6 kPa (2.2–21.3 kPa) 4.1 kPa (2.2–14.4 kPa)	7.8 kPa (males) 6.3 kPa (females)	LS was independently related to gender and ALT levels; 32% of those with LS values above the 95th percentile had liver disease
Chen et al. [23]	China	799 (all males)	N.A.	General population	5.2 ± 1.3 kPa (age ≤ 60) 5.9 ± 1.9 kPa (age > 60 years)	7.8 kPa (age ≤ 60) 9.7 kPa (age > 60)	LS was influenced by age and AST in but not by alcohol consumption and mass body index
Fung et al. [24]	Korea	530 (26% males)	37 (18–63)	General population, blood donors at low risk for liver disease	4.11 ± 0.89 kPa	5.9 kPa	Female gender and older age were associated with lower LS values
Corpechot et al. [25]	France	77 (42% males)	34 (18–79)	Healthy persons at low risk for liver disease	5.2 ± 0.7 kPa (males) 4.5 ± 1.0 kPa (females)	6.6 kPa (males) 6.5 kPa (females)	LS was not related with age, body weight, height, and BMI, but was significantly higher in men than in women
Roulot et al. [26]	France	429 (46% males)	45.1 ± 16.7	Apparently healthy subjects with normal liver enzyme	5.49 ± 1.59 kPa	8.67 kPa (all) 8.35 kPa (subjects without metabolic syndrome)	LS values were influenced independently by gender, BMI, and metabolic syndrome
Colombo et al. [27]	Italy	602 (56% males)	48 (22–66)	Blood donors without fatty liver	4.4 kPa (2.1–17.5 kPa)	6.7 kPa (males) 6.6 kPa (females)	Gender was the only influencing variable. LS by TE had a low false-positive rate for significant fibrosis and may have a role in screening for liver disease

Alsebaey et al. [28]	Egypt	50 (68% males)	28.4 ± 5.9	Living liver donors	4.3 ± 1.2 kPa	6.8 kPa	–
Das et al. [20]	India	418 (64% males)	37 ± 12	General population	5.4 kPa (2.2–10.4 kPa)	8.5 kPa	Both lean and obese healthy subjects have higher LS values compared with subjects with normal BMI. Liver stiffness begins to increase even before fibrosis appears in patients with liver disease
Kim et al. [29]	Korea	242 (50% males)	34.1 ± 11.8 (males) 40.5 ± 11.5 (females)	Living liver and kidney donors	5.2 ± 1.2 (males) 4.8 ± 1.1 (females)	7.0 kPa (males) 6.8 kPa (females)	Gender was independently related to LS
Sirli et al. [30]	Romania	152 (42% males)	45.3 ± 17.6	Healthy volunteers and patients hospitalized for non-hepatic conditions	5.1 ± 1.2 kPa (males) 4.6 ± 1.2 kPa (females)	7.5 kPa (males) 7 kPa (females)	LS not influenced by age and BMI, but significantly higher in men than in women
Basnet et al. [31]	Nepal	45 (66% males)	30.1 ± 5.0	Healthcare personnel	4.24 ± 0.70 kPa	5.64 kPa	Age, gender, and BMI were not significantly related to LS
Conti et al. [32]	Italy	331 (3.5% males)	47 ± 9	General population at low risk for liver disease	4.4 (3.7–5.2)	6.8 kPa	LS was influenced by insulin resistance

Data on LS measurement by TE in healthy children are limited. In a group of 270 children of age, the median value was 4.5 kPa, within a range of 2.5–8.9 kPa, and values did not vary significantly with age or gender; based on this distribution, an upper reference limit of about 6.5 kPa was also proposed [35]. Comparable results were obtained by Rowland et al. in 257 healthy children [36]. In the latter study, however, TE showed inadequate reproducibility, as suggested by low concordance between paired examinations. Thus, more evidence in the pediatric population is required to define healthy thresholds for LS measurement.

2.4 Conclusions

Probabilistic theories are extensively being used to summarize medical observations for diagnosis and to support clinical decisions. This approach facilitates the diagnosis and supports clinical decisions, but such an advantage is obtained at the price of some conceptual compromise. The "normal" thresholds that we use daily to separate health from disease are based on a process of statistical inference. It is, therefore, important to ensure that they are continuously updated and balanced to patient needs.

Over almost 20 years, sufficient data on LS measurement by TE in healthy individuals have been collected in several cohort studies and data synthesized in systematic review and individual participant data meta-analysis. On this basis, healthy thresholds have been proposed, improving the use of this technique in the screening and workup of liver disease. However, results should be interpreted critically and flexibly, taking into account the individual characteristics of the patients – gender, age, clinical history, risk factors for the disease, comorbidities, and possible confounders, as well as their personal preferences. Clinical decisions on the results of a single parameter should be avoided, especially when healthy thresholds are used to screen low-risk individuals.

References

1. Svevo I. Zeno's conscience: a novel. Translated by William Weaver. New York: Vintage International; 2003.
2. Colli A, et al. Elastographic measures: a methodological approach. In: Fraquelli M, editor. Elastography of the liver and beyond.
3. Link J, Hall MM. From the "power of the norm" to "flexible normalism": considerations after foucault. Cult Crit. 2004;57:14–32. https://doi.org/10.1353/cul.2004.0008.
4. How to read clinical journals: II. To learn about a diagnostic test. Can Med Assoc J. 1981;124(6):703–10.
5. Haynes RB, You JJ. The architecture of diagnostic research. In: Knottnerus JA, Buntinx F, editors. The evidence base of clinical diagnosis. Wiley; 2009.
6. Ritchie RF, Palomaki G. Selecting clinically relevant populations for reference intervals. Clin Chem Lab Med. 2004;42(7):702–9. https://doi.org/10.1515/CCLM.2004.120.
7. Prati D, Taioli E, Zanella A, Della Torre E, Butelli S, Del Vecchio E, et al. Updated definitions of healthy ranges for serum alanine aminotransferase levels. Ann Intern Med. 2002;137:1–10.

8. Takyar V, Nath A, Beri A, Gharib AM, Rotman Y. How healthy are the "healthy volunteers"? Penetrance of NAFLD in the biomedical research volunteer pool. Hepatology. 2017;66:825–33.
9. European Association for Study of Liver, Asociacion Latinoamericana para el Estudio del Higado. EASL-ALEH Clinical Practice Guidelines: Non-invasive tests for evaluation of liver disease severity and prognosis. J Hepatol. 2015;63:237–64.
10. Fraquelli M, Rigamonti C, Casazza G, Conte D, Donato MF, Ronchi G, Colombo M. Reproducibility of transient elastography in the evaluation of liver fibrosis in patients with chronic liver disease. Gut. 2007;56:968.
11. Castéra L, Foucher J, Bernard PH, Carvalho F, Allaix D, Merrouche W, et al. Pitfalls of liver stiffness measurement: a 5-year prospective study of 13,369 examinations. Hepatology. 2010;51:828.
12. Millonig G, Friedrich S, Adolf S, Fonouni H, Golriz M, Mehrabi A, et al. Liver stiffness is directly influenced by central venous pressure. J Hepatol. 2010;52:206.
13. Colli A, Pozzoni P, Berzuini A, Gerosa A, Canovi C, Molteni EE, et al. Decompensated chronic heart failure: increased liver stiffness measured by means of transient elastography. Radiology. 2010 Dec;257(3):872–8. https://doi.org/10.1148/radiol.10100013.
14. Tapper EB, Castera L, Afdhal NH. FibroScan (vibration-controlled transient elastography): where does it stand in the United States practice. Clin Gastroenterol Hepatol. 2015;13:27–36.
15. Huang R, Gao ZH, Tang A, Sebastiani G, Deschenes M. Transient elastography is an unreliable marker of liver fibrosis in patients with portal vein thrombosis. Hepatology. 2018;68:783–5.
16. Patel K, Sebastiani G. Limitations of non-invasive tests for assessment of liver fibrosis. JHEP Rep. 2020;2(2):100067. https://doi.org/10.1016/j.jhepr.2020.100067.
17. Gaia S, Carenzi S, Barilli AL, Bugianesi E, Smedile A, Brunello F, et al. Reliability of transient elastography for the detection of fibrosis in non-alcoholic fatty liver disease and chronic viral hepatitis. J Hepatol. 2011;54:64.
18. Petta S, Maida M, Macaluso FS, Di Marco V, Cammà C, Cabibi D, et al. The severity of steatosis influences liver stiffness measurement in patients with nonalcoholic fatty liver disease. Hepatology. 2015;62:1101.
19. Eddowes PJ, Sasso M, Allison M, Tsochatzis E, Anstee QM, Sheridan D, et al. Accuracy of FibroScan controlled attenuation parameter and liver stiffness measurement in assessing steatosis and fibrosis in patients with nonalcoholic fatty liver disease. Gastroenterology. 2019;156:1717.
20. Das K, Sarkar R, Ahmed SM, Mridha AR, Mukherjee PS, Das K, et al. "Normal" liver stiffness measure (LSM) values are higher in both lean and obese individuals: a population-based study from a developing country. Hepatology. 2012 Feb;55(2):584–93. https://doi.org/10.1002/hep.24694.
21. Prati D, Colli A, Berzuini A, Gerosa A, Duca P, Bonino F. Factors related to liver stiffness measurement by transient elastography among healthy individuals: results from a prospective study. J Hepatol. 2009;50:S370.
22. Colli A, Fraquelli M, Prati D, Riva A, Berzuini A, Conte D, et al. Deciding on interferon-free treatment for chronic hepatitis C: updating liver stiffness cut-off values to maximize benefit. PLoS One. 2016;11(10):e0164452. https://doi.org/10.1371/journal.pone.0164452.
23. Chen YP, Liang XE, Zhang Q, Dai M, Hou JL. Age influencing liver stiffness measurements in Chinese male general populations. J Hepatol. 2010;52:S162.
24. Fung J, Lee C-K, Chan M, Seto WK, Wong DK, Lai CL, et al. Defining normal liver stiffness range in a normal healthy Chinese population without liver disease. PLoS One. 2013;8:e85067.
25. Corpechot C, El Naggar A, Poupon R. Gender and liver: is the liver stiffness weaker in weaker sex? Hepatology. 2006;44:513–4.
26. Roulot D, Czernichow S, Le Clesiau H, Costes JL, Vergnaud AC, Beaugrand M. Liver stiffness values in apparently healthy subjects: influence of gender and metabolic syndrome. J Hepatol. 2008;48:606–13.
27. Colombo S, Belloli L, Zaccanelli M, Badia E, Jamoletti C, Buonocore M, et al. Normal liver stiffness and its determinants in healthy blood donors. Dig Liver Dis. 2011;43:231–6.

28. Alsebaey A, Allam N, Alswat K, Waked I. Normal liver stiffness: a study in living donors with normal liver histology. World J Hepatol. 2015;7:1149–53.
29. Kim BK, Kim SU, Choi GH, Han WK, Park MS, Kim EH, et al. "Normal" liver stiffness values differ between men and women: a prospective study for healthy living liver and kidney donors in a native Korean population. J Gastroenterol Hepatol. 2012;27:781–8.
30. Sirli R, Sporea I, Tudora A, Deleanu A, Popescu A. Transient elastographic evaluation of subjects without known hepatic pathology: does age change the liver stiffness? J Gastrointest Liver Dis. 2009;18:57–60.
31. Basnet BK, Kc S, Sharma D, Shrestha D. Transient elastographic values of healthy volunteers in a tertiary care hospital. JNMA J Nepal Med Assoc. 2014;52:661–7.
32. Conti F, Vukotic R, Foschi FG, Domenicali M, Giacomoni P, Savini S, et al. Transient elastography in healthy subjects and factors influencing liver stiffness in nonalcoholic fatty liver disease: an Italian community-based population study. Dig Liver Dis. 2016;48:1357–63.
33. Bazerbachi F, Haffar S, Wang Z, Cabezas J, Arias-Loste MT, Crespo J, et al. Range of normal liver stiffness and factors associated with increased stiffness measurements in apparently healthy individuals. Clin Gastroenterol Hepatol. 2019;17:54–64.
34. Motulsky HJ, Brown RE. Detecting outliers when fitting data with nonlinear regression - a new method based on robust nonlinear regression and the false discovery rate. BMC Bioinform. 2006;7(1):123.
35. Goldschmidt I, Streckenbach C, Dingemann C, Pfister ED, di Nanni A, Zapf A, et al. Application and limitations of transient liver elastography in children. J Pediatr Gastroenterol Nutr. 2013;57:109–13.
36. Rowland M, McGee A, Broderick A, Drumm B, Connolly L, Daly LE, et al. Repeatability of transient elastography in children. Pediatr Res. 2020;88:587–92.

The Role of Transient Elastography for Fibrosis Staging in HCV-Related Chronic Liver Disease

3

Marta Cilla and Emmanuel A. Tsochatzis

3.1 Introduction

Hepatitis C virus (HCV) infection is a major cause of chronic liver disease and constitutes a major public health concern, with 71.1 million (95% uncertainty interval 62.5–79.4) chronically infected individuals worldwide [1].

HCV transmission is most commonly associated with blood transfusions and health-care related injections in lower-income countries, while injection drug use is the primary transmission route in countries where other methods of transmission have mostly been eliminated [2].

The acute infection with HCV is generally asymptomatic and frequently it does not resolve spontaneously. Approximately 50–90% of the infected individuals become chronic carriers and may develop severe liver disease. The hepatic injury can range from minimal histological changes to rapid development of hepatic fibrosis and accelerated time to cirrhosis with or without hepatocellular carcinoma (HCC). Liver fibrosis is the excessive accumulation of extracellular matrix proteins, including collagen, and is considered as a wound healing response to chronic liver injury. Based on the natural history of chronic hepatitis C (CHC), it is estimated an overall annual risk for liver failure of 2.9%, HCC 3.2% and liver-related death 2.7% in patients with advanced fibrosis [3].

Chronic HCV infection is also accompanied by extra-hepatic manifestations reported in two-thirds of patients, including mixed cryoglobulinaemia-type vasculitis, renal disease, type 2 diabetes, cardiovascular disease (vasculitis, arterial hypertension), porphyria cutanea tarda, lichen planus, lymphoproliferative disorders and non-specific symptoms like fatigue, nausea, abdominal pain and weight loss. Therefore, HCV infection is considered a systemic disease.

M. Cilla · E. A. Tsochatzis (✉)
Sheila Sherlock Liver Centre, Royal Free Hospital, London, UK

UCL Institute for Liver and Digestive Health, Royal Free Hospital, UCL, London, UK
e-mail: e.tsochatzis@ucl.ac.uk

© Springer Nature Switzerland AG 2021
M. Fraquelli (ed.), *Elastography of the Liver and Beyond*,
https://doi.org/10.1007/978-3-030-74132-7_3

Treatment for HCV infection was revolutionized in 2014 with the development of direct-acting antivirals (DAAs). The goal of therapy is to cure HCV infection in order to prevent the complications of HCV-related liver and extra-hepatic diseases, improve quality of life, remove stigma and prevent onward transmission of HCV [4]. The endpoint of therapy is to achieve a sustained virological response (SVR) defined as undetectable HCV RNA 12 weeks (SVR12) or 24 weeks (SVR24) after treatment completion. An SVR corresponds to a cure of the HCV infection, with a very low chance of late relapse [4].

In 2017, WHO set targets to eliminate HCV infection globally as a public health threat by 2030. A decrease in both mortality and incidence in HCV could be possible through implementation of prevention, screening and treatment interventions.

Assessment of liver fibrosis is critical in the treatment decisions, prognosis and screening strategies of CHC patients. Non-invasive tests are increasingly included in new guidelines, leaving liver biopsy reserved for cases where there is uncertainty or potential additional aetiologies. Transient elastography (TE) is a useful tool for the detection of advanced fibrosis (F3) or cirrhosis (F4) and for the exclusion of significant fibrosis ($\geq$F2) [4].

In this review, we discuss the role of TE for fibrosis staging in CHC patients prior to therapy, after SVR, for monitoring disease progression and determining prognosis.

3.2 Assessment of Liver Disease Severity

Liver fibrosis is the main predictor of liver disease progression in patients with CHC. It is a dynamic non-linear process characterized by an excessive accumulation of extracellular matrix (ECM) proteins, such as collagen. It is considered as a wound healing reaction to chronic liver injury. HCV infection directly modulates signalling and metabolic pathways by viral proteins. Moreover, it indirectly induces host antiviral immune responses leading to chronic inflammation. Together, these events promote liver fibrogenesis [5].

Thus, assessment of liver fibrosis is necessary prior to therapy because it is critical for clinical management, prognosis and screening strategies of CHC patients. In fact, HCV treatment should be considered without delay in patients with significant fibrosis or cirrhosis (METAVIR score F2, F3 or F4), although it is probably cost-effective in all patients irrespective of their fibrosis stage [6]. In addition, patients with advanced fibrosis (F3) or cirrhosis (F4) who achieved SVR should undergo surveillance for HCC every 6 months by means of ultrasound and need to be assessed for portal hypertension, including the presence of gastro-oesophageal varices (GEV) [4].

3.2.1 Role of Liver Biopsy

Histopathological examination of a liver specimen obtained by percutaneous liver biopsy (LB) was until recently considered as the gold standard to diagnose and stage liver fibrosis. However, LB is a costly invasive procedure, and it is associated with complications including pain, serious bleeding, injury to other organs and, in rare cases, death [7]. Moreover, LB provides a static picture of the fibrogenic process, and, therefore, it does not permit clear prognostic indications, particularly on the rapidity of progression towards cirrhosis [5]. There is also a significant degree of inter- and intra-observer variability in the pathologic assessment of liver biopsy samples despite the development of staging criteria [8]. In addition, sampling error is common and many liver diseases do not affect the liver uniformly [9]. Finally, it is not practical for serially repeated assessment of disease progression.

These limitations have stimulated the search for non-invasive approaches that accurately measure the degree of liver fibrosis. Non-invasive methods for assessment of liver fibrosis are gradually being incorporated into new guidelines and are becoming standard of care, which significantly reduces the need for liver biopsy. Liver biopsy may be required in cases of known or suspected mixed aetiologies (e.g. metabolic syndrome, alcoholism or autoimmunity) [4].

3.2.2   Non-Invasive Assessment of Liver Fibrosis in CHC

Non-invasive methods should be used instead of liver biopsy to assess liver disease severity prior to therapy in patients with CHC [4]. Non-invasive tests can be divided into serum biomarkers and liver stiffness measurement (LSM) methods. The former include several, not closely liver-specific serum parameters that have been associated with fibrosis stage, as assessed by liver biopsies. The latter measure liver stiffness that corresponds to an intrinsic physical property of the liver parenchyma. The stiffer the tissue, the faster the shear wave propagates [10].

Both LSM and biomarkers perform well in the identification of cirrhosis or ruling out fibrosis; however, they perform less well in accurately identifying intermediate degrees of fibrosis [11, 12, 10].

3.3   Transient Elastography for the Assessment of Liver Fibrosis Prior to Antiviral Therapy

Transient elastography (TE), performed by using FibroScan (FS), is a non-invasive, rapid and reproducible method for assessment of liver fibrosis by measuring liver stiffness.

The diagnostic accuracy of TE is high for diagnosing advanced fibrosis (F3) or cirrhosis (F4); however, an important overlap in liver stiffness values is observed among patients with lower degrees of liver fibrosis (F0, F1 and F2) [13].

The recommended cut-off levels to diagnose advanced fibrosis (F3) and cirrhosis (F4) prior to therapy are, respectively, 10 kPa (area under the receiver operating characteristic curve (AUROC) 0.83, sensitivity (Se) 72%, specificity (Sp) 80%, positive predictive value (PPV) 62%, negative predictive value (NPV) 89%) and 13 kPa (AUROC 0.90–0.93, sensitivity 72–77%, specificity 85–90%, PPV 42–56%, NPV 95–98%) [4] (see Table 3.1).

Table 3.1 Non-invasive marker cut-offs for prediction of significant fibrosis (METAVIR ≥F2), advanced fibrosis (METAVIR ≥F3) and cirrhosis (METAVIR F4)

Test and algorithms	FibroScan		Castera		SAFE biopsy	
Stage of fibrosis (METAVIR)	≥F3	F4	≥F2	F4	≥F2	F4
Number of patients HCV+	560	1.855	302	302	302	302
Cut-off	10 kPa	13 kPa	FS ≥7.1 kPa and FT >0.48	FS ≥12.5 kPa and FT ≥0.75	APRI >1.5 and FT >0.48	APRI >2 and FT >0.75
AUROC (95% CI)	0.83	0.90–0.93	0.91 (0.86–0.96)	0.93 (0.90–0.96)	0.94 (0.90–0.98)	0.87 (0.84–0.90)
Se (%)	72	72–77	85.1	89.4	100	86.4
Sp (%)	80	85–90	97.2	98.2	87.3	89.7
PPV (%)	62	42–56	98.9	95	96.3	77.6
NPV (%)	89	95–98	66.9	95.9	100	94.1

APRI aspartate aminotransferase-to-platelet ratio index, *AUROC* area under the receiver operating characteristic curve, *FS* FibroScan, *FT* FibroTest, *HCV* hepatitis C virus, *SAFE* sequential algorithms for fibrosis evaluation, *Se* sensitivity, *Sp* specificity, *NPV* negative predictive value, *PPV* positive predictive value

Consideration must be given to factors that may adversely affect TE performance: risk factors of failure, risk factors of low quality and risk factors of false positive [5].

Risk factors of failure of LSM include obesity, narrow intercostal space and limited operator experience [14]. Myers et al. showed that in 276 patients with chronic liver disease (42% viral hepatitis, 46% NAFLD) and a BMI >28 kg/m^2, measurement failures were significantly less frequent with the XL probe than with the M probe (1.1% vs. 16%; $p < 0.00005$). However, stiffness values obtained with XL probe are probably lower than those obtained with the M probe (by a median of 1.4 kPa) [15].

Criteria of acceptable exam quality include at least ten valid measurements and interquartile range/median ratio (IQR/M) ≤0.30 [10].

Risk factors of false-positive results should also be carefully taken into account. Necro-inflammatory activity may limit the diagnostic accuracy of TE especially in patients with lower-intermediate stages of fibrosis. Indeed, necro-inflammatory activity increases LSM even after adjusting for fibrosis stage in patients who do not have cirrhosis [16]. Other confounding factors including extra-hepatic cholestasis [17], congestive heart failure [18], excessive alcohol intake [19] and food intake prior to the exam [20]. Instead, the extent of steatosis doesn't influence TE within each fibrosis stage [16].

3.3.1 Combination Algorithms

The accuracy of the different non-invasive methods developed in CHC may be improved when they are combined [4].

Serum markers range from simple routine laboratory tests such as the AST-to-platelet ratio index (APRI) [21] to more complex patented scores such as the FibroTest (FT) [22], which includes γ-glutamyl transpeptidase, total bilirubin, α2-macroglobulin, apolipoprotein A1 and haptoglobin levels.

Castèra et al. [23] evaluated paired combination of TE, FT and APRI, and all three markers together, for the diagnosis of fibrosis stage with liver biopsy examination results as the reference standard. The combined use of TE and FT offered the best diagnostic performance both for significant fibrosis ($\geq$F2, AUROC 0.88, 95% CI 0.82–0.92) and for severe fibrosis-cirrhosis ($\geq$F3, AUROC 0.95, 95% CI 0.91–0.97) (see Table 3.1).

In another study, Castèra et al. [24] prospectively compared, in a large population of CHC patients, the previous algorithm with the sequential algorithms for fibrosis evaluation (SAFE) algorithm (combining APRI and FT) using liver biopsy as the "gold standard" for staging fibrosis. Both algorithms were effective for the non-invasive staging of liver fibrosis in CHC. Their use in clinical practice could avoid the need for liver biopsy in 48–71% of cases for diagnosing significant fibrosis (72% with Castera vs. 48% with SAFE biopsy; $p < 0.0001$) and in 74–78% of cases for detecting cirrhosis (79% with Castera vs. 75% with SAFE biopsy; $p =$ NS). Although, for significant fibrosis, the Castera algorithm saved 23% more liver biopsies than the SAFE biopsy, its accuracy was significantly lower (88% vs. 97%, respectively; $p < 0.0001$). Instead, the number of saved liver biopsies for diagnosing cirrhosis did not differ between Castera and the SAFE biopsy algorithms, but the accuracy of Castera algorithm was significantly higher than that of the SAFE biopsy (96% vs. 89%, respectively; $p < 0.0001$) (Table 3.1).

Therefore, the use of combination algorithms with the aim of reducing liver biopsy represents a rational approach and results in higher diagnostic accuracy than the use of standalone diagnostic tests [25].

3.3.2 TE vs. Other Elastography Techniques

Several other liver elasticity-based imaging techniques are being developed, including ultrasound-based techniques and 3D magnetic resonance (MR) elastography. Ultrasound elastography methods are point shear wave elastography (pSWE), also known as acoustic radiation force impulse imaging (ARFI), and 2D-shear wave elastography (2D-SWE). Like TE, 2D-SWE and ARFI imaging measure shear wave velocities to provide a quantitative estimate of tissue stiffness. Different from TE, both methods are integrated in conventional ultrasound machines and can be performed with conventional ultrasound probes during an abdominal ultrasound scan. In addition, the latter methods enable the exact localization of a region of interest

(ROI) measurement site during B-mode ultrasound and are not limited by the presence of ascites [26].

A meta-analysis [27] including 13 studies ($n = 1163$ patients) comparing pSWE using ARFI with TE showed equivalent performance for detecting significant fibrosis and cirrhosis. The recommended cut-off levels to define an ARFI (VTQ®) positive test result for advanced fibrosis (F3) and cirrhosis (F4) prior to therapy are, respectively, 1.60–2.17 m/s (AUROC 0.94, sensitivity 84%, specificity 90%) and 2.19–2.67 m/s (AUROC 0.91, sensitivity 86%, specificity 84%) [4]. Reliability criteria for pSWE have recently been proposed [28].

2D-SWE seems to be at least equivalent to TE and pSWE/ARFI for non-invasive staging of liver fibrosis in CHC patients [29], but quality criteria for correct interpretation are not yet well defined.

Finally, comparison between MR elastography and TE has provided conflicting results [30, 31, 32]. MR elastography seems to provide a higher diagnostic performance than TE and pSWE for staging early stages of fibrosis [33]. However, widespread use of this method will depend on cost and availability.

3.4　Transient Elastography for the Assessment of Liver Fibrosis After SVR

The primary aim of HCV treatment is to achieve SVR; however, the main goal of HCV eradication is to reduce mortality and morbidity [4]. A major advantage of TE, compared with liver biopsy, is that it can be easily repeated over time and that it may be useful for monitoring fibrosis regression to identify those patients with a higher risk of developing complications during follow-up.

Several studies reported a significant decrease in LSM and non-invasive fibrosis biomarkers values, compared with baseline values, in patients with HCV who achieved SVR [34, 35, 36, 37]. However, it has to be taken into account that non-invasive methods to evaluate fibrosis regression have not been validated in non-viremic patients [10].

Pons et al. [34] demonstrated that LSM decrease very rapidly and significantly during the first 4 weeks of DAA treatment of HCV-infected compensated advanced chronic liver disease (cACLD) patients and that this improvement accounts for most of the stiffness improvement observed during follow-up (48 weeks). Moreover, a higher decrease in LSM was observed in patients with baseline ALT $\geq$ twofold upper limit normal (2 X ULN) than in those with ALT <2 X ULN.

These findings suggest that the improvement of LSM after SVR cannot be interpreted as a reduction of liver fibrosis (at least during the first year of follow-up) but as a suppression of liver inflammation, as a consequence of viral eradication.

D'Ambrosio et al. [35] examined reversal of cirrhosis in 33 cirrhotic patients with pre-treatment LB and post-SVR LB and TE, demonstrating that 21% of patients with LSM <12 kPa after 4 years of an SVR still has cirrhosis in LB. This pilot study indicated less accuracy of TE in excluding cirrhosis in patients with HCV clearance, as a consequence of its low sensitivity (61%), whereas its specificity remains high (95%).

Therefore, routine use of non-invasive tests after SVR in cirrhotic HCV patients has a high false-negative rate and cannot be used to establish which patients no longer need HCC screening or for the diagnosis of cirrhosis reversal. Moreover, TE cannot be used for staging liver fibrosis post-SVR in patients who did not have previous TE measurement. In addition, cut-off thresholds that predict low risk of liver-related events and the best timing for repeated assessment of LSM after therapy have not been established yet [10].

The topic is discussed in great depth in Chap. 9.

3.5 Transient Elastography for Diagnosing Liver-Related Complications

DAAs can cure CHC infection with a good safety profile; hence, most patients achieve an SVR regardless of the stage of chronic liver disease. Therefore, it is important to identify patients at risk of developing liver-related complications, such as liver decompensation or HCC.

Several studies have demonstrated that cirrhotic patients are at higher risk of complications than those without cirrhosis, although in patients with cirrhosis who have achieved SVR after DAA therapy the incidence of liver-related events and de novo HCC is significantly reduced [38, 39]. It is important to point out that patients at different stages of cirrhosis have different risks of developing complications and of dying. Accordingly, the Baveno VI workshop suggested the term "compensated advanced chronic liver disease (cACLD)" to better reflect that the spectrum of severe fibrosis and cirrhosis is a continuum in asymptomatic patients, and that distinguishing between the two is often not possible on clinical grounds [40]. The term cACLD refers to patients with LSM between 10 and 15 kPa (suggestive) and patients with LSM >15 kPa (highly suggestive).

The two major prognostic factors in cACLD are the presence of clinically significant portal hypertension (CSPH), defined by the Baveno VI workshop as a hepatic venous pressure gradient (HVPG) $\geq$10 mmHg [40], and the presence of GEV. Measurement of HVPG through hepatic vein catheterization and oesophagogastroduodenoscopy (OGD) are considered, respectively, the gold-standard tests for assessment of CSPH and GEV. However, these tests are invasive and impractical for frequent follow-up. Non-invasive methods can be used for the risk prediction of liver-related complications and for guiding the need of further evaluation with HVPG measurement and OGD [41].

This matter is further dealt with in Chap. 12.

3.5.1 Portal Hypertension

Portal hypertension is the haemodynamic abnormality associated with the most severe complications of cirrhosis, including variceal bleeding, hepatic encephalopathy and ascites [42, 43]. It is a consequence of the hepatic architectural remodelling of chronic liver diseases ("static component") in a tissue microenvironment characterized by a net predominance of vasoconstrictors ("dynamic component") [44]. In addition, an increased splanchnic vasodilatation and a state of hyperdynamic circulation contribute to the development of the "portal hypertensive syndrome" [45]. An HVPG $\geq$10 mmHg, defined by Baveno VI workshop as CPSH, is responsible for the formation of GEV, whereas clinical decompensation may develop when HVPG became severe ($\geq$12 mmHg).

Elastography has been extensively assessed in patients with portal hypertension [46]. According to the meta-analysis performed by Shi [47], TE has high accuracy for detection of CSPH in cACLD patients (AUROC 0.93, sensitivity 0.90, specificity 0.79, PPV 0.88, NPV 0.88). The cut-off values of LSM range from 13.6 to 34.9 kPa, with 81% probability of correct detection of CSPH over the threshold value and 11% probability of disease below the threshold value, when the pre-test probability was 50%. The absence of established cut-offs in this meta-analysis limits applicability in clinical practice.

Llop [48] demonstrated that in patients with cACLD and potentially resectable HCC, a LSM value <13.6 kPa was highly sensitive for ruling out CSPH (AUROC 0.84, sensitivity 0.91, specificity 0.57, PPV 0.59, NPV 0.90), and a value $\geq$21 kPa was highly specific for diagnosing CSPH (AUROC 0.84, sensitivity 0.53, specificity 0.91, PPV 0.81, NPV 0.74) (Table 3.2). Interestingly, in HCV-infected patients, the specificity of the information obtained by TE was 100%, suggesting that when LSM value is $\geq$21 kPa (AUROC 0.857, sensitivity 0.42, specificity 1.00, PPV 1.00, NPV 0.67), this exam might be sufficient to correctly diagnose CSPH in this subgroup of

Table 3.2 Performance of TE and Baveno VI criteria (TE and PLT) for ruling-in CSPH and ruling-out varices requiring treatment, respectively, in patients with compensated advanced chronic liver disease (cACLD)

Test	TE	Baveno VI criteria (TE and PLT)
Cut-off	LSM $\geq$21 kPa	LSM <20 kPa and PLT >150.000/mm^3
AUROC (95% CI)	0.840	0.746
Se (%)	53	87
Sp (%)	91	34
PPV (%)	81	6
NPV (%)	74	98
LR+	6.24	1.31
LR−	0.51	0.39
Ref.	[59]	[48]

AUROC area under the receiver operating characteristic curve, *LR+* positive likelihood ratio, *LR−* negative likelihood ratio, *LSM* liver stiffness measurement, *NPV* negative predictive value, *PPV* positive predictive value, *PLT* platelet, *Se* sensitivity, *Sp* specificity, *TE* transient elastography

patients. However, although the correlation between LSM and HVPG is excellent for HVPG values less than 12 mm Hg, it hardly reaches statistical significance for values $\geq$12 mmHg (r^2 = 0.17, P = 0.02) [49]. This important observation suggests that in advanced stages of cirrhosis, the degree of portal pressure becomes largely independent from fibrosis (and therefore LSM), while extra-hepatic components, such as the hyperdynamic circulation and the splanchnic vasodilatation, become more important [50]. Therefore, in patients with virus-related cACLD, non-invasive methods can be used to diagnose CSPH, defining the group of patients at higher risk of developing decompensation [40]. The Baveno VI workshop suggested that the LSM thresholds for CSPH are $\geq$20–25 kPa in at least two measurements on different days, alone or combined with platelets and spleen size [51].

This topic is analysed in great depth in Chap. 11.

3.5.2 Gastro-Oesophageal Varices (GEV)

GEV are a common consequence of portal hypertension and represent a major cause of morbidity and mortality due to the risk of bleeding. Their prevalence in cirrhosis is approximately 50% and is correlated with liver disease severity. Variceal bleeding occurs at a yearly rate of 5% and is related to the stage of cirrhosis, the size of varices and presence of red wale marks [52].

The utility of TE is mainly in patients with cACLD, where it can be used to spare OGDs in a subset of patients with no history of variceal bleeding. Currently, primary prophylaxis for variceal bleeding in cACLD is only recommended in patients with large varices. Patients with decompensated cirrhosis should receive primary prophylaxis irrespective of the size of varices.

A correlation between LSM values and the presence of GEV has been reported in several studies with AUROCs ranging from 0.74 to 0.85 and cut-offs from 13.9 to 21.5 kPa. Although the sensitivity for the prediction of the GEV was relatively high (76–95%), the specificity was poor (43–78%) [49, 53–58]. As a result, the diagnostic accuracy of TE alone has not been sufficient to replace OGD in the diagnosis of varices [4, 10].

The high sensitivity and NPV values of TE, especially in combination with other non-invasive criteria, can rule out high-risk varices in patients with Child-Pugh A cirrhosis, who can therefore avoid an unnecessary OGD. The Baveno VI criteria [40] define that cACLD patients with a LSM <20 kPa and a platelet count >150.000/mm^3 have a low risk of having varices requiring treatment and therefore can avoid screening endoscopy. They advise longitudinal follow-up of such patients by yearly repetition of TE and platelet count with the guidance that if LSM increases or platelet count declines, these patients should undergo screening OGD [40]. The retrospective study by Maurice et al. [59], which included 310 patients, reported that the Baveno VI criteria performed well correctly identifying 98% of patients who could safely avoid endoscopy (AUROC 0.746, sensitivity 0.87, specificity 0.34, PPV 0.06, NPV 0.98), but could incorrectly classify 2% of patients (Table 3.2). Application of the guidelines will have excluded the patients from endoscopic surveillance and delayed the introduction of appropriate primary prophylaxis. Therefore, careful consideration must be given to co-morbidities which may impact the validity of proposed platelet cut-off.

Three additional retrospective studies validated Baveno VI criteria for the detection of GEV and demonstrated that this strategy had acceptable rates of misdiagnosed patients, although the proportion of unnecessary gastroscopy was very high [60–62]. Expanded Baveno VI criteria have also been proposed [63].

In the last years, different studies evaluate the diagnostic performance of spleen stiffness measurement by TE in identifying patients with GEV and CSPH. Colecchia et al. [64] suggest that SS measurement, possibly associated with LSM, has a high diagnostic accuracy for the prediction of GEV and different degrees of PH in patients with CHC. Further validation is needed before the place of SS in clinical practice can be defined.

This topic is analysed in great depth in Chap. 11.

3.5.3 Hepatocellular Carcinoma (HCC)

HCC is the fifth most common cancer worldwide and the third most cause of cancer death [65]. CHC is the leading risk factor for HCC, with an annual HCC risk of 2–4% in patients with cirrhosis [66]. HCV-induced chronic inflammation is supposed to be a strong promoter of tumour development, and resolution of HCV infection should translate in a reduced incidence of HCC even in patients with liver cirrhosis [67]. Long-term post-SVR follow-up studies showed that the risk of HCC remains in patients with cirrhosis who clear HCV, although it is significantly reduced compared to untreated patients or patients who did not achieve an SVR [67, 68]. In addition, patients previously treated for HCC have still a high risk of tumour recurrence, despite DAA treatment [69]. Thus, guidelines recommend indefinite ultrasound surveillance every 6 months after SVR for patients with advanced fibrosis or cirrhosis before treatment [4]. Several studies identified that high LSM value measured by TE is significantly associated with the risk of presence of HCC [38, 69–71]. In a multicentre retrospective study of Conti et al. [69], patients with baseline LSM values $\geq$21.3 kPa were significantly more prone to develop HCC de novo ($p = 0.005$; OR, 4.24; 95% CI, 1.50–11.97) and HCC recurrence in those with a history of previous HCC ($p = 0.01$; OR, 11.91; 95% CI, 1.33–106.78). Degasperi et al. [70] demonstrated that baseline LSM was a predictor of de novo HCC as well (hazard ratio [HR], 1.03; 95% CI, 1.01–1.06; $P = 0.01$), with the best cut-off being an LSM $\geq$30 kPa. Take into account that both previous studies included patients with Child-Pugh class A and B liver cirrhosis, those patients with worse liver function also had higher LSM, which could lead to an overestimation of the effect of baseline LSM.

Ravaioli et al. [71] found that a LSM reduction <30% (HR, 5.360; 95% CI, 1.561–18.405; $p = 0.008$) during a median follow-up of 15 months after DAA treatment was an independent predictor of HCC development. A possible explanation of these results could be the persistence of greater fibrosis and portal hypertension after DAA therapy in patients who developed HCC compared to those who did not, in whom the lower reduction of LS might reflect an improvement in inflammation.

In contrast to what has been previously reported, a multicentre prospective study from Pons M et al. reported that neither baseline LSM nor LSM improvement predicted the occurrence of HCC. This study, including 572 patients with Child-Pugh class A, demonstrated that albumin levels at follow-up (HR 0.08; 95% CI 0.02–0.25; $p < 0.001$) and LSM <10 kPa at follow-up (HR 0.33; 95% CI 0.11–0.96; $p < 0.042$) were independently associated with the risk of HCC. Combining both predictors, they identified two groups with differing risk of HCC occurrence: those with LSM $\geq$20 kPa at follow-up or those with LSM between 10 and 20 kPa and albumin levels <4.4 g/dl were at the highest risk (IR $\geq$1.9/100 patient-years).

According to all these results, it can be concluded that TE could be useful to identify patients at risk of developing HCC, but more data are needed before it can be integrated into an HCC surveillance programme [10].

This matter is further dealt with in Chap. 12.

3.6   Transient Elastography to Determine Prognosis

There is increasing evidence for the prognostic value of non-invasive tests, particularly LS measurement using TE, in CHC patients [10]. Vergniol et al. [72] showed, in a cohort of 1457 CHC patients, the prognostic value of LSM for 5-year overall survival and survival without liver-related death, which remained after adjustment for treatment response, patient age and estimates of necro-inflammatory grade.

In another study, Vergniol et al. [73] demonstrated that survival decreased as delta of 3-year LSM increased, especially in patients with baseline LSM >7 kPa. According to these results, they proposed a clinical management algorithm, using baseline LSM (kPa, HR 5.76; 95% CI 3.74–8.87; $p < 0.001$), LSM evolution (kPa/ year, HR 1.19; 95% CI 1.11–1.28; $p < 0.001$) and SVR achievement (HR 0.19; 95% CI 0.05–0.80; $p = 0.023$) for the prediction of prognosis and patient management in CHC.

According to a meta-analysis [74] including 27 studies ($n = 5874$ treatment-naïve CHC patients), LSM progression rates were consistent with fibrosis progression rates derived from biopsy in predicting time-to-cirrhosis, although there was less consistency for early-stage progression (time-to-F2).

Therefore, the potential role of TE for predicting clinical outcomes seems to be greater than that of liver biopsy; probably LSM is consistent with pathophysiological processes that a biopsy cannot, but more studies are needed to obtain refined estimates [10].

This topic is further dealt with in Chap. 12.

3.7 Conclusions

Significant progress has been made in the field of non-invasive assessment of liver fibrosis, reducing the need of liver biopsies. The role of TE for fibrosis staging in CHC patients is crucial prior to therapy for predicting the presence of advanced fibrosis and cirrhosis and prioritizing patients for HCV therapy based on disease stage. Instead, for the diagnosis of significant fibrosis, the use of combination algorithms may provide the highest diagnostic accuracy. Therefore, TE can be used for the risk prediction of HCC and liver-related complications, like CSPH and GEV requiring treatment, and for guiding the need of further evaluation with more invasive tests. In addition, there is increasing evidence for the prognostic value of LS measurement using TE in patients with cirrhosis.

Routine use of TE after SVR in CHC patients, on the other hand, has a high false-negative rate and cannot be used to determine which patients no longer need HCC screening or for diagnosis of cirrhosis reversal. Finally, it remains to be seen the cut-off thresholds that predict low risk of liver-related events and the best timing for repeated assessment of LSM after therapy.

References

1. Blach S, Zeuzem S, Manns M, Altraif I, Duberg AS, Muljono DH, et al. Global prevalence and genotype distribution of hepatitis C virus infection in 2015: a modelling study. Lancet Gastroenterol Hepatol. 2017;2(3):161–76.
2. Alter MJ, Fabiani FL. Epidemiology of hepatitis C virus infection prevalence and incidence. World J Gastroenterol [Internet]. 2007;13(17):2436–41. Available from: www.wjgnet.comhttp://www.wjgnet.com/1007-9327/13/2436.asp
3. Singal AG, Volk ML, Jensen D, Di Bisceglie AM, Schoenfeld PS. A sustained viral response is associated with reduced liver-related morbidity and mortality in patients with hepatitis C virus. Clin Gastroenterol Hepatol. 2010;8(3):280–8.
4. European Association for the Study of the Liver. EASL recommendations on treatment of hepatitis C 2018. J Hepatol. 2018;69(2):461–511.
5. Sebastiani G, Gkouvatsos K, Pantopoulos K. Chronic hepatitis C and liver fibrosis. World J Gastroenterol. 2014;20:11033–53.
6. Tsochatzis EA, Crossan C, Longworth L, Gurusamy K, Rodriguez-Peralvarez M, Mantzoukis K, et al. Cost-effectiveness of noninvasive liver fibrosis tests for treatment decisions in patients with chronic hepatitis C. Hepatology. 2014;60(3):832–43.
7. Seeff LB, Everson GT, Morgan TR, Curto TM, Lee WM, Ghany MG, et al. Complication rate of percutaneous liver biopsies among persons with advanced chronic liver disease in the HALT-C trial. Clin Gastroenterol Hepatol. 2010;8(10):877–83.
8. Rousselet MC, Michalak S, Dupré F, Croué A, Bedossa P, Saint-André JP, et al. Sources of variability in histological scoring of chronic viral hepatitis. Hepatology. 2005;41(2):257–64.
9. Bedossa P, Dargère D, Paradis V. Sampling variability of liver fibrosis in chronic hepatitis C. Hepatology. 2003;38(6):1449–57.
10. Castera L, Yuen Chan HL, Arrese M, Afdhal N, Bedossa P, Friedrich-Rust M, et al. EASL-ALEH clinical practice guidelines: non-invasive tests for evaluation of liver disease severity and prognosis. J Hepatol. 2015;63(1):237–64.

11. Tsochatzis E, Gurusamy K, Ntaoula S, Cholongitas E, Davidson B, Burroughs A, et al. Elastography for the diagnosis of severity of fibrosis in chronic liver disease: a meta-analysis of diagnostic accuracy. J Hepatol. 2011;54(4):650–9.
12. Crossan C, Tsochatzis EA, Longworth L, Gurusamy K, Davidson B, Rodríguez-Perálvarez M, et al. Cost-effectiveness of non-invasive methods for assessment and monitoring of liver fibrosis and cirrhosis in patients with chronic liver disease: systematic review and economic evaluation. Health Technol Assess (Rockv). 2015;19(9):1–458.
13. Degos F, Perez P, Roche B, Mahmoudi A, Asselineau J, Voitot H, et al. Diagnostic accuracy of FibroScan and comparison to liver fibrosis biomarkers in chronic viral hepatitis: a multicenter prospective study (the FIBROSTIC study). J Hepatol. 2010;53(6):1013–21.
14. Sandrin L, Fourquet B, Hasquenoph JM, Yon S, Fournier C, Mal F, et al. Transient elastography: a new noninvasive method for assessment of hepatic fibrosis. Ultrasound Med Biol. 2003;29(12):1705–13.
15. Myers RP, Pomier-Layrargues G, Kirsch R, Pollett A, Duarte-Rojo A, Wong D, et al. Feasibility and diagnostic performance of the FibroScan XL probe for liver stiffness measurement in overweight and obese patients. Hepatology. 2020;55(1):199–208. Available from: http://doi.wiley.com/10.1002/hep.24624
16. Arena U, Vizzutti F, Abraldes JG, Corti G, Stasi C, Moscarella S, et al. Reliability of transient elastography for the diagnosis of advanced fibrosis in chronic hepatitis C. Gut. 2008;57(9):1288–93.
17. Millonig G, Reimann FM, Friedrich S, Fonouni H, Mehrabi A, Büchler MW, et al. Extrahepatic cholestasis increases liver stiffness (fibroScan) irrespective of fibrosis. Hepatology. 2008;48(5):1718–23.
18. Millonig G, Friedrich S, Adolf S, Fonouni H, Golriz M, Mehrabi A, et al. Liver stiffness is directly influenced by central venous pressure. J Hepatol. 2010;52(2):206–10.
19. Bardou-Jacquet E, Legros L, Soro D, Latournerie M, Guillygomarc'h A, Le Lan C, et al. Effect of alcohol consumption on liver stiffness measured by transient elastography. World J Gastroenterol. 2013;19(4):516–22.
20. Mederacke I, Wursthorn K, Kirschner J, Rifai K, Manns MP, Wedemeyer H, et al. Food intake increases liver stiffness in patients with chronic or resolved hepatitis C virus infection. Liver Int. 2009;29(10):1500–6.
21. Wai C. A simple noninvasive index can predict both significant fibrosis and cirrhosis in patients with chronic hepatitis C. Hepatology. 2003;38(2):518–26. Available from: http://doi.wiley.com/10.1053/jhep.2003.50346
22. Imbert-Bismut F, Ratziu V, Pieroni L, Charlotte F, Benhamou Y, Poynard T. Biochemical markers of liver fibrosis in patients with hepatitis C virus infection: a prospective study. Lancet. 2001;357(9262):1069–75.
23. Castéra L, Vergniol J, Foucher J, Le Bail B, Chanteloup E, Haaser M, et al. Prospective comparison of transient elastography, Fibrotest, APRI, and liver biopsy for the assessment of fibrosis in chronic hepatitis C. Gastroenterology. 2005;128(2):343–50.
24. Castéra L, Sebastiani G, Le Bail B, De Lédinghen V, Couzigou P, Alberti A. Prospective comparison of two algorithms combining non-invasive methods for staging liver fibrosis in chronic hepatitis. J Hepatol. 2010;52(2):191–8.
25. Majumdar A, Campos S, Gurusamy K, Pinzani M, Tsochatzis EA. Defining the minimum acceptable diagnostic accuracy of noninvasive fibrosis testing in cirrhosis: a decision analytic modeling study. Hepatology. 2020;71(2):627–42.
26. Gerber L, Kasper D, Fitting D, Knop V, Vermehren A, Sprinzl K, et al. Assessment of liver fibrosis with 2-D shear wave elastography in comparison to transient elastography and acoustic radiation force impulse imaging in patients with chronic liver disease. Ultrasound Med Biol. 2015;41(9):2350–9.
27. Bota S, Herkner H, Sporea I, Salzl P, Sirli R, Neghina AM, et al. Meta-analysis: ARFI elastography versus transient elastography for the evaluation of liver fibrosis. Liver Int. 2013;33:1138–47.

28. Roccarina D, Iogna Prat L, Buzzetti E, Guerrero Misas M, Aricó FM, Saffioti F, et al. Establishing reliability criteria for liver ElastPQ shear wave elastography (ElastPQ-SWE): comparison between 10, 5 and 3 measurements. Ultraschall Med. 2021;42:204–13.

29. Ferraioli G, Tinelli C, Dal Bello B, Zicchetti M, Filice G, Filice C. Accuracy of real-time shear wave elastography for assessing liver fibrosis in chronic hepatitis C: a pilot study. Hepatology. 2012;56(6):2125–33.

30. Huwart L, Sempoux C, Vicaut E, Salameh N, Annet L, Danse E, et al. Magnetic resonance elastography for the noninvasive staging of liver fibrosis. Gastroenterology. 2008;135(1):32–40. Available from: http://www.ncbi.nlm.nih.gov/pubmed/18471441

31. Ichikawa S, Motosugi U, Morisaka H, Sano K, Ichikawa T, Tatsumi A, et al. Comparison of the diagnostic accuracies of magnetic resonance elastography and transient elastography for hepatic fibrosis. Magn Reson Imaging. 2015;33(1):26–30.

32. Bohte AE, De Niet A, Jansen L, Bipat S, Nederveen AJ, Verheij J, et al. Non-invasive evaluation of liver fibrosis: a comparison of ultrasound-based transient elastography and MR elastography in patients with viral hepatitis B and C. Eur Radiol. 2014;24(3):638–48.

33. Lefebvre T, Wartelle-Bladou C, Wong P, Sebastiani G, Giard JM, Castel H, et al. Prospective comparison of transient, point shear wave, and magnetic resonance elastography for staging liver fibrosis. Eur Radiol. 2019;29(12):6477–88.

34. Pons M, Santos B, Simón-Talero M, Ventura-Cots M, Riveiro-Barciela M, Esteban R, et al. Rapid liver and spleen stiffness improvement in compensated advanced chronic liver disease patients treated with oral antivirals. Ther Adv Gastroenterol. 2017;10(8):619–29.

35. D'Ambrosio R, Aghemo A, Fraquelli M, Rumi MG, Donato MF, Paradis V, et al. The diagnostic accuracy of Fibroscan® for cirrhosis is influenced by liver morphometry in HCV patients with a sustained virological response. J Hepatol. 2013;59(2):251–6. Available from: http://www.ncbi.nlm.nih.gov/pubmed/23528378

36. Hézode C, Castéra L, Roudot-Thoraval F, Bouvier-Alias M, Rosa I, Roulot D, et al. Liver stiffness diminishes with antiviral response in chronic hepatitis C. Aliment Pharmacol Ther. 2011;34(6):656–63.

37. Rout G, Nayak B, Patel AH, Gunjan D, Singh V, Kedia S, et al. Therapy with oral directly acting agents in hepatitis c infection is associated with reduction in fibrosis and increase in hepatic steatosis on transient elastography. J Clin Exp Hepatol. 2019;9(2):207–14. Available from: http://www.ncbi.nlm.nih.gov/pubmed/31024203

38. Pons M, Rodríguez-Tajes S, Esteban JI, Mariño Z, Vargas V, Lens S, et al. Non-invasive prediction of liver-related events in patients with HCV-associated compensated advanced chronic liver disease after oral antivirals. J Hepatol. 2019;72(3):472–80.

39. Tateishi R, Masuzaki R, Enooku K, Kondo Y, Goto T, Ikeda H, et al. Liver stiffness measurement can predict overall survival in patients with chronic hepatitis C. Hepatol Int. 2012;6:149.

40. De Franchis R, Abraldes JG, Bajaj J, Berzigotti A, Bosch J, Burroughs AK, et al. Expanding consensus in portal hypertension report of the Baveno VI consensus workshop: stratifying risk and individualizing care for portal hypertension. J Hepatol. 2015;63:743–52.

41. Abraldes JG, Bureau C, Stefanescu H, Augustin S, Ney M, Blasco H, et al. Noninvasive tools and risk of clinically significant portal hypertension and varices in compensated cirrhosis: the "anticipate" study. Hepatology. 2016;64(6):2173–84. Available from: http://www.ncbi.nlm.nih.gov/pubmed/27639071

42. Tsochatzis EA, Bosch J, Burroughs AK. Liver cirrhosis. In: The lancet. Lancet Publishing Group; 2014. p. 1749–61.

43. Bosch J, García-Pagán JC. Complications of cirrhosis. I. Portal hypertension. J Hepatol. 2000;32(Suppl.1):141–56.

44. Iwakiri Y, Groszmann RJ. The hyperdynamic circulation of chronic liver diseases: from the patient to the molecule. Hepatology. 2006;43(2 Suppl 1):S121–31. Available from: http://www.ncbi.nlm.nih.gov/pubmed/16447289

45. Garcia-Tsao G. Portal hypertension. Curr Opin Gastroenterol. 2004;20:254–63. Available from: http://www.ncbi.nlm.nih.gov/pubmed/15703650

46. Roccarina D, Rosselli M, Genesca J, Tsochatzis EA. Elastography methods for the non-invasive assessment of portal hypertension. Exp Rev Gastroenterol Hepatol. 2018;12:155–64.
47. Shi KQ, Fan YC, Pan ZZ, Lin XF, Liu WY, Chen YP, et al. Transient elastography: a meta-analysis of diagnostic accuracy in evaluation of portal hypertension in chronic liver disease. Liver Int. 2013;33(1):62–71.
48. Llop E, Berzigotti A, Reig M, Erice E, Reverter E, Seijo S, et al. Assessment of portal hypertension by transient elastography in patients with compensated cirrhosis and potentially resectable liver tumors. J Hepatol. 2012;56(1):103–8.
49. Vizzutti F, Arena U, Romanelli RG, Rega L, Foschi M, Colagrande S, et al. Liver stiffness measurement predicts severe portal hypertension in patients with HCV-related cirrhosis. Hepatology. 2007;45(5):1290–7.
50. Reiberger T, Ferlitsch A, Payer BA, Pinter M, Homoncik M, Peck-Radosavljevic M. Non-selective β-blockers improve the correlation of liver stiffness and portal pressure in advanced cirrhosis. J Gastroenterol. 2012;47(5):561–8.
51. Abraldes JG, Bureau C, Stefanescu H, Augustin S, Ney M, Elène Blasco H, et al. Noninvasive tools and risk of clinically significant portal hypertension and varices in compensated cirrhosis: the 'anticipate' study. Hepatology. 2016;64(6):2173–84.
52. Garcia-Tsao G, Abraldes JG, Berzigotti A, Bosch J. Portal hypertensive bleeding in cirrhosis: risk stratification, diagnosis, and management: 2016 practice guidance by the American Association for the study of liver diseases. Hepatology. 2017;65(1):310–35. Available from: https://onlinelibrary.wiley.com/doi/abs/10.1002/hep.28906
53. Bureau C, Metivier S, Peron JM, Selves J, Robic MA, Gourraud PA, et al. Transient elastography accurately predicts presence of significant portal hypertension in patients with chronic liver disease. Aliment Pharmacol Ther. 2008;27(12):1261–8.
54. Lemoine M, Katsahian S, Ziol M, Nahon P, Ganne-Carrie N, Kazemi F, et al. Liver stiffness measurement as a predictive tool of clinically significant portal hypertension in patients with compensated hepatitis C virus or alcohol-related cirrhosis. Aliment Pharmacol Ther. 2008;28(9):1102–10.
55. Kazemi F, Kettaneh A, N'kontchou G, Pinto E, Ganne-Carrie N, Trinchet JC, et al. Liver stiffness measurement selects patients with cirrhosis at risk of bearing large oesophageal varices. J Hepatol. 2006;45(2):230–5.
56. Nguyen-Khac E, Saint-Leger P, Tramier B, Coevoet H, Capron D, Dupas JL. Noninvasive diagnosis of large esophageal varices by fibroscan: strong influence of the cirrhosis etiology. Alcohol Clin Exp Res. 2010;34(7):1146–53.
57. Pritchett S, Cardenas A, Manning D, Curry M, Afdhal NH. The optimal cut-off for predicting large oesophageal varices using transient elastography is disease specific. J Viral Hepat. 2011;18(4):e75–80.
58. Castera L, Pinzani M, Bosch J. Non invasive evaluation of portal hypertension using transient elastography. J Hepatol. 2012;56(3):696–703.
59. Maurice JB, Brodkin E, Arnold F, Navaratnam A, Paine H, Khawar S, et al. Validation of the Baveno VI criteria to identify low risk cirrhotic patients not requiring endoscopic surveillance for varices. J Hepatol. 2016;65(5):899–905.
60. Jangouk P, Turco L, De Oliveira A, Schepis F, Villa E, Garcia-Tsao G. Validating, deconstructing and refining Baveno criteria for ruling out high-risk varices in patients with compensated cirrhosis. Liver Int. 2017;37(8):1177–83.
61. Llop E, Lopez M, de la Revilla J, Fernandez N, Trapero M, Hernandez M, et al. Validation of noninvasive methods to predict the presence of gastroesophageal varices in a cohort of patients with compensated advanced chronic liver disease. J Gastroenterol Hepatol. 2017;32(11):1867–72.
62. Sousa M, Fernandes S, Proença L, Silva AP, Leite S, Silva J, et al. The Baveno VI criteria for predicting esophageal varices: validation in real life practice. Rev Esp Enferm Dig. 2017;109(10):704–7. Available from: http://www.ncbi.nlm.nih.gov/pubmed/28776387

63. Augustin S, Onica Pons M, Maurice JB, Bureau C, Stefanescu H, Ney M, et al. Expanding the Baveno VI criteria for the screening of varices in patients with compensated advanced chronic liver disease. Hepatology. 2017;66:1980–8.
64. Colecchia A, Montrone L, Scaioli E, Bacchireggiani ML, Colli A, Casazza G, et al. Measurement of spleen stiffness to evaluate portal hypertension and the presence of esophageal varices in patients with HCV-related cirrhosis. Gastroenterology. 2012;143(3):646–54.
65. Saab S, Hunt DR, Stone MA, McClune A, Tong MJ. Timing of hepatitis C antiviral therapy in patients with advanced liver disease: a decision analysis model. Liver Transplant. 2010;16(6):748–59.
66. Singal AG, Lim JK, Kanwal F. AGA clinical practice update on interaction between oral direct-acting antivirals for chronic hepatitis C infection and hepatocellular carcinoma: expert review. Gastroenterology. 2019;156:2149–57.
67. Bang CS, Song IH. Impact of antiviral therapy on hepatocellular carcinoma and mortality in patients with chronic hepatitis C: systematic review and meta-analysis. BMC Gastroenterol. 2017:1–19.
68. Waziry R, Hajarizadeh B, Grebely J, Amin J, Law M, Danta M, et al. Hepatocellular carcinoma risk following direct-acting antiviral HCV therapy: a systematic review, meta-analyses, and meta-regression. J Hepatol. 2017;67(6):1204–12.
69. Conti F, Buonfiglioli F, Scuteri A, Crespi C, Bolondi L, Caraceni P, et al. Early occurrence and recurrence of hepatocellular carcinoma in HCV-related cirrhosis treated with direct-acting antivirals. J Hepatol. 2016;65(4):727–33.
70. Degasperi E, D'Ambrosio R, Iavarone M, Sangiovanni A, Aghemo A, Soffredini R, et al. Factors associated with increased risk of de novo or recurrent hepatocellular carcinoma in patients with cirrhosis treated with direct-acting antivirals for HCV infection. Clin Gastroenterol Hepatol. 2019;17(6):1183–1191.e7.
71. Ravaioli F, Conti F, Brillanti S, Andreone P, Mazzella G, Buonfiglioli F, et al. Hepatocellular carcinoma risk assessment by the measurement of liver stiffness variations in HCV cirrhotics treated with direct acting antivirals. Dig Liver Dis. 2018;50(6):573–9.
72. Vergniol J, Foucher J, Terrebonne E, Bernard P, Le Bail B, Merrouche W, et al. Noninvasive tests for fibrosis and liver stiffness predict 5-year outcomes of patients with chronic hepatitis C. Gastroenterology. 2011;140(7):1970–1979.e3.
73. Vergniol J, Boursier J, Coutzac C, Bertrais S, Foucher J, Angel C, et al. Evolution of non-invasive tests of liver fibrosis is associated with prognosis in patients with chronic hepatitis C. Hepatology. 2014;60(1):65–76.
74. Erman A, Sathya A, Nam A, Bielecki JM, Feld JJ, Thein HH, et al. Estimating chronic hepatitis C prognosis using transient elastography-based liver stiffness: a systematic review and meta-analysis. J Viral Hepat. 2018;25(5):502–13.

The Role of Elastography in HBV: Assessing Liver Fibrosis

4

Barbara Coco, Gabriele Ricco, and Maurizia Rossana Brunetto

4.1 Introduction

Hepatitis B virus (HBV) infection is still a global public health problem with changing epidemiology due to several factors including vaccination policies and migration [1]. Approximately 250 million people are chronic HBV surface antigen (HBsAg) carriers, with a large regional variation between low (<2%) and high (>8%) endemicity levels [1]. The prevalence decreased from high to low-medium endemicity in several countries due to improvements in the socioeconomic status, universal vaccination programs, and effective antiviral treatments. However, population movements and migration are currently influencing the prevalence of the infection in several low-endemic countries in Europe (e.g., Italy, Germany), because of the high HBsAg prevalence rates in migrants from Central/Eastern Europe, Asia, and sub-Saharan Africa [2, 3].

Chronic HBV infection is a dynamic process reflecting the interaction between virus and host's immune response: in the presence of an effective immune control, a reduced transcriptional activity of the covalently closed circular viral DNA (cccDNA) is associated with persistently low-replicative levels and the absence of active liver disease; by converse when the immune system fails to control viral

B. Coco · G. Ricco
Hepatology Unit and Laboratory of Molecular Genetics and Pathology of Hepatitis Viruses, Reference Center of the Tuscany Region for Chronic Liver Disease and Cancer, University Hospital of Pisa, Pisa, Italy

M. R. Brunetto (✉)
Hepatology Unit and Laboratory of Molecular Genetics and Pathology of Hepatitis Viruses, Reference Center of the Tuscany Region for Chronic Liver Disease and Cancer, University Hospital of Pisa, Pisa, Italy

Department of Clinical and Experimental Medicine, University of Pisa, Pisa, Italy

Institute of Biostructure and Bioimaging, National Research Council, Naples, Italy
e-mail: maurizia.brunetto@unipi.it

© Springer Nature Switzerland AG 2021
M. Fraquelli (ed.), *Elastography of the Liver and Beyond*,
https://doi.org/10.1007/978-3-030-74132-7_4

infection, the presence of florid viral replication promotes hepatitis and its progression [4–6]. Accordingly, the natural history of chronic HBV infection can be described focusing on the presence or absence of liver inflammation, and the current nomenclature is based on the description of the two main conditions—infection and hepatitis—and distinguishes chronic HBV infection associated with HBV-induced liver disease, namely, chronic hepatitis B (CHB) (either HBeAg positive or negative), from chronic HBV infection without HBV-induced liver damage, namely, non-inflammatory HBeAg-positive and HBeAg-negative infection [2].

A correct identification of the phase of HBV infection is fundamental for the optimal management of HBV carriers in clinical practice as patients who have active disease require treatment intervention and more intensive monitoring, whereas patients who have infection without hepatitis do not require antiviral treatment [2, 7]. Diagnosis of the chronic HBV infection phase is based on virological and biochemical parameters, but in a significant number of patients, particularly in HBeAg-negative/anti-HBe-positive carriers, a single determination of HBV replication markers as well as serum transaminases does not allow an accurate classification into one of the two phases: HBeAg-negative chronic hepatitis B or infection (previously named inactive infection), because of the fluctuating profile of HBeAg-negative chronic hepatitis B (CHB) [2, 8]. Thus, in case of low viremia levels (<2000–20,000 IU/mL), a serial monitoring of serum HBV-DNA and alanine aminotransferase (ALT) levels is required for at least 12 months, unless additional markers are combined [2, 9, 10].

In patients with chronic hepatitis, the persistence of high replicative levels and liver necro-inflammation favors liver disease progression: the extent of fibrosis is a major prognostic factor which correlates with the risk of developing cirrhosis and liver-related complications [2]. In untreated CHB patients, the 5-year cumulative incidence of cirrhosis ranges from 8% to 20%, and, among those with cirrhosis, the 5-year cumulative risk of hepatic decompensation is 20%, with an annual risk of hepatocellular carcinoma (HCC) of 2–5% [6, 8, 11].

The current available antiviral therapy for CHB [short-term treatment with pegylated interferon (Peg-IFN) or long-term suppressive therapy with oral nucleos(t)ide analogues (NA)] prevents disease progression, reduces the risk of end-stage liver complication, and even reverses hepatitis B virus (HBV)-induced liver fibrosis [2]. However, because of the oncogenetic potential of HBV infection, mainly due to the random integration of HBV-DNA sequences into the hepatocyte genome, particularly in patients with cirrhotic de-arrangement of the liver acinus (persistence of porto-central fibrotic bridges), the risk of developing hepatocellular carcinoma (HCC) persists even after a sustained virological response to therapy [12]. Therefore, the definition of the stage of liver disease is crucial in the management of HBsAg carriers.

Liver biopsy is the reference standard for both grading and staging of liver damage. However, it is an invasive procedure, not suitable for tight monitoring, and minimal specimen's requirements are needed to allow a correct evaluation of the liver disease: minimum length 2–2.5 cm and presence of at least 11 portal tracts [13, 14]. Its diagnostic accuracy is significantly influenced by sampling errors and the high rate of intra- and inter-observer variability, leading to under-staging of fibrosis even in adequately sized specimens, with false-negative results in up to 30% of case [13, 14]. Therefore, major efforts had been made to identify noninvasive diagnostic tools providing a quantitative index of fibrosis for an appropriate diagnosis and management of CHB patients.

Liver fibrosis can be indirectly quantified by serum markers: fibrosis-4 (FIB-4) index (age x aspartate aminotransferase [AST])/(platelet square root of alanine aminotransferase [ALT]), direct serum markers related to extracellular matrix formation (e.g., hyaluronic acid), degradation, cytokines (e.g., transforming growth factor), or fibrinolytic pathways (e.g., tissue inhibitor of metalloproteinases-1) or a combination of several markers, such as the enhanced liver fibrosis or ELF-test [15]. Also ultrasound (US)-based tests including transient elastography (TE), acoustic radiation force impulse imaging (*ARFI*), and splenic Doppler impedance index have been implemented [15, 16]. Finally, transient elastography (TE) measured by FibroScan® (Echosens, Paris, France) provides a direct, rapid, and reproducible assessment of liver stiffness (LS) that is a reliable fibrosis index currently recommended by the European Association for the study of the liver (EASL), provided that its values are adequately contextualized [2, 17]. We briefly reviewed the use of TE in the management of chronic HBsAg carriers, providing evidences about the importance of combining the serum virologic and biochemical pattern with the liver stiffness value to achieve an accurate assessment of liver disease at the single patient level.

4.2   Liver Stiffness Cofactors and Confounders

Liver stiffness is a physical parameter that primarily results from liver fibrosis; however, its values are influenced also by other factors that modify liver elasticity, such as the inflammatory infiltrate, edema, vascular congestion, cholestasis, and, even if still controversial, steatosis [17, 18]. Therefore, for a proper interpretation of TE values, the interference of such factors, particularly of inflammation, has to be considered, given the disease profile of CHB. It is known that HBeAg-negative CHB patients frequently display fluctuations of necro-inflammation and biochemical activity (hepatitis flares) followed by prolonged spontaneous virological and biochemical remission that mimic the pattern of HBeAg-negative infection [8]. We firstly observed that in patients with CHB, there was a significant correlation between LS and ALT levels and significant fluctuations of TE values paralleled ALT values during hepatitis flares, in patients with acute or chronic hepatitis [19]. Independent studies [20–24] confirmed these observations in patients with acute liver damage of different etiology. Interestingly, in patients with acute hepatitis or CHB with ALT flare LS peak values frequently exceeded the threshold values proposed for cirrhosis even in patients with absent or mild fibrosis [19]. Thus, intrahepatic inflammation has important implications for LS values, and the ALT pattern has to be taken into account when interpreting the results of TE measurements to avoid an overestimation of liver fibrosis in patients with elevated ALT [17]. Chan et al. have proposed an algorithm which uses higher cutoffs in patients with elevated ALT levels, to avoid the overestimation of fibrosis because of the inflammation.

However, adapting cutoffs on ALT did not improve the overall percentage of patients correctly classified [24]. In agreement with the major interference of liver necro-inflammation on LS values is the rapid decline of LS paralleling that of ALT during the early phase of treatment [24].

The influence of steatosis on LS measured by FibroScan in chronic hepatitis B patients is still controversial, but it appears less relevant as compared to steatosis in CHC. Gaia et al. studied 219 patients with CHB with or without steatosis to determine the reliability of TE for the detection of fibrosis. In the subgroup of 72 patients with moderate steatosis ($\geq 33\%$) and advanced fibrosis, LS values were lower than expected and similar to fibrosis stages 1 and 2 [25]. Kim et al. recruited 162 CHB patients and demonstrated that mild to moderate steatosis (5–66%) did not have significant impact on LS values [26]. Cai et al. showed that in subjects with low-grade fibrosis (S0–S2/S0–S3), mean LS values were significantly higher in subjects with severe steatosis or controlled attenuation parameter (CAP) ≥ 287 dB/m compared with those without [27]. These findings are in agreement with the previously published data by Boursier et al. who found that, in chronic hepatitis C (CHC) patients, the influence of liver steatosis disappeared in patients with significant fibrosis [28]. The authors concluded that steatosis increases liver stiffness as measured by FibroScan only in patients without severe fibrosis, whereas the influence of steatosis disappears in the presence of severe fibrosis.

Finally, Fraquelli et al. made a comprehensive evaluation of the factors responsible for any discrepancies in diagnostic accuracy between TE and liver biopsy in both CHB and CHC patients [29]. The results of the study showed that *fibrosis stage and liver cell necro-inflammatory activity* were independently associated with LS values in both HBV and HCV patients, whereas steatosis was independently associated with TE only in HCV. Fibrosis overestimation was predicted by severe/moderate necro-inflammatory activity in HBV and by older age (41–60 years or >60 years vs <40 years), >2 upper limit of normal (ULN) AST and >2 ULN GGT, whereas severe/moderate necro-inflammatory activity and severe/moderate steatosis in CHC [29].

In conclusion, all these data demonstrate that LS results in multiple intrahepatic conditions, where fibrosis and necro-inflammation are the major drivers: therefore, as TE provide a quantitative index of fibrosis/inflammation, the relative impact of each of the two on the overall TE value at any given time point of the patient history has to be evaluated in strict relation with the time-specific clinical pathologic conditions.

4.3 TE in Untreated HBV Carriers

4.3.1 HBsAg Carriers Without Liver Disease

Individuals with HBeAg-negative infection are conventionally defined as HBsAg positive, hepatitis B e antigen (HBeAg) negative, anti-HBe-positive individuals with normal alanine aminotransferase (ALT), and HBV-DNA persistently

<2000 IU/mL [2]. Long-term follow-up studies showed that such virological profile is a favorable and benign condition, leading to a progressively control of HBV replication and fostering transition to occult hepatitis B infection (OBI) in a significant proportion of cases [7, 9, 10, 30–33]. Similarly, growing evidences suggest that carriers with viremia levels persistently <20,000 IU/mL have a benign outcome as well as high rate of transition to inactive infection (43% of subjects followed for 6 years, on our experience) [10]. Therefore, in this subset of HBeAg-negative carriers without active liver disease, there is not any need for an invasive assessment of liver histology. However, the diagnostic challenge remains to timely identify HBeAg-negative CHB patients who show a similar virological and biochemical profile because of a temporary remission of both viral replication and disease activity [8]. A tight monitoring of HBV-DNA for at least 1 year or a combination of different serum viral markers (HBsAg; total anti-HBc and HBcrAg) has been proposed [9, 10, 30–33]. Alternatively, to avoid a costly and time-consuming monitoring, several studies have investigated the accuracy of TE to discriminate between HBeAg-negative infection and CHB [10, 20, 34–36]. We firstly reported low LS values in 68 genotype D carriers of HBeAg-negative infection (TE = 5.0 ± 1.8 kPa), showing that in carriers with metabolic liver disease, mean LS values were significantly higher than in those without liver disease cofactors (6.9 ± 2.3 kPa in 17 patients with histologically proven steatohepatitis or steatosis vs 4.3 ± 1.0 kPa in 57 subjects with normal ALT and without cofactors) [20]. Many studies subsequently confirmed that carriers of HBeAg-negative infection have mean LS values comparable to those of normal controls and significantly lower than those of CHB patients [34–37]. Overall, all these studies confirmed that median TE values are less than 5 kPa in low-replicative HBeAg-negative carriers, with an upper range reaching 7.9 kPa values in some studies [34, 35]. Thus, high LS values (with or without serum ALT elevations) in carriers with viremia persistently <2000 IU/mL suggest the presence of liver damage due to causes other than HBV with the need for further investigations, eventually with liver biopsy.

Monitoring LS values can also contribute to confirm the benign course of infection. Castera et al. reported that LS measurements did not differ significantly over time in 82 low-replicative carriers (median follow-up, 21.7 months; range, 3.3–49.1 months) confirming the clinical usefulness of TE in these subjects [35]. Consistently with the previous reports, Wong et al. studied LS at baseline and after a 3-year follow-up in an Asian cohort of 361 HBeAg-negative HBV carriers: the liver disease progression (which was arbitrarily defined as "an increase in LS by at least 30% to a value suggestive of advanced fibrosis") appeared to be rare among patients with a HBV-DNA level <20,000 IU/mL (2.8%) and extremely rare in inactive carriers (0.8%) [36]. Similarly in our cohort of 133 low viremic carriers with uneventful outcome for over 60 months, liver stiffness values remained stable throughout the follow-up (baseline median stiffness values of HBeAg-negative carriers and low viremic carriers 4.9 (2.7–5.8) and 5.2 (3.1–6.1) kPa vs 4.6 (2.5–6.2) kPa vs 4.6 (3.2–5.9) kPa at the end of follow-up) [10].

4.3.2 Untreated CHB Patients

Both European and Asian studies showed that the natural course of HBV infection varies between geographical areas and is affected by several factors such as age at primary infection, gender, host genomics, HBV genotype, mutant strains, and presence of cofactors of liver disease [6, 7, 11]. However, high levels of HBV replication, independent of HBeAg status, and sustained disease activity are the strongest predictors of adverse clinical outcomes, increasing the risk of cirrhosis and liver-related mortality, due to the development of HCC and liver failure [2, 6, 8]. Therefore, in CHB patients, the assessment of the disease stage is crucially important to take appropriate therapeutic decisions, monitoring treatment response, and disease progression and to evaluate the need for HCC surveillance.

Several studies have analyzed the diagnostic accuracy of TE in predicting the stage of fibrosis in CHB patients; a summary of the most relevant studies is reported in Tables 4.1 and 4.2.

The proposed LS thresholds to diagnose significant fibrosis ($F \geq 2$ or $S \geq 3$) range from 5.2 to 8.7 kPa, with highly variable sensitivity (64–93%), specificity (38–92%), and AUROC ranging from 0.82 to 0.96. The range of the LS thresholds to identify cirrhosis ($F \geq 4$) is even higher, ranging from 9.4 to 17.5 kPa; nevertheless, many studies suggested values around 11 kPa, with AUROC >0.90 (Table 4.2).

The wide variations of LS thresholds are influenced by several factors: the heterogeneity of the different cohorts, with unbalanced distribution of patients in terms of phases of HBV infection, disease activity, and stages of fibrosis. Furthermore, in many studies, an accurate stratification according to the stage of portal hypertension is missing. Finally, since TE provide a fibrosis/inflammation index without

Table 4.1 Transient elastography performance for the diagnosis of significant fibrosis ($F \geq 2$) in CHB

Ref.	Country	Patients (n)	Cutoff (kPa)	Sensitivity (%)	Specificity (%)	AUROC (95% CI)
Oliveri et al. [20]	Italy	188	7.5	93	88	0.96 (0.94–0.99)
Marcellin et al. [38]	France	173	7.2	70	83	0.81 (0.73–0.86)
Chan et al. [24]	China	161	8.4	84	76	0.87 (0.82–0.93)
Degos et al. [39]	France	284	5.2	89	38	
Viganò et al. [37]	Italy	217	8.7	64	92	
Cardoso et al. [40]	France	202	7.2	74	88	0.86
Jia et al. [41]	China	486	7.3	66	83	0.82 (0.78–0.85)

Table 4.2 Transient elastography performance for the diagnosis of cirrhosis (F4) in CHB

Ref.	Country	Patients (n)	Cutoff (kPa)	Sensitivity (%)	Specificity (%)	AUROC (95% CI)
Oliveri et al. [20]	Italy	188	11.8	93	88	0.97 (0.95–0.99)
Marcellin et al. [38]	France	173	11.0	70	83	0.93 (0.82–0.98)
Chan et al. [24]	China	161	13.4	79	92	0.93 (0.89–0.97)
Viganò et al. [37]	Italy	217	9.4	100	82	
Kim et al. [42]	Korea	99	10.3	59	78	0.80
Cardoso et al. [40]	France	202	11.0	75	90	0.93
Jia et al. [41]	China	486	17.5	60	93	0.90 (0.87–0.94)

dissecting the relative values of these two components, the inclusion of patients during an ALT flare might have caused an overestimation of fibrosis in a subset of patients reducing the overall diagnostic performance of TE in predicting fibrosis.

A few studies have carried out direct comparisons between CHB and chronic hepatitis C (CHC) patients. Cardoso et al. and Verveer et al. have assessed—in a cross-sectional study—treatment-naive patients with CHB or CHC who underwent TE measurement and liver biopsy, showing that the overall TE diagnostic performance was similar in the two groups of patients [40, 43]. In a meta-analysis including 17 studies on CHC patients and ten studies on CHB patients, Tsochatzis et al. reported that LS cutoffs were globally lower in CHB as compared to CHC group (on average 7.0 vs 7.6 for $F \geq 2$, 8.2 vs 10.9 for $F \geq 3$, and 11.3 vs 15.3 for F4) [44]. Similar findings were reported by Chon et al. in another meta-analysis of 18 studies assessing HBV patients, which showed the estimated cutoff of 7.9 (range 6.1–11.8) kPa for $F \geq 2$, 8.8 (range 8.1–9.7) kPa for $F \geq 3$, and 11.7 (range 7.3–17.5) kPa for the identification of $F = 4$ [45]. A possible explanation for this finding is the evidence that fibrosis septa are usually thinner in CHB patients resulting in cirrhosis with larger nodules (macronodular cirrhosis) as compared to CHC [14, 46]. However, many additional cofactors can influence the LS values, and their different prevalence in CHC and CHB patients may well explain the results.

In clinical practice, TE contributes to identify chronic HBV carriers without liver disease (LS values ≤ 5 kPa and comparable to healthy subject) or patients without significant fibrosis (LS values ≤ 8 kPa). By converse, LS values ranging from 8 to 11 kPa are indicative of significant liver disease, but they need to be contextualized to rule out a possible interference of necro-inflammation. Similarly, values >11 kPa, in the absence of an ALT flare, are indicative of severe fibrosis (Fig. 4.1).

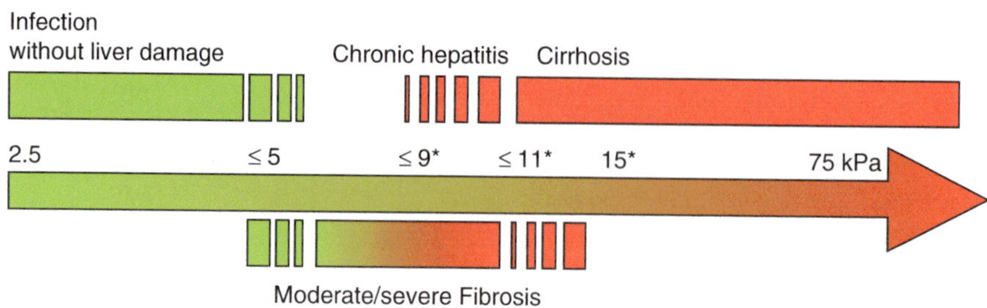

Fig. 4.1 FibroScan values and stage of liver disease in untreated HBV carriers. Schematic diagram of FibroScan values in untreated HBV carriers. For values in the range of 5–15 kPa, a correlation with the biochemical activity of disease is mandatory for the correct interpretation of the data. Adapted and modified from Bonino et al. [18]

4.4 TE in Treated CHB Patients

4.4.1 LS Kinetics During Antiviral Treatment

Antiviral therapy in CHB is aimed to prevent its progression to cirrhosis or, when cirrhosis is already present, to avoid or delay the development of the end-stage complications of liver disease and HCC [2]. Disease progression is promoted by persistent liver necro-inflammation that results from the inability of the host's immune system to control viral replication effectively. Two different therapeutic approaches can be attempted to suppress disease activity: (1) to shift the host-virus equilibrium from the pathogenic active to the nonpathogenic low-replicative phase with a time limited course of antiviral treatment capable of inducing a sustained off-therapy control of HBV replication and (2) to suppress viral replication persistently with continuous antiviral treatment [2]. Interferon (IFN) is the major player of the former strategy, even if also nucleos(t)ide analogues (NA) treatment can achieve a persistent control of the infection in a proportion of patients, usually after prolonged treatment. However, in many patients, mainly HBeAg negative with advanced fibrosis, a long-term, eventually lifelong, treatment is preferred to warrant a persistent pharmacological control of viral replication [2]. Since the early 1990s, several studies in IFN treated patients showed that an effective treatment is associated with the clearance of intrahepatic necro-inflammation and reduction of fibrosis, with an overall improvement of liver histology [8, 47–49]. More recently, the follow-up of patients in long-term NA treatment showed a similar picture, with the evidence of a significant reduction of fibrosis, eventually with cirrhosis reversal [50]. Actually, cirrhosis results not only from diffuse fibrosis but also from nodular parenchymal regeneration (architectural distortion) and major vascular derangements, including intrahepatic portosystemic shunts [51]. A full reversal of such alterations in patients with long-lasting cirrhosis is unlikely: even if resorption of fibrosis can occur, it remains to be clarified to which extent the plasticity of the vascular structures could favor the resolution of the abnormal vascular shunts [51]. Nevertheless, long-term NA treatment is associated with lower rates of liver decompensation, HCC development, and overall improvement of patients' survival [12, 50, 52, 53]. Therefore, mainly in patients with advanced fibrosis, it is mandatory to monitor antiviral therapy not only in terms of viral and biochemical response but also of liver disease improvement.

Liver biopsy, as discussed previously, is unsuitable for multiple evaluations that would be required to monitor the changes in liver disease during NAs. Therefore, alternative noninvasive and reliable tools for longitudinal follow-up of these patients are required in clinical practice. Accordingly, TE had been widely used to monitor treated CHB patients, and the LS dynamic changes in patients undergoing NAs treatment show a significant decrease of its values overtime. Nevertheless, since TE provides a combined fibrosis/inflammation index, it is difficult to differentiate the LS reduction resulting from the clearance of necro-inflammation from that due to the fibrosis regression. Several studies, mainly retrospective, investigated the role of necro-inflammation on LS changes during NAs, with conflicting results (Table 4.3). Some studies suggested that a decrease in LS values was a consequence of fibrosis regression because on-treatment LS decline was independent from baseline ALT levels or unrelated with ALT changes [54–56, 61, 64, 65]. On the contrary, other studies reported either a correlation between LS and ALT decline or a significant LS decline only in patients whose ALT levels were elevated at baseline [57, 58].

Interestingly, Wong et al. in their prospective study recruited 71 CHB patients with paired liver biopsy and transient elastography before and after week 48 of antiviral treatment in two randomized clinical trials. The authors reported ALT normalization in 82% of patients and LS decrease, defined as a decline >30% of baseline value, in 39%. Among patients with decreased LS values, only 11 (39%) had histological regression of fibrosis, while 14 and 3 had unchanged or progression of Metavir staging, suggesting that the decrease in LS values was more likely associated with the reduction of both intrahepatic necro-inflammation and ALT rather than a change in liver fibrosis [59].

More recently, Liang et al. studied the dynamics of LS every 6 months in 534 CHB patients treated with entecavir (ETV). Histological reassessment in a subset of 164 patients showed a regression of fibrosis in about 60% of cases after 2 years of ETV. Median LS values declined in parallel with ALT levels in the first 24 weeks; thereafter, from week 24 to 104, a slower but persisting decline of median LS was observed, in spite of stable ALT values. Interestingly, LS values declined independently of baseline ALT values, but their decline was greater in patients with more severe necro-inflammation and fibrosis at baseline as well as in patients with better virological response [63].

Overall, these findings and longitudinal studies with 3–5 years of follow-up confirm that LS is a measure of both liver inflammation and fibrosis: LS kinetics show a biphasic pattern with an initial phase of more rapid decline, followed by a subsequent slower decline [60, 62, 63]. The rapid-to-slow decline observed within the first 24–48 weeks of treatment suggests that in the early phase, the remission of biochemical activity and the progressive reduction of

Table 4.3 Studies on LS reduction following antiviral treatment with NAs

Ref.	Year	Study type	NAs	Time (years)	Patients (n)	bx	LS-BL (kPa)	LS-EOF (kPa)	P^a
Kim et al. [54]	2010	Retrospective	LAM/ADV	1	23	4	13.7 ± 8.0	11.3 ± 5.3	0.018
			ETV	2	18		12.1 ± 9.6	not given	0.017
Enomoto et al. [55]	2010	Retrospective	ETV	1	20	2	11.2 (7.0–15.2)	7.8 (5.1–11.9)	0.0090
Osakabe et al. [56]	2011	Retrospective	LAM/ETV	3	29	/	12.9 (6.2–17.9)	4.7 (3.1–7.9)	0.006
Fung et al. [57]	2011	Prospective	LAM/ADV ETV/TDF	3	110	/	7.3	6.1	<0.001
Lim et al. [58]	2011	Retrospective	ETV	1	62	/	15.1 (5.6–75.0)	8.8 (3.0–33.8)	<0.001
Wong et al. [59]	2011	Prospective	CLV/ADV	1	71	71	8.8 (3.1–26.3)	6.6 (3.3–18.8)	<0.001
Ogawa et al. [60]	2011	Retrospective	LAM/ETV	3	22	/	8.2 (4.2–28.5)	5.3 (2.5–18.0)	<0.001
Kim et al. [61]	2014	Prospective	ETV	3	121	/	14.3 (9.0–23.5)	7.3 (5.3–11.8)	<0.001
Chon et al. [62]	2017	Prospective	LAM/ETV	5	120	/	14.5	8.3	<0.001
Liang et al. [63]	2018	Prospective	LdT/ LdT + ADV	2	534	164	8.6 (2.6–49.5)	5.3 (2.7–36.8)	<0.001
Rinaldi et al. [64]	2018	Retrospective	ETV/TDF	2	149	/	12.4 ± 9.3	8.2 ± 4.9	<0.001
Li et al. [65]	2018	Retrospective	ETV	3	104	/	8.2 (5.9–9.7)	5.6 (4.5–8.5)	<0.001

ADV adefovir; bx, liver biopsy, *CLV* clevudine, *ETV* entecavir, *LAM* lamivudine, *LdT* telbivudine, *LS-BL* liver stiffness at baseline, *LS-EOF* liver stiffness at end of follow-up, *NAs* nucleos(t)ide analogues, *TDF* tenofovir disoproxil fumarate
aComparison between baseline and follow-up LS values

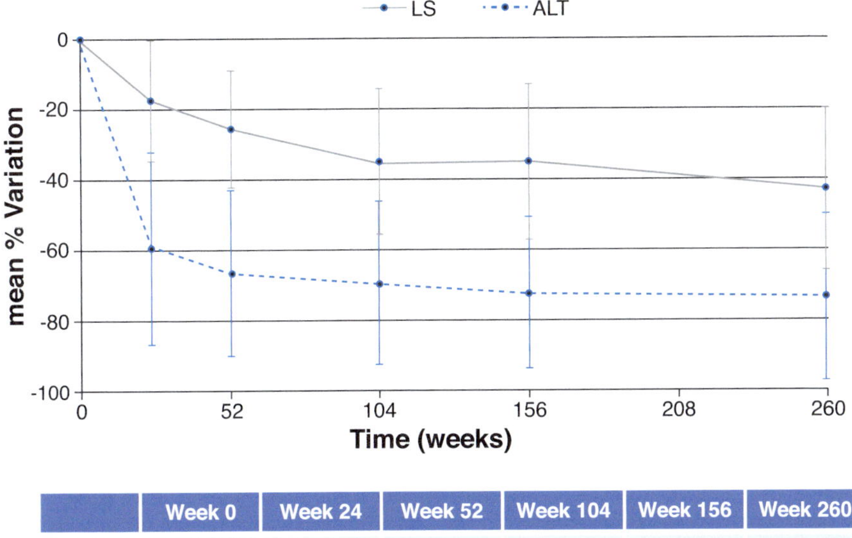

	Week 0	Week 24	Week 52	Week 104	Week 156	Week 260
ALT (U/L)	212 ± 452.6	33 ± 22.3	24.8 ± 9.1	21.2 ± 8.0	19.6 ± 7.5	18.3 ± 5.53
LS (kPa)	10.6 ± 6.6	8.7 ± 5.3	7.6 ± 3.4	6.1 ± 2.6	5.4 ± 1.4	5.2 ± 1.9

Data are expressed as mean values $\pm$ SD

Fig. 4.2 Dynamic changes in liver necro-inflammation and liver stiffness in CHB patients undergoing NAs. Dynamic changes of ALT and liver stiffness values in 50 CHB patients on long-term (>5 years) antiviral therapy with NAs. Personal unpublished data

intrahepatic necro-inflammation play a major role in LS values variation. Later during treatment, particularly after ALT normalization, the more gradual LS reduction reflects the regression of fibrosis (Fig. 4.2). Since fibrosis is more likely to regress if it is recent (such as in case of the unregulated wound-healing response induced by active necro-inflammation) [66], it remains to be demonstrated whether a greater LS decline could reflect mainly a regression of a more recent fibrosis.

In our previous experience of 35 treated patients monitored with TE for 48 months, LS showed a mean yearly decline of about 0.2-folds reaching values below the cirrhosis cutoff (11.8 kPa) in patients who maintained the histologic evidence of cirrhosis [20]. As a consequence, it remains open the question whether the LS thresholds currently used to identify the different stages of fibrosis in patients with active liver disease can be automatically applied to patients with a complete and long-lasting resolution of disease activity (i.e., necro-inflammation). In fact, studies where LS values are compared with the histological picture, in an adequate number of both patients with active and inactive cirrhosis, are missing. Therefore, in patients on long-term NA treatment, without a baseline characterization of liver disease stage, the LS values must be always interpreted on the light of the other biochemical and instrumental information, to rule out the presence of cirrhosis.

4.4.2 Correlation Between LS Changes During Treatment and CHB Outcomes

Chronic HBV infection, as previously discussed, is a major cause of HCC worldwide with an annual incidence of 2–3% for HBsAg-positive carriers with compensated cirrhosis and less than 1% for those without cirrhosis [11]. It is now widely accepted that the risk of HCC development is reduced by an effective and prolonged viral load suppression such as that obtained under NAs. However, the risk of HCC is not eliminated, probably due to pathophysiological events that occurred before therapy start or to oncogenetic mechanisms that are not influenced by antivirals [12]. Therefore, surveillance for HCC is recommended in CHB patients, but reliable tools for risk stratification are of crucial importance in order to sustain cost-effectiveness [67]. Accordingly, several risk prediction scores have been developed in the past decade, initially in untreated cohorts of Asian patients, based on multiple factors that were found associated with HBV-related HCC, such as gender, age, fibrotic stage, and HBV-DNA levels [68]. Most of them in addition to demographic and biochemical parameters include HBV-DNA as the major prediction variable: the CU (Chinese University)-HCC score, which was derived from 1005 untreated CHB patients (38% with cirrhosis), utilizes age, albumin, bilirubin, HBV-DNA levels, and presence or absence of cirrhosis [69], and the REACH-B score (risk estimation for HCC in CHB), derived from 3584 non-cirrhotic CHB patients, is based on sex, age, ALT, HBeAg, and HBV-DNA levels [70]. However, since high genetic barrier NAs were introduced in the treatment of CHB, the prognostic significance of serum HBV-DNA levels loses power because most of the treated patients achieve and maintain a complete virological response. Actually, several studies demonstrated that a stratification according to fibrotic burden could be more prognostic, since the degree of fibrosis was associated with HCC development [71], hepatic decompensation [72], and portal hypertension-related complications [73].

In 2014, Wong et al. refined the CU-HCC score in a training cohort of 1035 subjects, including 390 patients under antiviral treatment, where the clinical definition of cirrhosis was replaced by a stratification of the population in three groups according to the increasing levels of LS ($\leq$8.0 kPa, 8.1–12.0 kPa, and >12.0 kPa). The new score (LSM-HCC) was superior in predicting the 3- and 5-year risk of HCC development, with an AUROC in the validation cohort of 0.89 at 3 years and 0.83 at 5 years. Using a cutoff of 11 points to stratify the population, the HCC rates at 5 years were 0.3% and 7.6% in the low- and high-risk group, respectively [74]. In same year, Lee et al. demonstrated that a reduction $\geq$25% in LS values from BL at complete virological response was associated with favorable outcomes in CHB patients treated with ETV. Therefore, they developed a modified REACH-B score (mREACH-B) in which the HBV-DNA level of the original score was substituted with the LS value stratified into three groups (<8.0 kPa, 8.0–13.0 kPa, and >13.0 kPa) [75]. Finally, the authors compared all the available predictive scores in a cohort of 1308 patients (848 undergoing antiviral treatment) and found that the AUROC of mREACH-B at 3 and 5 years in the prediction of HCC development were higher than those of the other models, both overall and in the subgroup of treated patients [76]. More recently, the same group developed another LS-based HCC prediction model, including US features of cirrhosis, age, gender, platelet count, albumin, and LS ≥ 11 kPa (CAMPAS), in 1511 patients receiving NAs. The CAMPAS model was validated in an external independent cohort of 252 treated patients and showed a significantly higher prognostic performance compared to the mREACH-B [77]. Overall, these findings are very promising; however, the modified score using LS needs to be validated in non-Asian cohorts, to rule out possible bias from confounding factors that can influence LS values in different patients' populations [68]. Currently, the HCC predictive score developed in Caucasian patients treated with ETV or TDF, the PAGE-B, does not take into account the cirrhosis or LS values [16]. Therefore, additional prospective studies are needed to investigate the role of LS in the prediction of HCC development in Western CHB patients. In addition, liver rehashing during NA therapy is a multistep process where clearance of necro-inflammation is the first and early one, whereas fibrosis regression is a later and slower process that could have a different impact on liver anatomical structure depending on the extent of vascular alterations. Therefore, future prospective studies should more accurately analyze the kinetics of LS during NA therapy to identify not only absolute LS values but also their on-treatment delta variation possibly correlating with different HCC risk.

4.5 Conclusions

In carriers with chronic HBV infection, the noninvasive measure of LS provides a reliable noninvasive index of liver disease burden that combines both fibrosis and inflammation. In carriers of HBeAg-negative infection, who do not have active liver disease, LS values are comparable with those of normal controls and significantly lower than in CHB patients. Therefore, in this subset of chronic HBsAg carriers, elevated LS values suggest the presence of liver disease due to factors different from HBV. In untreated CHB patients, ALT flares (and the extent of necro-inflammation at histology) are factors that significantly influence LS in addition to fibrosis. Therefore, LS values should be interpreted with caution in patients with elevated ALT, especially in those with significant ALT flare (>10 × ULN). TE appears to be a reliable method to identify CHB patients with advanced fibrosis or cirrhosis. Interestingly, LS cutoff associated with cirrhosis in CHB is lower than in CHC patients, possibly because of a different cirrhotic derangement.

In CHB patients responding to antivirals, the LS decline shows a biphasic pattern that might be explained by the combined kinetics of an earlier and faster decline of necro-inflammation and a later and slower decline of fibrosis. Lower LS values achieved during antiviral therapy are associated with a lower risk of HCC development, at least in Asian cohorts. Future studies should validate the finding in Western CHB patients and investigate whether the lack of a significant second-phase long-term decline of LS would predict a higher residual HCC risk in responders to antiviral therapy.

References

1. Scweitzer A, Horn J, Mykolajczyk RT, Krause G, Ott J. Estimation of worldwide prevalence of chronic hepatitis B virus infection: a systematic review of data published between 1965 and 2013. Lancet. 2015;386:1546–55.
2. EASL. 2017 Clinical Practice Guidelines on the management of hepatitis B virus infection. J Hepatol. 2017;67:370–98.
3. The Polaris Observatory Collaborators. Global prevalence, treatment and prevention of hepatitis B virus infection in 2016: a modeling study. Lancet Gastroenterol Hepatol. 2018;3:383–403.
4. Cox AL, El-Sayed MH, Kao JH, Lazarus JV, Lemoine M, Lok AS, Zoulim F. Progress towards elimination goals for viral hepatitis. Nat Rev Gastroenterol Hepatol. 2020;17(9):533–42.
5. Bertoletti A, Ferrari C. Adaptive immunity in HBV infection. J Hepatol. 2016;64:571–83.
6. Fattovich G, Bortolotti F, Donato F. Natural history of chronic-hepatitis-B: special emphasis on disease progression and prognostic factors. J Hepatol. 2008;48(2):335–52.
7. Manno M, Cammà C, Schepis F, Bassi F, Gelmini R, Giannini F, et al. Natural history of chronic HBV carriers in northern Italy: morbidity and mortality after 30 years. Gastroenterology. 2004;127(3):756–63.
8. Brunetto MR, Oliveri F, Coco B, Leandro G, Colombatto P, Gorin JM, Bonino F. Outcome of anti-HBe positive chronic hepatitis B in alpha-interferon treated and untreated patients: a long term cohort study. J Hepatol. 2002;36(2):263–70.
9. Brunetto MR, Oliveri F, Colombatto P, Moriconi P, Ciccorossi P, Coco B, et al. Hepatitis B Surface antigen serum levels help to distinguish active from inactive hepatitis B virus genotype D carriers. Gastroenterology. 2010;2:483–94.
10. Oliveri F, Surace L, Cavallone D, Colombatto P, Ricco G, Salvati N, et al. Long-term outcome of inactive and active low viraemic HBeAg-negative hepatitis B virus infection: benign course towards HBeAg clearance. Liver Int. 2017;37(11):1622–31.
11. Liaw YF, Brunetto MR, Hadziyannis S. The natural history of chronic-HBV-infection and geographical differences. Antivir Ther. 2010;15(S3):25–33.
12. Papatheodoris GV, Sypsa V, Dalekos G, Yurdaydin C, Buti M, Goulis J, et al. PAGE-B predicts the risk of developing hepatocellular carcinoma in Caucasian chronic hepatitis B on 5-year antiviral therapy. J Hepatol. 2016;64(4):800–6.
13. Colloredo G, Guido M, Sonzogni A, Leandro G. Impact of liver biopsy size on histological evaluation of chronic viral hepatitis: the smaller the sample, the milder the disease. J Hepatol. 2003;39(2):239–44.
14. Bedossa P, Dargere D, Paradis V. Sampling variability of liver fibrosis in chronic hepatitis C. Hepatology. 2003;38(6):1449–57.
15. Parikh P, Ryan JD, Tsochatzi E. Fibrosis assessment in patients with chronic hepatitis B virus (HBV) infection. Ann Transl Med. 2017;5(3):40.
16. Ferraioli G, Wong VW, Casterà L, Berzigotti A, Sporea I, Dietrich CF, et al. Liver Ultrasound elastography: an update to the world federation for ultrasound in medicine and biology guidelines and recommendations. Ultrasound Med Biol. 2018;44(12):2419–40.
17. EASL-ALEH Clinical Practice Guidelines: non-invasive tests for evaluation of liver disease severity and prognosis. J Hepatol. 2015;63(1):237–64.
18. Bonino F, Arena U, Brunetto MR, Coco B, Fraquelli M, Oliveri F, et al. Liver stiffness, a non invasive marker of liver disease: a core study group report. Antivir Ther. 2010;15(Suppl 3):69–78.
19. Coco B, Oliveri F, Maina AM, Ciccorossi P, Sacco R, Colombatto P, et al. Transient elastography: a new surrogate marker of liver fibrosis influenced by major changes of transaminases. J Viral Hepat. 2007;14(5):360–9.
20. Oliveri F, Coco B, Ciccorossi P, Colombatto P, Romagnoli V, Cherubini B, et al. Liver stiffness in the hepatitis B virus carrier: a non-invasive marker of liver disease influenced by the pattern of transaminases. World J Gastroenterol. 2008;14(40):6154–62.

21. Viganò M, Massironi S, Lampertico P, Iavarone M, Paggi S, Pozzi R, et al. Transient elastography assessment of the liver stiffness dynamics during acute hepatitis B. Eur J Gastroenterol Hepatol. 2010;22(2):180–4.
22. Arena U, Vizzutti F, Corti G, Ambu S, Stasi C, Bresci S, et al. Acute viral hepatitis increases liver stiffness values measured by transient elastography. Hepatology. 2008;47(2):380–4.
23. Sagir A, Erhardt A, Schmitt M, Häussinger D. Transient elastography is unreliable for detection of cirrhosis in patients with acute liver damage. Hepatology. 2008;47(2):592–5.
24. Chan HL, Wong GL, Choi PC, Chan AW, Chim AM, Yiu KK, et al. Alanine aminotransferase-based algorithms of liver stiffness measurement by transient elastography (Fibroscan) for liver fibrosis in chronic hepatitis B. J Viral Hepat. 2009;16:36–44.
25. Gaia S, Carenzi S, Barilli AL, Bugianesi E, Smedile A, Brunello F, et al. Reliability of transient elastography for the detection of fibrosis in non-alcoholic fatty liver disease and chronic viral hepatitis. J Hepatol. 2011;54:64–7.
26. Kim SU, Kim DY, Ahn SH, Kim HM, Lee JM, Chon CY, et al. The impact of steatosis on liver stiffness measurement in patients with chronic hepatitis B. Hepatogastroent. 2010;57(101):832–8.
27. Cai YJ, Dong JJ, Wang XD, Huang SS, Chen RC, Chen Y, et al. A diagnostic algorithm for assessment of liver fibrosis by liver stiffness measurement in patients with chronic hepatitis B. J Viral Hepat. 2017;24(11):1005–15.
28. Boursier J, de Ledinghen V, Sturm N, Amrani L, Bacq Y, Sandrini J, et al. Precise evaluation of liver histology by computerized morphometry shows that steatosis influences liver stiffness measured by transient elastography in chronic hepatitis C. J Gastroenterol. 2014;49(3):527–37.
29. Fraquelli M, Rigamonti C, Casazza G, Donato MF, Ronchi G, Conte D, et al. Etiology-related determinants of liver stiffness values in chronic viral hepatitis B or C. J Hepatol. 2011;54(4):621–8.
30. Brower WP, Chan HL, Brunetto MR, Martinot-Peignoux M, Arends P, Cornberg M, et al. Repeated measurements of HBsAg identify carriers of inactive HBV during long-term follow up. Clin Gastroenterol Hepatol. 2016;14(10):1481–9.
31. Han ZG, Qie ZH, Qiao WZ. HBsAg spontaneous clearance in hepatitis B-e-antigen-negative chronic hepatitis B patients. J Med Virol. 2016;88(1):79–85.
32. Papatheodoris GV, Manolakopoulos S, Liaw YF, Lok A. Follow-up and indication for liver biopsy in HBeAg-negative chronic hepatitis B virus infection with persistently normal ALT: a systematic review. J Hepatol. 2012;57(1):196–202.
33. Yuan Q, Song LW, Cavallone D, Moriconi F, Cherubini B, Colombatto P, et al. Total Hepatitis B-Core Antigen Antibody, a quantitative non-invasive marker of Hepatitis B-Virus induced liver disease. PLoS One. 2015;10(6):e130209.
34. Maimone S, Calvaruso V, Pleguezuelo M, Squadrito G, Amaddeo G, Jacobs M, et al. An evaluation of transient elastography in the discrimination of HBeAg negative disease from inactive hepatitis B carriers. J Viral Hepat. 2009;16(11):769–74.
35. Castéra L, Bernard PH, Le Bail B, Foucher J, Trimoulet P, Merrouche W, et al. Transient elastography and biomarkers for liver fibrosis assessment and follow-up of inactive hepatitis B carriers. Aliment Pharmacol Ther. 2011;33(4):455–65.
36. Wong GL, Chan HL, Yu Z, Chan HY, Tse CH, Wong VW. Liver fibrosis progression is uncommon in patients with inactive chronic hepatitis B: a prospective cohort study with paired transient elastography examination. J Gastroenterol Hepatol. 2013;28(12):1842–8.
37. Viganò M, Paggi S, Lampertico P, Fraquelli M, Massironi S, Ronchi G, et al. Dual cut off transient elastography to assess liver fibrosis in chronic hepatitis B: a cohort study with internal validation. Aliment Pharmacol Ther. 2011;34(3):353–62.
38. Marcellin P, Ziol M, Bedossa P, Douvin C, Poupon R, de Lédinghen V, Beaugrand M. Non-invasive assessment of liver fibrosis by stiffness measurement in patients with chronic hepatitis B. Liver Int. 2009;29(2):242–7.
39. Degos F, Perez P, Roche B, Mahmoudi A, Asselineau J, Voitot H, et al. Diagnostic accuracy of Fibroscan and comparison to liver fibrosis biomarkers in chronic viral hepatitis: a multicenter prospective study (the FIBROSTIC study). J Hepatol. 2010;53(6):1013–21.

40. Cardoso AC, Carvalho-Filho RJ, Stern C, Dipumpo A, Giuily N, Ripault MP, et al. Direct comparison of diagnostic performance of transient elastography in patients with chronic hepatitis B and chronic hepatitis C. Liver Int. 2012;32(4):612–21.

41. Jia J, Hou J, Ding H, Chen G, Xie Q, Wang Y, et al. Transient elastography compared to serum markers to predict liver fibrosis in a cohort of Chinese patients with chronic hepatitis B. J Gastroenterol Hepatol. 2015;30(4):756–62.

42. Kim DY, Kim SU, Ahn SH, Park JY, Lee JM, Park YN, et al. Usefulness of Fibroscan and ultrasonography to detection of early compensated liver cirrhosis in chronic hepatitis B. Dig Dis Sci. 2009;54(8):1578–63.

43. Verveer C, Zondervan PE, ten Kate FJ, Hansen BE, Janssen HL, de Knegt RJ. Evaluation of transient elastography for fibrosis assessment compared with large biopsies in chronic hepatitis B and C. Liver Int. 2012;32(4):622–8.

44. Tsochatzis EA, Gurusamy KS, Ntaoula S, Cholongitas E, Davidson BR, Burroughs AK. Elastography for the diagnosis of severity of fibrosis in chronic liver disease: a meta-analysis of diagnostic accuracy. J Hepatol. 2011;54(4):650–9.

45. Chon YE, Choi EH, Song KJ, Park JK, Kim DY, Han KH, et al. Performance of transient elastography for the staging of liver fibrosis in patients with chronic hepatitis B: a meta-analyses. PLoS One. 2012;7(9):e44930.

46. Rousselet MC, Michalak S, Dupre F, Croué A, Bedossa P, Saint-André JP, et al. Sources of variability in histological scoring of chronic viral hepatitis. Hepatology. 2005;41(2):257–64.

47. Brunetto MR, Oliveri F, Rocca G, Criscuolo D, Chiaberge E, Capalbo M, David E, Verme G, Bonino F. Natural course and response to interferon of chronic hepatitis B accompanied by antibody to hepatitis B e antigen. Hepatology. 1989;10(2):198–202.

48. Lampertico P, Del Ninno E, Viganò M, Romeo R, Donato MF, Sablon E, et al. Long-term suppression of hepatitis B e antigen negative chronic hepatitis B by 24 months interferon therapy. Hepatology. 2003;37(4):756–63.

49. Papatheodoridis GV, Petraki K, Cholongitas E, Kanta E, Ketikoglou I, Manesis EK. Impact of interferon-alpha therapy on liver fibrosis progression in patients with HBeAg-negative chronic hepatitis B. J Viral Hepat. 2005;12(2):199–206.

50. Marcellin P, Gane E, Buti M, Afdhal N, Sievert W, Jacobson IM, et al. Regression of cirrhosis during treatment with tenofovir disoproxil fumarate for chronic hepatitis B: a 5-year open-label follow-up study. Lancet. 2013;381(9865):468–75.

51. Desmet VJ. Roskams. Cirrhosis reversal: a duel between dogma and myth. J Hepatol. 2004;40(5):860–7.

52. Chang TT, Liaw YF, Wu SS, Schiff E, Han KH, Lai CL, et al. Long-term entecavir therapy results in the reversal of fibrosis/cirrhosis and continued histological improvement in patients with chronic hepatitis B. Hepatology. 2010;52(3):886–93.

53. Schiff ER, Lee SS, Chao YC, Kew Yoon S, Bessone F, Wu SS, et al. Long-term treatment with entecavir induces reversal of advanced fibrosis or cirrhosis in patients with chronic hepatitis B. Clin Gastroenterol Hepatol. 2011;9(3):274–6.

54. Kim SU, Park JY, Kim DY, Ahn SH, Choi EH, Seok JY, et al. Non-invasive assessment of changes in liver fibrosis via liver stiffness measurement in patients with chronic hepatitis B: impact of antiviral treatment on fibrosis regression. Hepatol Int. 2010;4(4):673–80.

55. Enomoto M, Mori M, Ogawa T, Fujii H, Kobayashi S, Iwai S, et al. Usefulness of transient elastography for assessment of liver fibrosis in chronic hepatitis B: regression of liver stiffness during entecavir therapy. Hepatol Res. 2010;40(9):853–61.

56. Osakabe K, Ichino N, Nishikawa T, Sugiyama H, Kato M, Kitahara S, et al. Reduction of liver stiffness by antiviral therapy in chronic hepatitis B. J Gastroenterol. 2011;46(11):1324–34.

57. Fung J, Lai CL, Wong DK, Seto WK, Hung I, Yuen MF. Significant changes in liver stiffness measurements in patients with chronic hepatitis B: 3-year follow-up study. J Viral Hepat. 2011;18(7):e200–5.

58. Lim SG, Cho SW, Lee YC, Jeon SJ, Lee MH, Cho YJ, et al. Changes in liver stiffness measurement during antiviral therapy in patients with chronic hepatitis B. Hepato-Gastroenterology. 2011;58(106):539–45.

59. Wong GL, Wong VW, Choi PC, Chan AW, Chim AM, Yiu KK, et al. On-treatment monitoring of liver fibrosis with transient elastography in chronic hepatitis B patients. Antivir Ther. 2011;16(2):165–72.
60. Ogawa E, Furusyo N, Murata M, Ohnishi H, Toyoda K, Taniai H, et al. Longitudinal assessment of liver stiffness by transient elastography for chronic hepatitis B patients treated with nucleoside analog. Hepatol Res. 2011;41(12):1178–88.
61. Kim MN, Kim SU, Kim BK, Park JY, Kim DY, Ahn SH, Han KH. Long-term changes of liver stiffness values assessed using transient elastography in patients with chronic hepatitis B receiving entecavir. Liver Int. 2014;34(8):1216–23.
62. Chon YE, Park JY, Myoung SM, Jung KS, Kim BK, Kim SU, et al. Improvement of Liver Fibrosis after Long-Term Antiviral Therapy Assessed by Fibroscan in Chronic Hepatitis B Patients With Advanced Fibrosis. Am J Gastroenterol. 2017;112(6):882–91.
63. Liang X, Xie Q, Tan D, Ning Q, Niu J, Bai X, et al. Interpretation of liver stiffness measurement-based approach for the monitoring of hepatitis B patients with antiviral therapy: a 2-year prospective study. J Viral Hepat. 2018;25(3):296–305.
64. Rinaldi L, Ascione A, Messina V, Rosato V, Valente G, Sangiovanni V, et al. Influence of antiviral therapy on the liver stiffness in chronic HBV hepatitis. Infection. 2018;46(2):231–8.
65. Li Q, Chen L, Zhou Y. Changes of FibroScan, APRI, and FIB-4 in chronic hepatitis B patients with significant liver histological changes receiving 3-year entecavir therapy. Clin Exp Med. 2018;18(2):273–82.
66. Bedossa P. Reversibility of hepatitis B virus cirrhosis after therapy: who and why? Liver Int. 2015;35(Suppl 1):78–81.
67. Liang LY, Wong GL. Unmet need in chronic Hepatitis B management. Clin Mol Hepatol. 2019;25(2):172–80.
68. Wong VW, Janssen HLA. Can we use HCC risk score to individualize surveillance in chronic hepatitis B infection. J Hepatol. 2015;63(3):722–32.
69. Wong VW, Chan SL, Mo F, Chan TC, Loong HH, Wong GL, et al. Clinical scoring system to predict hepatocellular carcinoma in chronic hepatitis B carriers. J Clin Oncol. 2010;28(10):1660–5.
70. Yang HI, Yuen MF, Chan HL, Han KH, Chen PJ, Kim DY, et al. Risk estimation for hepatocellular carcinoma in chronic hepatitis B (REACH-B): development and validation of a predictive score. Lancet Oncol. 2011;12(6):568–74.
71. Jung KS, Kim SU, Ahn SH, Park YN, Kim DY, Park JY, et al. Risk assessment of hepatitis B virus-related hepatocellular carcinoma development using liver stiffness measurement (FibroScan). Hepatology. 2011;53(3):885–94.
72. Kim BK, Park YN, Kim DY, Park JY, Chon CY, Han KH, Ahn SH. Risk assessment of development of hepatic decompensation in histologically proven hepatitis B viral cirrhosis using liver stiffness measurement. Digestion. 2012;85(3):219–27.
73. Kim BK, Kim DY, Han KH, Park JY, Kim JK, Paik YH, et al. Risk assessment of esophageal variceal bleeding in B-viral liver cirrhosis by a liver stiffness measurement-based model. Am J Gastroenterol. 2011;106(9):1654–62.
74. Wong GL, Chan HL, Wong CK, Leung C, Chan CY, Ho PP, et al. Liver stiffness-based optimization of hepatocellular carcinoma risk score in patients with chronic hepatitis B. J Hepatol. 2014;60(2):339–45.
75. Lee HW, Yoo EJ, Kim BK, Kim SU, Park JY, Kim DY, et al. Prediction of development of liver-related events by transient elastography in hepatitis B patients with complete virological response on antiviral therapy. Am J Gastroenterol. 2014;109(8):1241–9.
76. Jung KS, Kim SU, Song K, Park JY, Kim DY, Ahn SH, et al. Validation of hepatitis B virus-related hepatocellular carcinoma prediction models in the era of antiviral therapy. Hepatology. 2015;62(6):1757–66.
77. Lee HW, Park SY, Lee M, Lee EJ, Lee J, Kim SU, et al. An optimized hepatocellular carcinoma prediction model for chronic hepatitis B with well-controlled viremia. Liver Int. 2020;40(7):1736–43.

The Role of Transient Elastography in NAFLD

5

Grazia Pennisi, Antonina Giammanco, and Salvatore Petta

5.1 Fibrosis in NAFLD: The Burden

On the ground of its rising prevalence, nonalcoholic fatty liver disease (NAFLD) is nowadays the most relevant liver disease worldwide, affecting about 25% of the general population [1].

Liver fibrosis represents a milestone of the progression toward end-stage liver disease in NAFLD, and it is currently the strongest predictor of liver-related complications [2–5], including hepatocellular carcinoma (HCC) [6–8], and of all-cause mortality [2–4, 9–14]. However, natural history studies of patients who underwent paired liver biopsies did not show a linear rate of fibrosis progression while observing patients with stable disease, patients with impairment of liver fibrosis, and also patients with improvement in fibrosis stage [15–17]. Furthermore, a recent meta-analysis, among patients with fibrosis progression, also discriminated slow versus rapid progressors [17].

Moreover, liver fibrosis progresses in patients with simple fatty liver and with nonalcoholic steatohepatitis (NASH) [17–19].

Consistently, stratification of fibrosis at baseline and its changes during follow-up are required to predict clinical outcomes in NAFLD.

Despite histology holding the "gold standard" diagnostic tool, liver stiffness measurement (LSM) assessed by FibroScan (vibration controlled transient elastography, VCTE, also commonly known as transient elastography, TE) was validated

G. Pennisi · S. Petta (✉)
Section of Gastroenterology and Hepatology, PROMISE, University of Palermo, Palermo, Italy
e-mail: salvatore.petta@unipa.it

A. Giammanco
Department of Health Promotion Sciences Maternal and Infantile Care, Internal Medicine and Medical Specialities, University of Palermo, Palermo, Italy

© Springer Nature Switzerland AG 2021
M. Fraquelli (ed.), *Elastography of the Liver and Beyond*,
https://doi.org/10.1007/978-3-030-74132-7_5

as accurate to exclude the presence of advanced liver fibrosis in NAFLD [20], and its changes over time have been also found reliable to noninvasively predict fibrosis progression during follow-up having histology as standard [15].

5.2 Transient Elastography: The Technique

Transient elastography, developed in 1992, was the first ultrasound-based elastography technique [21]. TE measures the velocity of an elastic shear wave via propagation of ultrasound waves through the liver. Transient elastography is a noninvasive, simple, highly reproducible method and allows examination of at least 100 times larger volume of liver tissue compared to a liver sample obtained through liver biopsy [22], with consequent sampling error less than with liver biopsy [23].

TE requires a one-dimensional probe and an ultrasonic transducer. The probe is placed between two intercostal spaces, inducing the propagation of an elastic shear wave from the probe to the liver. The mechanical pulse is transmitted with a low amplitude (50 Hz). The propagation velocity measured is positively related to the liver stiffness, within the range of 1.5 to 75 kPa [24].

5.2.1 The Procedure

TE is assessed using FibroScan® equipment (Echosens, Paris, France). The exam is conducted after a fasting of at least 3 h. The procedure is performed in a supine position with the right arm abducted and placed under the patient's head. The probe was applied on the skin surface overlying the right liver lobe (Fig. 5.1a, b). After pressing the button on the probe, a pulse wave is transmitted across the liver parenchyma. The velocities of the propagation of two waves in the liver parenchyma are calculated using the Doppler technique (Fig. 5.1c) [25, 26], and, as it is known from physical principles, it increases with the stiffness of the liver parenchyma, correlating with severity of fibrosis (Fig. 5.1d).

A minimum of ten measurements are required to obtain a reliable liver stiffness measurement. They will be considered valid if the interquartile range (which reflects the variability of measurements) is <30% of the median LSM [27].

5.2.2 Probes

The probe utilizes pulse-echo ultrasound to follow the shear wave propagation to measure velocity (m/s) and to provide a liver stiffness measurement [28].

Three different probes can be used to make measurements under various circumstances. A standard M probe (3.5 MHz) and XL probe (2.5 MHz) are frequently used for adults, and an S probe (5.0 MHz) is used for children. Since lower-frequency probes are suitable to reduce wave attenuation in patients with a high degree of abdominal adiposity or a long distance between the skin and liver surface, XL probe

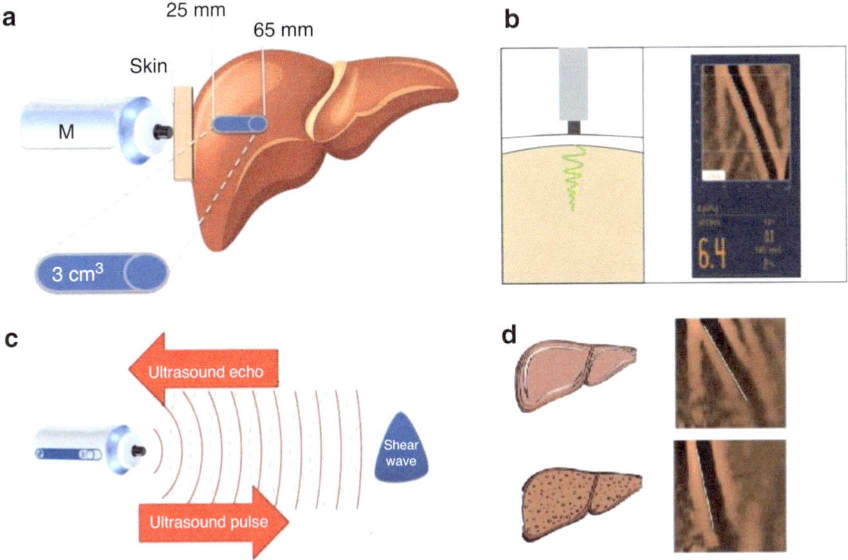

Fig. 5.1 (**a**) The probe analyzes a little quote of liver tissue overlying the skin surface. (**b**) After pressing buttons on the probe, the pulse wave is transmitted across the liver parenchyma. (**c**) The ultrasound pulse propagates in the liver and its echo will be recorded and processed. (**d**) Liver stiffness increases progressively with severity of fibrosis

could be used for overweight patients with a similar diagnostic accuracy [29]. The AUROC values using FibroScan M and XL probes for diagnosing advanced fibrosis are 0.88 and 0.85, respectively [30].

5.2.3 The Role of Controlled Attenuation Parameter (CAP)

The amplitude of ultrasound waves decreases more rapidly in a steatotic liver.

This explains why deeper tissues are less clear when one uses ultrasonography to examine a patient with NAFLD. Controlled attenuation parameter (CAP) by vibration-controlled transient elastography makes use of this physical phenomenon to measure the attenuation of ultrasound waves and thereby estimates the severity of hepatic steatosis. Overall, CAP has moderate accuracy in detecting fatty liver, but there is considerable overlap of CAP values among steatosis grades [31].

Because vibration-controlled transient elastography is a point-of-care test, its role as a monitoring tool during NASH treatment deserves further evaluation. Similar to ultrasonography, CAP is affected by obesity. Above all, failed examinations are more common in obese patients [32], though this problem is largely mitigated by the development of the XL probe [33]. Studies from Malaysia and Japan suggest that the accuracy of CAP for the detection of hepatic steatosis was also lower in obese patients [34, 35]. Moreover, significant liver fibrosis may affect ultrasound attenuation and lower the diagnostic performance of CAP [35]. Although food intake and active hepatitis are well-known causes of false-positive liver stiffness measurement, these factors do not appear to affect CAP [36, 37].

5.2.4 Limitations

As expected, TE has some limitations. First of all, some of these are insite of procedure, such as normal measurements' variability and operator inexperience. However, TE cannot be used in the presence of significant fat or fluid between the chest wall and the liver. Failures or unreliable results were found in 5% of patients, particularly in people with obesity and with narrow intercostal spaces. Furthermore, results should be interpreted with caution in case of high transaminase levels, sinusoidal congestion, and extrahepatic cholestasis [38]. Limitations are summarized in Table 5.1.

5.3 Transient Elastography in NAFLD: The Quote

In 2007, Yoneda et al. [39] first reported the usefulness of TE for estimating the severity of liver fibrosis in patients with NAFLD. Then, TE became the first Food and Drug Administration-approved US-based elastography technique in a few years.

As discussed above, in patients with NAFLD, repeated measurements of liver stiffness could be useful for long-term monitoring and the prediction of liver-related complications and cardiovascular events [40, 41]. Furthermore, repeated measurements of liver stiffness can reduce false-positive diagnosis of advanced fibrosis [42, 43]. The benefits of TE are its extensive validation, availability, high patient acceptance due to non-invasiveness, and good intra- and interobserver reproducibility (intra-class correlation coefficient (ICC) = 0.98) [44].

Table 5.1 Advantages and limitations of TE in patients with nonalcoholic fatty liver disease

Advantages	Limitations
Painless	No discriminations of different etiologies
Rapid and low-cost procedure	Confounders (obesity, inflammation, ascites, cholestasis, hepatic congestion)
Lower inter- and intraobserver variability	Narrow intercostal space
Good availability	Technical failure (<5% by using both M and XL probes)
Straightforward and rapid training of operators	Operator inexperience
Samples a volume 100 times larger than biopsy	Samples a volume lower than MR-based techniques

5.3.1 Diagnostic Accuracy

Tsochatzis et al. [45], in a meta-analysis of 40 studies based on liver biopsy as a reference standard, reported a sensitivity and specificity of 0.79 (95% CI 0.74–0.82) and 0.78 (95% CI 0.72–0.83) for F2 stage and 0.83 (95% CI 0.79–0.86) and 0.89 (95% CI 0.87–0.91) for cirrhosis. Authors concluded that TE performed with a good sensitivity and specificity profile for cirrhosis although it was not possible to confirm the same for the lower degrees of fibrosis.

Wong et al. have performed a large study in 246 patients with confirmed NAFLD by liver biopsy (128 French and 118 Chinese patients) and have identified the best LSM cutoff values to discriminate significant fibrosis, severe fibrosis, and cirrhosis (respectively 7.0 kPa, 8.7 kPa, and 10.3 kPa), with AUROC of 0.84 for the identification of moderate fibrosis, 0.93 for severe fibrosis, and 0.84 for cirrhosis [46]. In addition, FibroScan has shown a good diagnostic performance for both significant and severe fibrosis (AUC = 0.84 and 0.94, respectively) in another meta-analysis [11], and it has been considered the best performing and predictive test together with FibroMeter (V2G) compared to blood fibrosis tests, as exhibited in a cross-sectional study of 452 biopsy-proven NAFLD patients [38].

In 2014, a meta-analysis of 50 studies [47] has evaluated the performance of TE according to the stage of fibrosis, showing mean AUROC of 0.84, 0.89, and 0.94 for the diagnosis of significant fibrosis, severe fibrosis, and cirrhosis, respectively. As predicted, the diagnostic accuracy progressively decreased in the differentiation of severe fibrosis (stages 3 and 4) and significant fibrosis (stages 2, 3, and 4) from milder stage of fibrosis. The diagnostic achievement of TE for advanced fibrosis and cirrhosis in NAFLD was higher than AST/ALT ratio, APRI, FIB-4, BARD and NAFLD fibrosis scores, and other noninvasive serum markers, with AUROC values of TE for significant liver fibrosis (stages 2, 3, and 4) being 0.84, 0.93, and 0.95, respectively.

Kwok et al. [48] performed the first systematic review and meta-analysis of 854 patients studied with M probe. Sensitivity and specificity for the diagnosis of stages 2, 3, and 4 fibrosis were 0.79 and 0.75, 0.85 and 0.85, and 0.92 and 0.92, respectively. In 2017, Xiao et al. [20] performed a meta-analysis of the use of the XL probe. The meta-analysis included three studies involving 318 patients with NAFLD and showed that the AUROC for the diagnosis of stages 2, 3, and 4 fibrosis were 0.82, 0.86, and 0.94, respectively.

Jiang et al., in a recent meta-analysis of TE (M probe), based on 11 studies and 1753 patients with NAFLD, showed an AUROC for the diagnosis of stages 2, 3, and 4 fibrosis of 0.85, 0.92, and 0.94, respectively [49]. The authors concluded that TE is useful for the staging of liver fibrosis in patients with NAFLD, particularly for those with advanced fibrosis and cirrhosis. Meta-analyses of TE with sensitivity, specificity, and AUROC for the diagnosis of liver fibrosis are summarized in Table 5.2.

Table 5.2 Meta-analyses of transient elastography for the diagnosis of liver fibrosis in patients with nonalcoholic fatty liver disease

Authors	Year	Studies	Fibrosis stage	Sensitivity	Specificity	AUROC
Tsochatzis et al. [45]	2011	40	≥2	0.74–0.82	0.72–0.83	
			≥3	0.78–0.86	0.82–0.89	
			≥4	0.79–0.86	0.87–0.91	
Musso et al. [11]	2011	32	≥3	0.88–0.99	0.89–0.99	0.90–0.99
Kwok et al. [48]	2014	8	≥2	0.67–0.94	0.61–0.84	0.79–0.87
			≥3	0.65–1.00	0.75–0.97	0.76–0.98
			≥4	0.78–1.00	0.82–0.98	0.91–0.99
Xiao et al. [20]	2017	16	≥2	0.90–0.94	0.42–0.80	0.79–0.86
			≥3	0.76–0.88	0.63–0.88	0.83–0.90
			≥4	0.78–1.00	0.82–0.90	0.90–0.94
Jiang et al. [49]	2018	11	≥2	0.60–0.94	0.61–1.00	0.79–0.88
			≥3	0.57–1.00	0.76–0.97	0.76–0.99
			≥4	0.65–1.00	0.76–0.98	0.87–0.99

5.3.2 The Issue of Rule-In and Rule-Out

Ideally, the diagnostic cutoff values of noninvasive diagnosis should have a high negative predictive value (NPV) and low negative likelihood ratio (LR−) to rule out a diagnosis as well as a high positive predictive value (PPV) and high positive likelihood ratio (LR+) to confirm a diagnosis. So, it should be necessary to adopt cutoffs (low and high) to exclude or to confirm the diagnosis. The main problem of liver stiffness measurement occurs when values fall in the gray zone and liver biopsy is still necessary [50, 51]. In a meta-analysis of 40 studies, the LR- was 0.12 at a cutoff value of 7.9 kPa for the diagnosis of F3 fibrosis and 0.09 at a cutoff value of 10.3 kPa for the diagnosis of cirrhosis. The LR+ was 8.9 at a cutoff value of 9.6 kPa for the diagnosis of F3 fibrosis [46].

In another recent study that included 104 patients, considering three different cutoff values (7.9, 8.7, and 9.6 kPa), TE showed the highest sensitivity values (95%, 90%, and 85% respectively), and the highest NPV (98%, 96.4%, and 95.1% respectively) for the diagnosis of advanced fibrosis, with a high AUROC (0.87; CI 95% 0.78–0.97) [52].

These evidence shed a light on the most relevant diagnostic limit of the procedure. It should be surely used as a noninvasive diagnostic tool in patients with advanced fibrosis, especially in the presence of cirrhosis, and it could be considered a reliable rule-out.

Very recently, Newsome et al. [53] have developed and suggested a score to identify, in a noninvasive manner, patients with NAFLD at risk of progressive NASH, elevated NAFLD activity score (NAS ≥ 4), and advanced fibrosis (stage 2 or higher [$F \geq 2$]): the FibroScan-AST (FAST) score. This tool is based on the combination of liver stiffness measurement (LSM) by vibration-controlled transient elastography and controlled attenuation parameter (CAP) measured by FibroScan device with aspartate aminotransferase (AST), alanine aminotransferase (ALT), or AST/ALT ratio. FAST was tested in a large prospective study on 350 patients, was subsequently validated in seven cohorts, and seemed able to avoid unnecessary liver biopsy in subjects unlikely to have significant fibrosis. Furthermore, the FAST score was configured to have two thresholds, a rule-out (LR− 0·2) and a rule-in (LR+ 5) cutoff showing a good performance in testing more than 70% patients eligible for clinical trials or new pharmacotherapies.

5.3.3 Confounding Factors

Although these results demonstrated a very interesting role of FibroScan for the assessment of liver fibrosis in NAFLD, several factors might influence the performance and the reliability of LSM in clinical practice. Indeed, it has been shown in a cohort of 253 biopsy-proven NAFLD patients that the presence of severe steatosis could overestimate LSM values, mainly in patients with low stages of fibrosis (F0–F1 and F0–F2). In these patients, median LSM values were significantly higher in those with severe steatosis ($\geq$66% at liver biopsy) compared to those without, and this observation was also confirmed when liver steatosis was defined by ultrasound instead of histology [54]. In this line, the use of controlled attenuation parameter (CAP), a parameter associated with steatosis and provided by the same machine used for LSM, should be taken into account in the interpretation of LSM values. It has been demonstrated that among patients with F0–F2 fibrosis, mean LSM values significantly increased according to CAP tertiles, leading to an increase of the rate of false-positive LSM results for F3–F4 fibrosis according to CAP tertiles [55]. At the same time, AUROC of LSM for F3–F4 fibrosis was progressively reduced from lower to higher CAP tertiles, suggesting that steatosis assessed by CAP has a significant impact on the diagnostic accuracy and reliability of TE.

Moreover, in a prospective study were analyzed 79 chronic liver disease patients who performed liver biopsy, FibroScan, ultrasonography, and hepatic steatosis index (HSI): as previously, it was confirmed the importance of CAP in ascertaining steatosis, even in the early stages, with reliable results strongly accordant with histological data [56].

More recently, a cross-sectional study assessed the diagnostic accuracy of LSM by TE for fibrosis and of CAP for steatosis in 450 histologically proven NAFLD patients [57]. Although steatosis was associated with LSM by univariate analysis, multivariate analysis demonstrated an independent association between fibrosis stage and LSM and did not confirm the independent association between steatosis and LSM. However, it should be considered that fibrosis was evaluable with NASH CRN scoring system in only 373 patients. Chi-Wang Loong et al. evaluated 215 patients with NAFLD, and they have proven that liver stiffness measurement alone can reliably exclude significant and advanced fibrosis [58]. The use of FM VCTE in patients with high liver stiffness might raise the positive predictive value to rule in F2–F4 and F3–F4.

Body mass index (BMI) represents another factor which decreases the diagnostic performance of FibroScan, since obesity is very frequent in patients with NAFLD. In details, TE didn't result reliable in 5–15% of patients with NAFLD using the standard probe. A possible way to reduce the impact of obesity on the feasibility and on the reliability of FibroScan is the use of XL probe. In a multicenter study of 276 patients with chronic liver disease (46% with NAFLD), FibroScan failure was less frequent using XL probe, and AUROC for F2–F4 fibrosis and cirrhosis were similar. However, median LSM values were significantly lower in comparison with M probe, suggesting that lower liver stiffness cutoffs should be necessary in the interpretation of LSM values obtained with XL probe [59]. For this reason, the XL probe is a useful tool to improve the limitations of FibroScan [60]. A newer version of VCTE (FibroScan 502 Touch, Echosens™) overcomes some of its prior limitations, and it was assessed in a cross-sectional study of 992 patients with histological diagnosis of NAFLD, using both M+ and XL+ probes [61].

A cross-sectional study on 496 biopsy-diagnosed NAFLD patients analyzed the chance of a unified interpretation of VCTE by M and XL probe when used according to BMI [62]. The AUROC of M and XL probe for the diagnosis of F3–F4 fibrosis were similar (0.86 and 0.84, respectively), and in the same patient, LSM by XL probe resulted lower than that by M probe. Using M probe in nonobese patients and XL probe in obese patients, they yielded nearly identical median LSM at each fibrosis stage and similar diagnostic performance. However, cutoffs used for rule-in and rule-out F3–F4 fibrosis (10 and 15 Kpa, respectively) were different from those proposed by the same group in another study, which requires further validation. It has been recently reported by Petta et al. that LSM by FibroScan is better than FIB-4 and NFS for diagnosis of F3–F4 fibrosis, but only in nonobese patients and in subjects with ALT increase [63].

Petta et al. suggested a serial approach consisting in the execution of FibroScan as second-line exam in patients with FIB-4 or NFS values falling in the gray zone, which could be better than a single tool strategy also in patients with high ALT and obesity, although the accuracy in obese patients is poor. Hence, the consecutive combination of LSM by FibroScan with other noninvasive biomarkers of fibrosis (i.e., blood tests) could represent an interesting way to overcome some of the limitations of FibroScan in the prediction of fibrosis. A cross-sectional study conducted on 938 patients with biopsy-proven NAFLD confirmed the diagnostic accuracy for F3–F4 fibrosis of LSM by VCTE and noninvasive scores (NFS, FIB4, FibroTest, Hepascore, FibroMeter) and combination in a single score of FibroMeter and LSM (FibroMeterVCTE) [64]. LSM by TE resulted significantly more accurate than blood test with an AUROC of 0.840, but, more interestingly, the combination of FibroMeter with VCTE outperformed LSM and blood tests (AUROC 0.866, $p \leq 0.005$), and the sequential combination of FIB-4 with FibroMeterVCTE or LSM and then with FibroMeterVCTE provided a diagnostic accuracy of 90% for advanced fibrosis, decreasing the need for liver biopsy to confirm the diagnosis to only 20% of cases. These data suggest that these sequential algorithms could be more accurate than the pragmatic algorithms currently proposed. Similar results were obtained in 3202 biopsy-proven NAFLD patients who underwent screening for STELLAR trials (2262 with F3–F4 fibrosis): the sequential use of FIB-4 and then LSM by VCTE reduced the misclassification rate of F3–F4 fibrosis stage to 20%, although it should be considered that the prevalence of F3–F4 patients was extremely high [65].

In addition, Kao et al. have recently developed an easy, clinical scoring system combining FibroScan and aspartate aminotransferase/platelet ratio index (APRI) to predict significant liver fibrosis in severe obese patients [66]. Furthermore, age and diabetes represent two other factors potentially limiting the diagnostic accuracy of FibroScan [67, 68] as well as cholestasis, heart failure, ascites, and post-meal [69].

5.3.4   Liver Stiffness as Predictor of Liver Events

Patients with NAFLD and chronic liver diseases progressing to advanced fibrosis and cirrhosis may often undergo development of liver-related events (LREs) including HCC, hepatic decompensation (variceal bleeding, ascites, hepatic encephalopathy, spontaneous bacterial peritonitis, hepatorenal syndrome), and liver-related death: in this context, liver stiffness measurement (LSM) using TE has been used as a surveillance strategy to evaluate the severity of the liver disease and to appraise consequently the risk of LREs. In a recent study, Kim SU et al. [70] have analyzed 128 chronic hepatitis B (CHB) patients showing advanced (F3) liver fibrosis on LB with a high viral load: the authors reported that LSM represents a significant predictor of LREs and performs better than liver biopsy alone, especially in chronic hepatitis B patients undergoing antiviral therapy. However, another study has evaluated 1772 hepatitis C patients with advanced fibrosis or cirrhosis and treated with telaprevir-based triple therapy in the context of the telaprevir Early Access Program HEP3002: the authors reported that although FibroScan exhibited a low prediction profile of safety and efficacy in HCV patients, it can be used in addition to other clinical and biochemical data to support the detection of patients who will benefit from the triple therapy [71].

In a recent multicenter study, 1039 patients with NAFLD and F3–F4 fibrosis, baseline LSM was independently associated with occurrence of hepatic decompensation (HR 1.03; 95% CI, 1.02–1.04; $P < 0.001$), HCC (HR, 1.03; 95% CI, 1.00–1.04; $P = 0.003$), and liver-related death (HR, 1.02; 95% CI, 1.02–1.03; $P = 0.005$). In addition, in patients with availability of LSMs during the follow-up period, change in LSM was independently associated with hepatic decompensation (HR, 1.56; 95% CI, 1.05–2.51; $P = 0.04$), HCC (HR, 1.72; 95% CI, 1.01–3.02; $P = 0.04$), overall mortality (HR, 1.73; 95% CI, 1.11–2.69; $P = 0.01$), and liver-related mortality (HR, 1.96; 95% CI, 1.10–3.38; $P = 0.02$) [72].

Moreover, subjects with NAFLD are often characterized by insulin resistance (IR) which correlates with severe hepatocyte inflammation and cardiovascular diseases. Considering the prevalence of NAFLD and its association with possible systemic consequences, Hanafy et al. [73] have analyzed 272 patients with NAFLD and cardio-metabolic risk factors by evaluating some blood parameters such HOMA-IR, mean platelet volume (MPV), neutrophil-lymphocyte ratio

(NLR), uric acid, ferritin, and lipid profile, and then they correlated these results to liver stiffness measurement (LSM), controlled attenuation parameter (CAP) by FibroScan, and carotid intima media thickness (CIMT): significant fibrosis and cardiovascular risk in NAFLD were independently associated with AST/ALT ratio, GGT, CIMT, uric acid, VLDL, HOMA-IR, ferritin, CAP, and LSM. By this method, a new noninvasive tool was identified to assess the severity of NAFLD and cardiovascular risk.

5.4   Conclusions

Due to its noninvasiveness, good accuracy, and reproducibility, TE is strongly recommended in patients with NAFLD. In this setting, TE can be used to assess fibrosis at baseline and to identify patients at risk of liver-related events during follow-up. When looking at the general population, a suggested strategy could be screening at-risk patients by easy noninvasive scores like FIB-4 and then using TE for further stratifying the risk of fibrosis severity in patients at medium-high risk by FIB-4.

Evaluation of CAP can help to detect steatosis and to parse LSM results in the presence of higher hepatic fat.

However, TE may not replace hepatic biopsy that is still considered the "gold standard" to diagnose NAFLD and to stage fibrosis.

References

1. Younossi ZM, Koenig AB, Abdelatif D, Fazel Y, Henry L, Wymer M. Global epidemiology of non-alcoholic fatty liver disease-meta-analytic assessment of prevalence. Inciden Outcom Hepatol. 2016;64(1):73–84.
2. Adams LA, Lymp JF, St Sauver J, Sanderson SO, Lindor KD, Feldstein A, et al. The natural history of nonalcoholic fatty liver disease: a population-based cohort study. Gastroenterology. 2005;129(1):113–21.
3. Ekstedt M, Franzén LE, Mathiesen UL, Thorelius L, Holmqvist M, Bodemar G, et al. Long-term follow-up of patients with NAFLD and elevated liver enzymes. Hepatology. 2006;44(4):865–73. https://doi.org/10.1002/hep.21327.
4. Angulo P, Kleiner DE, Dam-Larsen S, Adams LA, Bjornsson ES, Charatcharoenwitthaya P, et al. Liver fibrosis, but no other histologic features, is associated with long-term outcomes of patients with nonalcoholic fatty liver disease. Gastroenterology. 2015;149(2):389–97.e10.
5. Bhala N, Angulo P, van der Poorten D, Lee E, Hui JM, Saracco G, et al. The natural history of nonalcoholic fatty liver disease with advanced fibrosis or cirrhosis: an international collaborative study. Hepatology. 2011;54(4):1208–16.
6. Ascha MS, Hanouneh IA, Lopez R, Tamimi TA, Feldstein AF, Zein NN. The incidence and risk factors of hepatocellular carcinoma in patients with nonalcoholic steatohepatitis. Hepatology. 2010;51(6):1972–8.
7. White DL, Kanwal F, El-Serag HB. Association between nonalcoholic fatty liver disease and risk for hepatocellular cancer, based on systematic review. Clin Gastroenterol Hepatol. 2012;10(12):1342–59.e2.
8. Younossi ZM, Otgonsuren M, Henry L, Venkatesan C, Mishra A, Erario M, et al. Association of nonalcoholic fatty liver disease (NAFLD) with hepatocellular carcinoma (HCC) in the United States from 2004 to 2009. Hepatology. 2015;62(6):1723–30.

9. Adams LA, Harmsen S, St Sauver JL, Charatcharoenwitthaya P, Enders FB, Therneau T, et al. Nonalcoholic fatty liver disease increases risk of death among patients with diabetes: a community-based cohort study. Am J Gastroenterol. 2010;105(7):1567–73.

10. Ekstedt M, Hagström H, Nasr P, Fredrikson M, Stål P, Kechagias S, et al. Fibrosis stage is the strongest predictor for disease-specific mortality in NAFLD after up to 33 years of follow-up. Hepatology. 2015;61(5):1547–54. https://doi.org/10.1002/hep.27368.

11. Musso G, Gambino R, Cassader M, Pagano G. Meta-analysis: natural history of non-alcoholic fatty liver disease (NAFLD) and diagnostic accuracy of non-invasive tests for liver disease severity. Ann Med. 2011;43(8):617–49.

12. Wu S, Wu F, Ding Y, Hou J, Bi J, Zhang Z. Association of non-alcoholic fatty liver disease with major adverse cardiovascular events: a systematic review and meta-analysis. Sci Rep. 2016;6:33386.

13. Vilar-Gomez E, Calzadilla-Bertot L, Wai-Sun Wong V, Castellanos M, Aller-de la Fuente R, Metwally M, et al. Fibrosis severity as a determinant of cause-specific mortality in patients with advanced nonalcoholic fatty liver disease: a multi-national cohort study. Gastroenterology. 2018;155(2):443–57.e17.

14. Dulai PS, Singh S, Patel J, Soni M, Prokop LJ, Younossi Z, et al. R. Increased risk of mortality by fibrosis stage in nonalcoholic fatty liver disease: systematic review and meta-analysis. Hepatology. 2017;65(5):1557–65.

15. Siddiqui MS, et al. Diagnostic accuracy of noninvasive fibrosis models to detect change in fibrosis stage. Clin Gastroenterol Hepatol. 2019;17(9):1877–85.e5.

16. Pelusi S, Cespiati A, Rametta R, et al. Prevalence and risk factors of significant fibrosis in patients with nonalcoholic fatty liver without steatohepatitis. Clin Gastroenterol Hepatol. 2019;17(11):2310–19.e6.

17. Singh S, Allen AM, Wang Z, Prokop LJ, Murad MH, Loomba R. Fibrosis progression in non-alcoholic fatty liver vs nonalcoholic steatohepatitis: a systematic review and meta-analysis of paired-biopsy studies. Clin Gastroenterol Hepatol. 2015;13(4):643–e40.

18. McPherson S, Henderson E, Burt AD, Day CP, Anstee QM. Serum immunoglobulin levels predict fibrosis in patients with non-alcoholic fatty liver disease. J Hepatol. 2014;60(5):1055–62.

19. Pais R, Charlotte F, Fedchuk L, et al. A systematic review of follow-up biopsies reveals disease progression in patients with non-alcoholic fatty liver. J Hepatol. 2013;59(3):550–6.

20. Xiao G, Zhu S, Xiao X, Yan L, Yang J, Wu G. Comparison of laboratory tests, ultrasound, or magnetic resonance elastography to detect fibrosis in patients with nonalcoholic fatty liver disease: a meta-analysis. Hepatology. 2017;66(5):1486–501.

21. Talwalkar JA. Elastography for detecting hepatic fibrosis: options and considerations. Gastroenterology. 2008;135:299–302.

22. de Ledinghen V, Barreiro P, Foucher J, Labarga P, Castera L, Vispo ME, et al. Liver fibrosis on account of chronic hepatitis C is more severe in HIV-positive than HIV-negative patients despite antiretroviral therapy. J Viral Hepat. 2008;15(6):427–33.

23. Ingiliz P, Chhay KP, Munteanu M, et al. Applicability and variability of liver stiffness measurements according to probe position. World J Gastroenterol. 2009;15(27):3398–404. https://doi.org/10.3748/wjg.15.3398.

24. Sandrin L, Tanter M, Gennisson JL, Catheline S, Fink M. Shear elasticity probe for soft tissues with 1-D transient elastography. IEEE Trans Ultrason Ferroelectr Freq Control. 2002;49:436–46.

25. Sandrin L, Fourquet B, Hasquenoph JM, Yon S, Fournier C, Mal F, Christidis C, Ziol M, Poulet B, Kazemi F, et al. Transient elastography: a new noninvasive method for assessment of hepatic fibrosis. Ultrasound Med Biol. 2003;29:1705–13.

26. Nahon P, Kettaneh A, Lemoine M, et al. Liver stiffness measurement in patients with cirrhosis and hepatocellular carcinoma: a case-control study. Eur J Gastroenterol Hepatol. 2009;21:214–9.

27. Tapper EB, Challies T, Imad Nasser I, Afdhal NH, Lai M. The performance of vibration controlled transient elastography in a US cohort of patients with nonalcoholic fatty liver disease. Am J Gastroenterol. 2016;111:677–84.

28. European Association for Study of Liver, Asociación Latinoamericana para el Estudio del Higado, Castera L, Chan H, Arrese M, Afdhal N, Bedossa P, Friedrich-Rust M, Han KH, Pinzani M. EASL-ALEH clinical practice guidelines tests for evaluation of on-invasive tests for liver disease severity and prognosis. J Hepatol. 2015;63:237–64.
29. Ferraioli G, Wong VW, Castera L, Berzigotti A, Sporea I, Dietrich CF, Choi BI, Wilson SR, Kudo M, Barr RG. Liver ultrasound elastography: an update to the world federation for ultrasound in medicine and biology guidelines and recommendations. Ultrasound Med Biol. 2018;44:2419–40.
30. Piazzolla VA, Mangia A. Noninvasive diagnosis of NAFLD and NASH. Cell. 2020;9:1005.
31. Karlas T, Petroff D, Sasso M, et al. Individual patient data meta-analysis of controlled attenuation parameter (CAP) technology for assessing steatosis. J Hepatol. 2017;66:1022–30.
32. Wong GL, Wong VW, Chim AM, et al. Factors associated with unreliable liver stiffness measurement and its failure with transient elastography in the Chinese population. J Gastroenterol Hepatol. 2011;26:300–5.
33. Wong VW, Vergniol J, Wong GL, et al. Liver stiffness measurement using XL probe in patients with nonalcoholic fatty liver disease. Am J Gastroenterol. 2012;107:1862–71.
34. Chan WK, Nik Mustapha NR, Mahadeva S. Controlled attenuation parameter for the detection and quantification of hepatic steatosis in nonalcoholic fatty liver disease. J Gastroenterol Hepatol. 2014;29:1470–6.
35. Fujimori N, Tanaka N, Shibata S, et al. Controlled attenuation parameter is correlated with actual hepatic fat content in patients with non-alcoholic fatty liver disease with none-to-mild obesity and liver fibrosis. Hepatol Res. 2016;46:1019–27.
36. Jung KS, Kim BK, Kim SU, et al. Factors affecting the accuracy of controlled attenuation parameter (CAP) in assessing hepatic steatosis in patients with chronic liver disease. PLoS One. 2014;9:e98689.
37. Silva M, Costa Moreira P, Peixoto A, et al. Effect of meal ingestion on liver stiffness and controlled attenuation parameter. GE Port J Gastroenterol. 2019;26:99–104.
38. Boursier J, Vergniol J, Guillet A, Hiriart JB, Lannes A, Le Bail B, Michalak S, Chermak F, Bertrais S, Foucher J, et al. Diagnostic accuracy and prognostic significance of blood fibrosis tests and liver stiffness measurement by FibroScan in non alcoholic fatty liver disease. J Hepatol. 2016;65:570–8.
39. Yoneda M, Fujita K, Inamori M, Nakajima A, Yoneda M, Tamano M, Hiraishi H. Transient elastography in patients with non-alcoholic fatty liver disease (NAFLD). Gut. 2007;56:1330–1.
40. Kamarajah SK, Chan WK, Nik Mustapha NR, Mahadeva S. Repeated liver stiffness measurement compared with paired liver biopsy in patients with non-alcoholic fatty liver disease. Hepatol Int. 2018;12:44–55.
41. Nogami A, Yoneda M, Kobayashi T, Kessoku T, Honda Y, Ogawa Y, Suzuki K, Tomeno W, Imajo K, Kirikoshi H, et al. Assessment of 10-year changes in liver stiffness using vibration-controlled transient elastography in non-alcoholic fatty liver disease. Hepatol Res. 2019;49:872–80.
42. Chow JC, Wong GL, Chan AW, Shu SS, Chan CK, Leung JK, Choi PC, Chim AM, Chan HL, Wong VW. Repeating measurements by transient elastography in non-alcoholic fatty liver disease patients with high liver stiffness. J Gastroenterol Hepatol. 2019;34:241–8.
43. Chuah KH, Lai LL, Vethakkan SR, Nik Mustapha NR, Mahadeva S, Chan WK. Liver stiffness measurement in non-alcoholic fatty liver disease: two is better than one. J Gastroenterol Hepatol. 2020;35(8):1404–11.
44. Fraquelli M, Rigamonti C, Casazza G, Conte D, Donato MF, Ronchi G, Colombo M. Reproducibility of transient elastography in the evaluation of liver fibrosis in patients with chronic liver disease. Gut. 2007;56:968–73.
45. Tsochatzis EA, Gurusamy KS, Ntaoula S, Cholongitas E, Davidson BR, Burroughs AK. Elastography for the diagnosis of severity of fibrosis in chronic liver disease: a meta-analysis of diagnostic accuracy. J Hepatol. 2011;54(4):650–9.
46. Wong VW, Vergniol J, Wong GL, et al. Diagnosis of fibrosis and cirrhosis using liver stiffness measurement in non-alcoholic fatty liver disease. Hepatology. 2010;51:454–62.

47. Expert Panel on Liver Stiffness Measurement. Clinical application of transient elastography in the diagnosis of liver fibrosis: an expert panel review and opinion. J Clin Transl Hepatol. 2014;2:110–6.
48. Kwok R, Tse YK, Wong GL, Ha Y, Lee AU, Ngu MC, Chan HL, Wong VW. Systematic review with meta-analysis: non-invasive assessment of non-alcoholic fatty liver disease–the role of transient elastography and plasma cytokeratin-18 fragments. Aliment Pharmacol Ther. 2014;39:254–69.
49. Jiang W, Huang S, Teng H, Wang P, Wu M, Zhou X, Ran H. Diagnostic accuracy of point shear wave elastography and transient elastography for staging hepatic fibrosis in patients with non-alcoholic fatty liver disease: a meta-analysis. BMJ Open. 2018;8:e021787.
50. Sebastiani G, Alberti A. Non-invasive fibrosis biomarkers reduce but not substitute the need for liver biopsy. World J Gastroenterol. 2006;12:3682–94.
51. Manning DS, Afdhal NH. Diagnosis and quantitation of fibrosis. Gastroenterology. 2008;134:1670–81. https://doi.org/10.1053/j.gastro.2008.03.001.
52. Tovo CV, Villela-Nogueira CA, Leite NC, et al. Transient hepatic elastography has the best performance to evaluate liver fibrosis in non-alcoholic fatty liver disease (NAFLD). Ann Hepatol. 2019;18(3):445–9. https://doi.org/10.1016/j.aohep.2018.09.003.
53. Newsome PN, Sasso M, Deeks JJ, Paredes A, Boursier J, Chan WK, et al. FibroScan-AST (FAST) score for the non-invasive identification of patients with non-alcoholic steatohepatitis with significant activity and fibrosis: a prospective derivation and global validation study. Lancet Gastroenterol Hepatol. 2020;5(4):362–73.
54. Petta S, Maida M, Macaluso FS, Marco VD, Cammà C, Cabibi D, Craxì A. The severity of steatosis influences liver stiffness measurement in patients with non-alcoholic fatty liver disease. Hepatology. 2015;62(4):1101–10.
55. Petta S, Wong VW, Cammà C, Hiriart JB, Wong GL, Marra F, Vergniol J, Chan AW, Di Marco V, Merrouche W, Chan HL, Barbara M, Le-Bail B, Arena U, Craxì A, de Ledinghen V. Improved noninvasive prediction of liver fibrosis by liver stiffness measurement in patients with nonalcoholic fatty liver disease accounting for controlled attenuation parameter values. Hepatology. 2017;65(4):1145–55.
56. Jun BG, Park WY, Park EY, Jang JY, Jeong SW, Lee SH, et al. A prospective comparative assessment of the accuracy of the FibroScan in evaluating liver steatosis. PLoS One. 2017;12(8):e0182784.
57. Eddowes PJ, Sasso M, Allison M, Tsochatzis E, Anstee QM, Sheridan D, Guha IN, Cobbold JF, Deeks JJ, Paradis V, Bedossa P, Newsome PN. Accuracy of FibroScan controlled attenuation parameter and liver stiffness measurement in assessing steatosis and fibrosis in patients with nonalcoholic fatty liver disease. Gastroenterology. 2019;156(6):1717–30.
58. Chi-Wang Loong T, Lok Wei J, Chung-Fai Leung J, Lai-Hung Wong G, She-Ting Shu S, Mei-Ling Chim A, et al. Application of the combined FibroMeter vibration-controlled transient elastography algorithm in Chinese patients with non-alcoholic fatty liver disease. J Gastroenterol Hepatol. 2017;32(7):1363–9.
59. Myers RP, Pomier-Layrargues G, et al. Feasibility and diagnostic performance of the FibroScan XL probe for liver stiffness measurement in overweight and obese patients. Hepatology. 2012;55:199–208.
60. de Lédinghen V, Wong VW, Vergniol J, et al. Diagnosis of liver fibrosis and cirrhosis using liver stiffness measurement: comparison between M and XL probe of FibroScan®. J Hepatol. 2012;56:833–9.
61. Vuppalanchi R, Siddiqui MS, Van Natta ML, Hallinan E, Brandman D, Kowdley K, Neuschwander-Tetri BA, Loomba R, Dasarathy S, Abdelmalek M, Doo E, Tonascia JA, Kleiner DE, Sanyal AJ, Chalasani N, NASH Clinical Research Network. Performance characteristics of vibration-controlled transient elastography for evaluation of nonalcoholic fatty liver disease. Hepatology. 2018;67(1):134–44.
62. Wong VW, Irles M, Wong GL, Shili S, Chan AW, Merrouche W, Shu SS, Foucher J, Le Bail B, Chan WK, Chan HL, de Ledinghen V. Unified interpretation of liver stiffness measurement by M and XL probes in non-alcoholic fatty liver disease. Gut. 2019;68(11):2057–64.

63. Petta S, Wai-Sun Wong V, Bugianesi E, Fracanzani AL, Cammà C, Hiriart JB, Lai-Hung Wong G, Vergniol J, Wing-Hung Chan A, Giannetti A, Merrouche W, Lik-Yuen Chan H, Le-Bail B, Lombardi R, Guastella S, Craxì A, de Ledinghen V. Impact of obesity and alanine aminotransferase levels on the diagnostic accuracy for advanced liver fibrosis of noninvasive tools in patients with nonalcoholic fatty liver disease. Am J Gastroenterol. 2019;114(6):916–28.

64. Boursier J, Guillaume M, Leroy V, Irlès M, Roux M, Lannes A, Foucher J, Zuberbuhler F, Delabaudière C, Barthelon J, Michalak S, Hiriart JB, Peron JM, Gerster T, Le Bail B, Riou J, Hunault G, Merrouche W, Oberti F, Pelade L, Fouchard I, Bureau C, Calès P, de Ledinghen V. New sequential combinations of non-invasive fibrosis tests provide an accurate diagnosis of advanced fibrosis in NAFLD. J Hepatol. 2019;71(2):389–96.

65. Anstee QM, Lawitz EJ, Alkhouri N, Wong VW, Romero-Gomez M, Okanoue T, Trauner M, Kersey K, Li G, Han L, Jia C, Wang L, Chen G, Subramanian GM, Myers RP, Djedjos CS, Kohli A, Bzowej N, Younes Z, Sarin S, Shiffman ML, Harrison SA, Afdhal NH, Goodman Z, Younossi ZM. Noninvasive tests accurately identify advanced fibrosis due to NASH: baseline data from the STELLAR trials. Hepatology. 2019;70(5):1521–30.

66. Kao WY, Chang IW, Chen CL, Su CW, Fang SU, Tang JH, et al. Fibroscan-based score to predict significant liver fibrosis in morbidly obese patients with nonalcoholic fatty liver disease. Obes Surg. 2020;30(4):1249–57.

67. McPherson S, Hardy T, Dufour JF, Petta S, Romero-Gomez M, Allison M, Oliveira CP, Francque S, Van Gaal L, Schattenberg JM, Tiniakos D, Burt A, Bugianesi E, Ratziu V, Day CP, Anstee QM. Age as a confounding factor for the accurate non-invasive diagnosis of advanced NAFLD fibrosis. Am J Gastroenterol. 2017;112(5):740–51.

68. Bertot LC, Jeffrey GP, de Boer B, MacQuillan G, Garas G, Chin J, Huang Y, Adams LA. Diabetes impacts prediction of cirrhosis and prognosis by non-invasive fibrosis models in non-alcoholic fatty liver disease. Liver Int. 2018;38(10):1793–802.

69. Chang PE, Goh GBB, Ngu JH, Tan HK, Tan CK. Clinical applications, limitations and future role of transient elastography in the management of liver disease. World J Gastrointest Pharmacol Ther. 2016;7(1):91–106.

70. Kim SU, Lee JH, Kim DY, Ahn SH, Jung KS, Choi EH, et al. Prediction of liver-related events using fibroscan in chronic hepatitis b patients showing advanced liver fibrosis. PLoS One. 2012;7(5):e36676.

71. Lepida A, Colombo M, Fernandez I, Abdurakhmanov D, Ferreira PA, Strasser SI, et al. Final results of the telaprevir access program: fibroscan values predict safety and efficacy in hepatitis c patients with advanced fibrosis or cirrhosis. PLoS One. 2015; https://doi.org/10.1371/journal.pone.0138503.

72. Petta S, Sebastiani G, Viganò M, et al. Monitoring occurrence of liver-related events and survival by transient elastography in patients with nonalcoholic fatty liver disease and compensated advanced chronic liver disease. Clin Gastroenterol Hepatol. 2020;2020. S1542-3565(20)30908-3.

73. Hanafy AS, Seleem WM, El-Kalla F, Basha MA, Abd-Elsalam S. Efficacy of a non-invasive model in predicting the cardiovascular morbidity and histological severity in non-alcoholic fatty liver disease. Diabetes Metab Syndr. 2019;13(3):2272–8.

Elastography in Liver-Transplanted Patients

6

Cristina Rigamonti, Carla De Benedittis, and Maria Francesca Donato

Liver transplantation (LT) is one of the most complex and fascinating surgical procedures: it represents the best curative treatment option for patients with decompensated end-stage liver disease, hepatocellular carcinoma and acute liver failure. The success of LT over the last decades has meant that there is a growing cohort of LT recipients throughout the world at risk of complications due to graft rejection, recurrence of the underlying liver disease and a long-life use of immunosuppressive drugs. The management of adult recipients of LT aims at maintaining graft and patient health and best preventing the occurrence of complications. Causes of graft damage after LT include immune-mediated disease (rejection and de novo autoimmune hepatitis), recurrent liver disease (viral, primary biliary cholangitis, autoimmune hepatitis, primary sclerosing cholangitis and others), drug toxicity (including immunosuppressive drugs), alcohol and other toxins, de novo infection (including de novo HBV and HCV), space-occupying lesion (recurrent cancer) and de novo or recurrent non-alcoholic fatty liver disease (NAFLD) and biliary and vascular disease [1].

Liver biopsy (LB) remains the reference standard for assessing graft damage. However, non-invasive tests for assessing liver fibrosis have gained popularity as an adjunct and substitution to LB in the longitudinal surveillance of LT patients. Among them, vibration-controlled transient elastography (VCTE, FibroScan®), which measures liver stiffness (LS), has been the most validated method also in the LT setting.

C. Rigamonti (✉) · C. De Benedittis
Department of Translational Medicine, Università del Piemonte Orientale UPO, Novara, Italy
e-mail: cristina.rigamonti@uniupo.it

M. F. Donato
C.R.C. "A.M. & A. Migliavacca" Center for Liver Disease and Division of Gastroenterology and Hepatology, Fondazione IRCCS Ca' Granda Ospedale Maggiore Policlinico and University of Milan, Milan, Italy

© Springer Nature Switzerland AG 2021
M. Fraquelli (ed.), *Elastography of the Liver and Beyond*,
https://doi.org/10.1007/978-3-030-74132-7_6

This chapter will discuss VCTE performance in assessing graft damage and its applicability in the management of recipients after liver transplantation.

6.1   Acute Rejection

Acute cellular rejection (ACR) is a common complication of LT, characterized by a lymphocyte-mediated immune reaction against the graft with an inflammatory response directed to endothelial and bile epithelial cells.

The diagnosis of acute cellular rejection is based on liver histology. Nevertheless, the presence of ACR may be suspected by increased TE values during post-transplant follow-up. In fact, the inflammatory process that takes place in ACR may increase liver stiffness. A pilot study on 27 LT recipients has shown that patients with moderate/severe ACR had higher liver stiffness measurement (LSM) than patients with mild ACR, thus suggesting an association between liver stiffness and severity of rejection [2]. Similar results were achieved by Nacif et al., who observed a significant correlation between the presence of ACR and liver stiffness assessed by VCTE in 25 LT recipients [3].

In the study by Crespo et al. a longitudinal evaluation by VCTE demonstrated an improvement of LSM with respect to baseline measurements in 66% of patients with moderate/severe ACR after a successful treatment of rejection, while a progressive increase of LSM during follow-up was observed in one patient who developed an histologically proven chronic rejection [2]. Similarly, in a study on 27 recipients in the early post-LT period, liver stiffness changes predicted the development and resolution of ACR in three patients, who presented a sharp rise in LSM followed by a decrease after successful immunosuppression [4].

These studies, even if limited by a small sample size, highlight the ability of VCTE to select patients to undergo LB for suspicion of rejection, since it is clear that LSM by itself cannot replace LB for the diagnosis of ACR.

6.2   Recurrent Hepatitis C

Liver cirrhosis and hepatocellular carcinoma due to chronic hepatitis C virus (HCV) infection have been the leading causes for LT worldwide until 2014, and recurrent HCV infection post-LT has been a major challenge to successful LT, because of a rapid progression to hepatic fibrosis, cirrhosis, graft failure and shortened patient survival in the majority of HCV-re-infected LT recipients [5–7]. The first attempts to modify the course of recurrent HCV with standard interferon (IFN)-based therapies and subsequently with pegylated IFN and ribavirin yielded unsatisfactory results in terms of successful HCV eradication after LT [8, 9]. The advent of anti-HCV IFN-free all-oral direct antiviral agents (DAAs)-based regimens with a very favourable safety profile and high rates of sustained virological response (SVR) of over 95% has provided an unprecedented opportunity to cure HCV before and after LT [10, 11]. After the introduction of DAAs in 2014, a dramatic decline was observed in the number of liver transplants performed in patients with end-stage liver disease due to HCV [12]. At the same time, the survival of LT recipients with recurrent hepatitis C dramatically improved [12]. Historically, the management of LT patients with recurrent hepatitis C has relied on repeated protocol liver biopsies for assessing liver fibrosis progression and graft disease severity. As non-invasive tests for diagnosing liver fibrosis have been introduced as a complementary tool in the management of chronic liver diseases in the non-transplant setting [13], they have then been validated in the setting of recurrent hepatitis C. Their diagnostic performance has been validated with protocol LB performed during post-LT follow-up. The first study assessing VCTE performance in liver-transplanted patients with recurrent hepatitis C showed by cross-sectional analysis a good correlation of liver stiffness with both histological scores of liver fibrosis and hepatic vein pressure gradient (HVPG) (Table 6.1) [14]. In LT recipients with recurrent hepatitis C, Rigamonti et al. replicated these results by showing a strong correlation between VCTE results and histological scores of liver fibrosis, together with a high rate of test applicability (95%) (i.e. the proportion of patients with a successful examination) [15].

The diagnostic performance of VCTE in diagnosing the stage of fibrosis was good for significant fibrosis (stage ≥ 2 by Metavir, $F \geq 2$), excellent for advanced fibrosis (stage ≥ 3 by Metavir, $F \geq 3$) and definite cirrhosis (stage 4 by Metavir, F4) with VCTE having a greater negative than positive predictive power for the diagnosis of cirrhosis (Table 6.1) [14, 15]. Also, in patients who received living donor liver transplantation, VCTE performance resulted excellent in diagnosing liver fibrosis (Table 6.1) [16]. In the study by Rigamonti et al. [15], necroinflammatory activity not only positively correlated with VCTE results, but also it turned out to be an independent predictor of VCTE values. Perisinusoidal fibrosis, which is a determinant of portal hypertension in LT patients [17], emerged as an influencer of VCTE values at univariate analysis; steatosis did not appear to influence LS [15]. The importance of histological activity as an influencer of LS has emerged in previous studies in the non-transplant setting and might be due to tissue oedema accompanying liver cell necrosis and swelling of liver cells as occurring in the course of the necroinflammatory process [18, 19].

Besides being correlated with liver fibrosis in cross-sectional studies, LSM has proven to be useful to assess histological progression after transplantation, as shown in a prospective longitudinal study in 40 liver graft recipients with recurrent hepatitis C, who underwent sequential paired LB and VCTE examinations (Table 6.1) [15]. LS changes were dynamically correlated not only with the changes in the liver fibrosis stage but also with changes in necroinflammatory features or the occurrence of such other concomitant complications as cellular rejection, intra- or extra-hepatic cholestasis and de novo autoimmune hepatitis, therefore being predictive of an additional cause of graft damage [15].

With this background, on evaluating 49 untreated recipients with recurrent hepatitis C with yearly repeated LSM coupled with a baseline assessment and a LB after 2 years, it was demonstrated that VCTE examinations possibly enable to prolong the time interval between protocol liver biopsies for recipients with mild/stable

C. Rigamonti et al.

Table 6.1 VCTE performance in LT recipients with recurrent hepatitis C

Author, year	End-point	Patient #	Cut-off kPa	Sensitivity, %	Specificity, %	LR−	LR+	AUROC
Carrion (2006)	$F \geq 2$	124 (169 LB)	8.7	88	81	0.15	4.6	0.90
	F4	124 (169 LB)	12.5	100	87	0	7.7	0.98
	HVPG $\geq$6 mmHg	124 (129 HVPG)	8.7	90	81	0.12	4.7	0.93
Rigamonti (2008)	$F \geq 2$	90	7.9	81	76	0.25	3.4	0.85
	$F \geq 3$	90	11.9	82	96	0.19	19.0	0.90
	F4	90	12.0	93	93	0.07	14.0	0.93
	$\geq$1 point Ishak's score increase	40	$\geq$30% of TE baseline value increase	86	92	0.15	11.1	–
Harada (2008)	$F \geq 2$	56	9.9	90	91	0.10	10.0	0.92
	F4	56	26.5	100	98	0	50.0	0.98

VCTE vibration-controlled transient elastography, *LB* liver biopsy, *HVPG* hepatic venous pressure gradient, *F* fibrosis stage by Metavir score

recurrent hepatitis C, from yearly to every other year or even longer, thus sparing more than one third of protocol LB [20]. Furthermore, two prospective longitudinal studies demonstrated that early repeated VCTE examinations in the first year following LT were able to discriminate between patients with rapidly progressive and those with slowly progressive recurrent hepatitis C [21, 22]. The results from a longitudinal mixed model for repeated measurements (VCTE examinations performed at 3, 6, 9 and 12 months after LT) showed that the slope of LS variations was significantly greater in "rapid" than in "slow" *fibrosers*: respectively, 0.42 and 0.05 kPa/month in rapid and slow *fibrosers* as of the study by Carrion et al. [21] and 0.40 and 0.05 kPa/month in rapid and slow *fibrosers* as of the study by Rigamonti et al. [22]. Interestingly, the $\geq$7.9 kPa TE cut-off value at month 6 after LT could identify 67% of rapid *fibrosers* [21, 22].

In another study that evaluated 173 patients who had mild recurrent hepatitis C, as defined by absent or minimal fibrosis at LB or LSM <8.7 kPa 1 year after LT, and were followed up for 80 months, the cumulative risk of cirrhosis was 13% and 30% at 5 and 10 years after LT, respectively [23]. Early changes in LSM over time resulted very helpful to identify LT recipients at risk of cirrhosis: the slope of liver stiffness progression throughout the first 2 years after LT was significantly steeper in patients who developed cirrhosis (0.331 kPa/month) compared to patients who did not develop cirrhosis during follow-up (0.091 kPa/month, $P = 0.038$). Interestingly, none of the patients followed up for 18 months after LT with LS <7.8 kPa progressed to liver cirrhosis [23].

As previously stated, a successful viral eradication and, by consequence, an increased survival [12] are nowadays achievable following the administration of safe and highly effective DAAs in more than 95% of graft recipients with recurrent hepatitis C; however, whether HCV eradication in such transplanted population also determines such crucial clinical outcomes as fibrosis and/or cirrhosis regression remains to be demonstrated. In addition, HCV LT recipients may still need hepatic fibrosis surveillance despite HCV eradication with DAAs, since such non-viral comorbidities as non-alcoholic fatty liver, de novo autoimmune hepatitis, allograft rejection or other injuries may affect the liver graft.

In the non-transplant setting, several studies have shown that VCTE values decrease after antiviral treatment in patients with chronic hepatitis C. In the pre-DAAs era, VCTE dynamics were described in patients treated with pegylated IFN plus ribavirin [24, 25]. More recently, some papers have shown that approximately half of the cirrhotics who had achieved SVR after DAAs had a significant LS decrease (>30% from baseline) at week 24 of follow-up [26–28]. In the study by Mandorfer et al. [26], the relative change in LSM was a predictor of a HVPG decrease $\geq$10% among patients with a clinically significant baseline portal hypertension. However, the meaning of VCTE decrease in terms of improvement of inflammatory activity, fibrosis regression and portal hypertension improvement, which might be mainly related not only to regression of septal fibrosis/cirrhosis but also to perisinusoidal fibrosis remodelling, has not been fully elucidated.

As showed in a retrospective study conducted on 30 liver-transplanted HCV patients, who had undergone both LSM and LB before and post-DAAs treatment,

LS value decreased for $\geq 30\%$ with respect to baseline in 14 patients (47%), increased in 4 (13%) and remained stable in 12 (40%). SVR induced significant improvement in perisinusoidal fibrosis for more than 50% of the treated recipients, and this improvement was detected from the significant LS decrease following DAAs [29].

In a longitudinal study, 46 LT recipients with recurrent hepatitis C and liver stiffness ≥ 8.8 kPa before DAA treatment underwent VCTE examination 12 and 18 months after achieving SVR [30]. Over an 18-month follow-up period, 80% showed improvement in LS (defined as a LS reduction compatible with a change in at least one Metavir stage) and 20% did not [30]; however, liver biopsies were not performed in this study; therefore, no conclusions could be drawn regarding the meaning of LS decrease after SVR (i.e. regression of fibrosis or necroinflammatory activity).

Mauro et al. [31] investigated 112 hepatitis C virus-infected LT recipients who achieved SVR between 2001 and 2015. A LB was performed before treatment and 12 months following SVR: 67% of the cohort presented fibrosis regression (i.e. a decrease of ≥ 1 stage in the Metavir score at follow-up LB) and 31% stabilization, and only 2% saw their stage worsened. In 84 patients, TE examination was also performed concomitantly with LB: 67% of patients showed a significant LS decrease (defined as $\geq 30\%$ decrease compared to pre-treatment evaluation). A decrease of 50% from baseline LS obtained a positive predictive value of 78% for fibrosis regression [31]. In the 34 patients with cirrhosis, LS decreased more in those patients with fibrosis regression. Parenthetically, post-treatment LS <10 kPa was observed in some patients who remained with advanced fibrosis [31]. This study emphasized the concept that the higher the liver stiffness before DAA treatment (i.e. the more advanced the disease before treatment), the lower the probability of fibrosis regression after SVR.

Even if it is not fully clear yet how structural, inflammatory and haemodynamic processes affect liver stiffness and which of such processes is mostly and earliest affected by HCV eradication, it seems clear that LS decrease after antiviral treatment is advantageous, as it carries a general meaning of liver improvement, whatever it is, that may in turn translate into better prognosis.

6.3 "Non-viral" Graft Disease After Transplantation

Liver stiffness is not disease-specific and simply reflects an ongoing intra-hepatic process, which can be related to several conditions—other than fibrosis—and produces itself an increase in liver stiffness. In the non-transplant setting, VCTE was validated in a variety of liver disease [32].

There is limited data regarding the clinical application of VCTE in patients transplanted for end-stage liver diseases other than hepatitis C. In these patients, histological abnormalities of the graft are commonly present in protocol liver biopsies even in the absence of abnormal liver function tests [33]. In a prospective study which investigated, by concurrent VCTE and protocol or on-demand LB examinations, 65 liver graft recipients transplanted for non-HCV-related end-stage liver disease, LS was an accurate and independent predictor of graft damage, unrelated of the aetiology [34]. This is not an unexpected finding since liver stiffness measured by VCTE was previously shown to correlate not only with liver fibrosis but also with necroinflammatory activity, cholestasis and steatosis [19, 35–37].

In 28 patients (43% of the overall series), the liver graft was impaired by multiple aetiologic factors at both protocol ($n = 19$) and on-demand LB ($n = 9$) [34]. At ROC curve analysis, two different VCTE cut-offs were identified able to correctly classify patients regarding the presence or absence of graft damage [34]. A higher than 7.4 kPa VCTE cut-off was found in 56% with graft damage, but in none of the 37 patients without liver graft damage, and it provided a clinical approach to confirm the presence of liver graft damage [34]. By contrast, none of the patients with VCTE results lower than 5.4 kPa had histological features of graft damage, providing the best approach to exclude graft damage [34]. In the "diagnostic grey area" of VCTE results spanning between 5.4 and 7.4 kPa, VCTE was not able to help in the diagnosis of graft damage [34]. However, the diagnostic performance of VCTE may be slightly further improved by taking into the account serum levels of liver function tests (transaminases and gamma-glutamyl transpeptidase). Indeed, if liver function tests were increased ≥ 2 upper limit of normal (ULN), 50% of patients would show graft damage, calling for a liver biopsy to confirm and define the graft disease in this subgroup [34]. Actually, VCTE was able to detect mild graft damage, thus supporting the use of VCTE as a tool to guide the decision-making process for histological evaluation of non-hepatitis C liver-transplanted patients, including patients with normal liver function tests.

The role of longitudinal LS examination in monitoring LT patients, detecting the presence of graft damage and selecting those requiring liver biopsy, has been recently explored in a multicentre study which involved 162 patients (37% transplanted for HCV), investigated with at least three longitudinal LSMs, each at a maximum 6-month interval [38]. In 35 patients (among them 28 with HCV), LS increased over time (defined as a 20% LS change in three or more measurements performed at least 3 months apart); in two patients with normal liver function tests, the LS increase during follow-up suggested a liver graft injury, and a liver biopsy showed severe fibrosis, and in one patient, the LSM increase reflected the occurrence of severe or chronic rejection, which was diagnosed at histology [38].

The use of VCTE as a guide for the selection of patients in need of histological assessment of the graft improves the management of LT recipients: it increases the early recognition of clinically unsuspected liver graft damage, which needs to be further assessed by LB. In fact, the detection of histological abnormalities in the graft may have an impact on the clinical management of the patients. VCTE detects the presence of graft damage early, ultimately being more reliable than blood tests in the LT setting.

6.4 Non-alcoholic Fatty Liver Disease (NAFLD)

Non-alcoholic fatty liver disease (NAFLD) is nowadays a leading cause of chronic liver disease: it has an estimated worldwide prevalence of about 25%, which is even higher in Central Europe (32%) [39]. NAFLD is defined by the presence at liver histology of macrovesicular steatosis in $\geq$5% hepatocytes, in the absence of a secondary cause, such as alcohol or drugs. It can range across a wide spectrum of diseases, from non-alcoholic fatty liver (NAFL) to non-alcoholic steatohepatitis (NASH), fibrosis and cirrhosis [40]. NAFLD and NASH-related end-stage cirrhosis are increasingly recognized as an indication for LT, mainly in industrialized countries. Although the gold standard for the diagnosis of NAFLD and NASH is liver biopsy [41], several studies have investigated the potential role of non-invasive methods in predicting liver fibrosis in patients with NAFLD.

In the non-transplant setting, VCTE is validated and widely used for assessing the presence of fibrosis in NAFLD patients: a meta-analysis has shown that its operative characteristics are excellent for diagnosing advanced fibrosis (85% sensitivity, 82% specificity) and cirrhosis (92% sensitivity, 92% specificity) and fair for significant fibrosis (79% sensitivity, 75% specificity) [42].

More recently, a new parameter called controlled attenuation parameter (CAP) has been introduced for hepatic steatosis estimation [43]. CAP can be measured concurrently with liver stiffness using the same instrument, i.e. FibroScan® (VCTE), and allows the non-invasive measurement of liver fat content, based on the principle that the attenuation of ultrasound signals is greater in fat than water [44]. CAP provides an immediate and standardized non-invasive measurement of hepatic steatosis, as shown in a meta-analysis which included data from 2735 patients [45] and in a large study on 5323 adult patients with suspected chronic liver disease [46]. Despite good sensitivity and specificity for detecting hepatic steatosis as compared to liver biopsy, a meta-analysis demonstrated that CAP was not an excellent test for the detection of steatosis severity in chronic liver disease due to the low ability of CAP to exclude the presence of steatosis in the presence of a negative test [47].

In the transplant setting, the concomitant measurement of LS and CAP is possibly applicable to the assessment of hepatic steatosis and fibrosis in a donor graft and for evaluating recurrent or de novo NAFLD [48]. With the aim of optimal graft selection, Mancia et al. [49] performed a pilot study on 23 donors with brain death, assessing the performance of VCTE and CAP compared to liver biopsy (as the reference standard), and found that the combination of CAP and LS could successfully quantify steatosis and fibrosis in the preoperative selection of liver grafts from brain-dead subjects. In the study by Hong and colleagues [50], 55 potential living donors were evaluated by CAP and liver biopsy, with CAP showing an AUROC of 78% for detecting mild steatosis and 88% for moderate steatosis.

In 2018, Yen et al. [51] compared CAP to intraoperative LB for detecting steatosis in 54 living donors: a cut-off value of 257 dB/m achieved a 100% sensitivity for hepatic steatosis, though only 58% of patients with CAP >257 dB/m had biopsy-proven steatosis.

De novo NAFLD/NASH after LT is associated with metabolic syndrome, which seems to have a higher incidence among LT patients than in the general population. This can be partially explained by the use of immunosuppressive drugs, as both corticosteroids and calcineurin inhibitors promote arterial hypertension, hyperlipidaemia, diabetes and weight gain. Necroinflammation related to NASH might influence graft survival because of the development of fibrosis and cirrhosis; thus, it is important to make a prompt diagnosis of NASH in the LT setting, as well as managing risk factors for metabolic syndrome [52, 53].

LT recipients are at risk of developing hepatic graft steatosis, recurrence of NASH after LT or de novo NAFLD occurrence [54].

Non-invasive steatosis monitoring in this setting has not been widely studied yet. The vast majority of studies, in fact, are based on liver histology alone. One possible limitation is that VCTE accuracy is impaired by obesity, which is obviously very common among this type of patients.

In 2015, Karlas and colleagues [55] prospectively evaluated 204 patients by ultrasonography and VCTE with CAP measurement and confirmed a high prevalence of graft steatosis, being 36% at US evaluation and rising to 44% when considering CAP measurement. They also found a high rate of graft fibrosis (31%, defined by LS >7.9 kPa) and cirrhosis (13%, defined by LS >12 kPa); the higher the CAP, the worse the fibrosis stage. Interestingly, these authors [55] found that the graft steatosis was associated with neither immunosuppressive treatment regimen nor the post-transplant interval, while it was significantly associated with BMI, diabetes mellitus and alcoholic aetiology of cirrhosis.

The high prevalence of post-LT steatosis has also been demonstrated in the study by Chayanupatkul et al. [56] covering 150 post-LT subjects, who underwent CAP measurement: a 70% and 40% prevalence of any steatosis (CAP ≥222 dB/m) and severe steatosis (CAP ≥290 dB/m) were demonstrated, respectively. Bhati et al. [57] carried out a long-term follow-up of 90 patients liver-transplanted for cirrhosis due to confirmed NASH or cryptogenic cirrhosis suspected to be NASH: 56 patients underwent VCTE with CAP measurement, and 34 had liver biopsy. Post-transplant NAFLD recurrence was 88% based on LB and 87% based on CAP (87.5%); similarly, the prevalence of advanced fibrosis was 21% in the patients evaluated histologically and 27% in those tested by VCTE [57]. In a recent paper evaluating 99 liver transplant recipients [58], a CAP cut-off value of 270 dB/m showed an AUROC of 0.88 (95% CI, 0.78–0.93) for detecting any hepatic steatosis; however, CAP was less accurate in differentiating grades of steatosis having overlapping cut-off values.

Due to the high prevalence of NAFLD after LT, the availability of a user-friendly, reliable and non-invasive technique for steatosis and fibrosis assessment would be greatly relevant. However, more data is necessary for assessing the diagnostic performance of CAP in the LT setting and incorporating it into a definite diagnostic workup of LT recipients in order to identify those with suspected NAFLD for closer follow-up.

6.5   Elastography Outcome After Liver Transplantation

Since the stage of hepatic fibrosis significantly influences outcome, the assessment of liver fibrosis is a cornerstone of the management of liver diseases and a key step to the estimation of prognosis. In the non-transplant setting, non-invasive methods, including vibration-controlled transient elastography, can ably predict patients' survival with higher accuracy than LB staging in large cohorts of patients with chronic hepatitis C [58]. Equally, the prognostic value of VCTE has been shown in patients with NAFLD. In an observational cohort study of 2245 NAFLD patients followed up for a median time of 27 months, baseline LS emerged as an independent predictor of overall survival; also, the occurrence of cardiovascular events and liver complications could be predicted by high LS [59].

In the LT setting, some studies have investigated the ability of liver stiffness to predict clinical outcomes, including graft and patient survival.

Liver stiffness value at 1 year after LT has been shown to be predictive of clinical decompensation and graft loss in 144 HCV-infected LT recipients [60]. The presence of LS $\geq$8.7 kPa 1 year after LT was significantly associated with all-cause-related graft loss. Indeed, the 8.7 kPa cut-off value stratified patients in two different categories of risk of clinical decompensation, graft loss and death: the cumulative probabilities of clinical decompensation, graft loss and death 5 years after LT were 8%, 10% and 8% for patients with LS <8.7 kPa versus 47%, 37% and 36% for patients with LSM $\geq$8.7 kPa, respectively (log-rank <0.001) [60]. In addition, LS at 1 year after LT was independently associated with graft loss and patient survival at multivariate analysis [60].

In 173 patients with mild recurrent hepatitis C (as defined by absent or minimal fibrosis at LB or LS <8.7 kPa 1 year after LT), after a median follow-up of 92 months, cumulative HCV-related graft survival rates at 5 and 10 years after LT were respectively 97% and 90% versus 64% and 51% in 200 patients with severe hepatitis C recurrence ($P < 0.001$), this suggesting that a LS <8.7 kPa 1 year after LT might be predictive of better graft survival over time [23].

Liver stiffness measured at 3 months after LT in 137 liver-transplanted patients with different aetiologies of liver disease emerged as an independent risk factor of reduced survival after LT (OR = 1.080, 95% CI 1.001–1.166, $p = 0.047$), along with platelets (OR = 0.992, 95% CI 0.986–0.999, $p = 0.020$) and metabolic syndrome (OR = 0.250, 95% CI 0.070–0.895, $p = 0.033$) [61].

In the multicentre study by Rinaldi et al. [38] on 162 patients investigated with at least three longitudinal VCTE examinations, a stable LS over time had a very high negative predictive value for both clinical events (including liver decompensation) and death.

Overall, these studies support the concept that the non-invasive assessment by vibration-controlled transient elastography may help to identify recipients at risk of poor outcome: the higher the liver stiffness during first year after LT, the poorer the clinical outcome over time. In this setting, clinicians can use VCTE as a complementary tool for differentiating the intensity of follow-up in the clinical practice, each patient's clinical history remaining also crucial.

6.6   Spleen Stiffness and Liver Transplant

The measurement of spleen stiffness is a further possible application of elastography that might be useful to assess portal hypertension dynamics after LT.

With this regard, Chin et al. [62] evaluated spleen stiffness at 2–8 weeks after LT: spleen stiffness significantly decreased comparing pre- and post-LT, being 75.0 kPa (63.9–75.0) vs. 28.4 kPa (22.0–37.5) ($P < 0.0001$). In 14 patients studied at all time points, the stiffness of the spleen progressively reduced from a median of 75.0 (62.0–75.0) kPa before LT to 41.9 (27.0–47.4) kPa at 2 weeks after transplant and 32.9 (29.1–38.0) kPa in the subsequent weeks (4–8 weeks after LT) ($P < 0.0001$) [62]. Similar encouraging results were also found by Bayramov et al. [63], who measured spleen stiffness before LT and at 1, 3 and 6 months after LT and demonstrated a significant decrease of spleen stiffness over time.

Although it needs further validation in larger studies, all this data is encouraging: in the near future, spleen stiffness measurement might become the predictor of portal hypertension changes or resolution after LT.

In conclusion, VTCE is a reliable tool for detecting liver graft damage, whatever the aetiology, and its introduction in the clinical management of LT recipients may ultimately provide added clinical benefits in terms of prediction of liver fibrosis, sparing of unnecessary liver biopsies and early detection of graft damage with selection of patients in need of prompt histological evaluation.

References

1. Lucey MR, Terrault N, Ojo L, Hay JE, Neuberger J, Blumberg E, Teperman LW. Long-term management of the successful adult liver transplant: 2012 practice guideline by the american association for the study of liver diseases and the American Society of Transplantation. Liver Transpl. 2013;19:3–26. https://doi.org/10.1002/lt.23566.
2. Crespo G, Castro-Narro G, García-Juárez I, Benítez C, Ruiz P, Sastre L, et al. Usefulness of liver stiffness measurement during acute cellular rejection in liver transplantation. Liver Transpl. 2016;22:298–304. https://doi.org/10.1002/lt.24376.
3. Nacif LS, de Cassia GC, Paranaguá-Vezozzo D, Flores Cassenote AJ, Pinheiro RS, Waisberg DR, et al. Liver elastography in acute cellular rejection after liver transplantation. Transplant Proc. 2020;52:1340–3. https://doi.org/10.1016/j.transproceed.2020.02.026.
4. Inoue Y, Sugawara Y, Tamura S, Ohtsu H, Taguri M, Makuuchi M, et al. Validity and feasibility of transient elastography for the transplanted liver in the peritransplantation period. Transplantation. 2009;88:103–9. https://doi.org/10.1097/TP.0b013e3181aacb7f.
5. Forman LM, Lewis JD, Berlin JA, Feldman HI, Lucey MR. The association between hepatitis C infection and survival after orthotopic liver transplantation. Gastroenterology. 2002;122:889–96. https://doi.org/10.1053/gast.2002.32418.
6. Berenguer M. What determines the natural history of recurrent hepatitis C after liver transplantation? J Hepatol. 2005;42:448–56. https://doi.org/10.1016/j.jhep.2005.01.011.
7. Gane EJ. The natural history of recurrent hepatitis C and what influences this. Liver Transpl. 2008;14:S36–44. https://doi.org/10.1002/lt.21646.
8. Berenguer M, Xavier L-L, Wright T. Hepatitis C recurrence and liver transplantation. J Hepatol. 2001;35:666–8. https://doi.org/10.1016/s0168-8278(01)00179-9.

9. Berenguer M. Systematic review of the treatment of established recurrent hepatitis C with pegylated interferon in combination with ribavirin. J Hepatol. 2008;49:274–87. https://doi.org/10.1016/j.jhep.2008.05.002.

10. Liao HT, Tan P, Huang JW, Yuan KF. Ledipasvir + sofosbuvir for liver transplant recipients with recurrent hepatitis c: a systematic review and meta-analysis. Transplant Proc. 2017;49:1855–63. https://doi.org/10.1016/j.transproceed.2017.04.014.

11. Liu J, Ma B, Cao W, Li M, Bramer WM, Peppelenbosch MP, et al. Direct-acting antiviral agents for liver transplant recipients with recurrent genotype 1 hepatitis C virus infection: systematic review and meta-analysis. Transpl Infect Dis. 2019;21:e13047. https://doi.org/10.1111/tid.13047.

12. Belli LS, Perricone G, Adam R, Cortesi PA, Strazzabosco M, Facchetti R, et al. Impact of DAAs on liver transplantation: major effects on the evolution of indications and results. An ELITA study based on the ELTR registry. J Hepatol. 2018;69:810–7. https://doi.org/10.1016/j.jhep.2018.06.010.

13. Castéra L, Vergniol J, Foucher J, Le Bail B, Chanteloup E, Haaser M, et al. Prospective comparison of transient elastography, Fibrotest, APRI, and liver biopsy for the assessment of fibrosis in chronic hepatitis C. Gastroenterology. 2005;128:343–50. https://doi.org/10.1053/j.gastro.2004.11.018.

14. Carrion JA, Navasa M, Bosch J, Bruguera M, Gilabert R, Forns X. Transient elastography for diagnosis of advanced fibrosis and portal hypertension in patients with hepatitis C recurrence after liver transplantation. Liver Transpl. 2006;12:1791–8. https://doi.org/10.1002/lt.20857.

15. Rigamonti C, Donato MF, Fraquelli M, Agnelli F, Ronchi G, Casazza G, et al. Transient elastography predicts fibrosis progression in patients with recurrent hepatitis C after liver transplantation. Gut. 2008;57:821–7. https://doi.org/10.1136/gut.2007.135046.

16. Harada N, Soejima Y, Taketomi A, Yoshizumi T, Ikegami T, Yamashita Y, et al. Assessment of graft fibrosis by transient elastography in patients with recurrent hepatitis C after living donor liver transplantation. Transplantation. 2008;85:69–74. https://doi.org/10.1097/01.tp.0000297248.18483.16.

17. Blasco A, Forns X, Carrión JA, García-Pagán JC, Gilabert R, Rimola A, et al. Hepatic venous pressure gradient identifies patients at risk of severe hepatitis C recurrence after liver transplantation. Hepatology. 2006;43:492–9. https://doi.org/10.1002/hep.21090.

18. Fraquelli M, Rigamonti C, Casazza G, Conte D, Donato MF, Ronchi G, et al. Reproducibility of transient elastography in the evaluation of liver fibrosis in patients with chronic liver disease. Gut. 2007;56:968–73. https://doi.org/10.1136/gut.2006.111302.

19. Fraquelli M, Rigamonti C, Casazza G, Donato MF, Ronchi G, Conte D, et al. Etiology-related determinants of liver stiffness values in chronic viral hepatitis B or C. J Hepatol. 2011;54:621–8. https://doi.org/10.1016/j.jhep.2010.07.017.

20. Donato MF, Rigamonti C, Colombo M. Can protocol liver biopsy be avoided to evaluate post-transplant hepatitis C recurrence? Transient elastography makes it possible. Dig Liver Dis. 2010;42:307. https://doi.org/10.1016/j.dld.2009.07.015.

21. Carrion JA, Torres F, Crespo G, et al. Liver stiffness identifies two different patterns of fibrosis progression in patients with hepatitis C virus recurrence after liver transplantation. Hepatology. 2010;51:23–34. https://doi.org/10.1002/hep.23240.

22. Rigamonti C, Donato MF, Colombo M. Transient elastography in the early prediction of progressive recurrent hepatitis C following liver transplantation. Hepatology. 2010;52:800–1. https://doi.org/10.1002/hep.23607.

23. Gambato M, Crespo G, Torres F, LLovet L, Carrión J, Londoño M, et al. Simple prediction of long-term clinical outcomes in patients with mild hepatitis C recurrence after liver transplantation. Transpl Int. 2016;29:698–706. https://doi.org/10.1111/tri.12730.

24. Hézode C, Castéra L, Roudot-Thoraval F, Bouvier-Alias M, Rosa I, Roulot D, et al. Liver stiffness diminishes with antiviral response in chronic hepatitis C. Aliment Pharmacol Ther. 2011;34:656–63. https://doi.org/10.1111/j.1365-2036.2011.04765.x.

25. Stasi C, Arena U, Zignego AL, Corti G, Monti M, Elisa Triboli E, et al. Longitudinal assessment of liver stiffness in patients undergoing antiviral treatment for hepatitis C. Dig Liver Dis. 2013;45:840–3. https://doi.org/10.1016/j.dld.2013.03.023.
26. Mandorfer M, Kozbial K, Freissmuth C, Schwabl P, Stättermayer AF, Reiberger T, et al. Interferon-free regimens for chronic hepatitis C overcome the effects of portal hypertension on virological responses. Aliment Pharmacol Ther. 2015;42:707–18. https://doi.org/10.1111/apt.13315.
27. Knop V, Hoppe D, Welzel T, Vermehren J, Herrmann E, Vermehren A, et al. Regression of fibrosis and portal hypertension in HCV-associated cirrhosis and sustained virologic response after interferon-free antiviral therapy. J Viral Hepat. 2016;23:994–1002. https://doi.org/10.1111/jvh.12578.
28. Rigamonti C, Tran Minh M, Minisini R, Guaschino G, Pirisi M. Dynamics of liver stiffness and serum IP10 levels among patients with chronic hepatitis C who achieved SVR with DAA treatment. J Hepatol. 2017;66:S666.
29. Donato MF, Rigamonti C, Invernizzi F, Colucci G, Fraquelli M, Maggioni M, et al. Paired Liver biopsy, Fibrotest and FibroScan® before and after treatment with DAA in liver transplanted recipients with recurrent hepatitis C: diagnostic accuracy and concordance. Hepatology. 2016;64(S1):134A.
30. Omar H, Said M, Eletreby R, Mehrez M, Bassam M, Abdellatif Z, et al. Longitudinal assessment of hepatic fibrosis in responders to direct-acting antivirals for recurrent hepatitis C after liver transplantation using noninvasive methods. Clin Transpl. 2018;32:e13334. https://doi.org/10.1111/ctr.13334.
31. Mauro E, Crespo G, Montironi C, Londono MC, Hernandez-Gea V, Ruiz P, et al. Portal pressure and liver stiffness measurements in the prediction of fibrosis regression after SVR in recurrent hepatitis C. Hepatology. 2018;67:1683–94. https://doi.org/10.1002/hep.29557.
32. European Association for Study of Liver, Asociacion Latinoamericana para el Estudio del Higado, Castera L, HLY C, Arrese M, Afdhal N, Bedossa P, Friedrich-Rust M, et al. EASL-ALEH Clinical Practice Guidelines: non-invasive tests for evaluation of liver disease severity and prognosis. J Hepatol. 2015;63:237–64. https://doi.org/10.1016/j.jhep.2015.04.006.
33. Hübscher SG. What is the long-term outcome of the liver allograft? J Hepatol. 2011;55:702–17. https://doi.org/10.1016/j.jhep.2011.03.005.
34. Rigamonti C, Fraquelli M, Bastiampillai AJ, Caccamo L, Reggiani P, Rossi G, et al. Transient elastography identifies liver recipients with nonviral graft disease after transplantation: a guide for liver biopsy. Liver Transpl. 2012;18(5):566–76. https://doi.org/10.1002/lt.23391.
35. Lupşor M, Badea R, Stefanescu H, Grigorescu M, Sparchez Z, Serban A, et al. Analysis of histopathological changes that influence liver stiffness in chronic hepatitis C. Results from a cohort of 324 patients. J Gastrointestin Liver Dis. 2008;17:155–63.
36. Corpechot C, El Naggar A, Poujol-Robert A, Ziol M, Wendum D, Chazouillères O, et al. Assessment of biliary fibrosis by transient elastography in patients with PBC and PSC. Hepatology. 2006;43:1118–24. https://doi.org/10.1002/hep.21151.
37. Millonig G, Reimann FM, Friedrich S, Fonouni H, Mehrabi A, Büchler MW, et al. Extrahepatic cholestasis increases liver stiffness (FibroScan) irrespective of fibrosis. Hepatology. 2008;48:1718–23. https://doi.org/10.1002/hep.22577.
38. Rinaldi L, Valente G, Piai G. Serial liver stiffness measurements and monitoring of liver-transplanted patients in a real-life clinical practice. Hepat Mon. 2016;16:e41162. https://doi.org/10.5812/hepatmon.41162.
39. Younossi ZM, Koenig AB, Abdelatif D, Fazel Y, Henry L, Wymer M. Global epidemiology of nonalcoholic fatty liver disease-meta-analytic assessment of prevalence, incidence, and outcomes. Hepatology. 2016;64:73–84. https://doi.org/10.1002/hep.28431.
40. European Association for the Study of the Liver (EASL), European Association for the Study of Diabetes (EASD), European Association for the Study of Obesity (EASO). EASL-EASD-EASO Clinical Practice Guidelines for the management of non-alcoholic fatty liver disease. J Hepatol. 2016;64:1388–402. https://doi.org/10.1016/j.jhep.2015.11.004.

41. Ratziu V, Charlotte F, Heurtier A, Gombert S, Giral P, Bruckert E, et al. Sampling variability of liver biopsy in nonalcoholic fatty liver disease. Gastroenterology. 2005;128:1898–906. https://doi.org/10.1053/j.gastro.2005.03.084.

42. Kwok R, Tse YK, Wong GL, Ha Y, Lee AU, Ngu MC, et al. Systematic review with meta-analysis: non-invasive assessment of non-alcoholic fatty liver disease--the role of transient elastography and plasma cytokeratin-18 fragments. Aliment Pharmacol Ther. 2014;39:254–69. https://doi.org/10.1111/apt.12569.

43. Controlled attenuation parameter (CAP): a novel VCTE™ guided ultrasonic attenuation measurement for the evaluation of hepatic steatosis: preliminary study and validation in a cohort of patients with chronic liver disease from various causes. Ultrasound Med Biol. 2010;36:1825–35. https://doi.org/10.1016/j.ultrasmedbio.2010.07.005.

44. Wong GL, Wong VW. Fat and fiber: how the controlled attenuation parameter complements noninvasive assessment of liver fibrosis. Dig Dis Sci. 2015;60:9–12. https://doi.org/10.1007/s10620-014-3429-3.

45. Karlas T, Petroff D, Sasso M, Fan JG, Mi YQ, de Lédinghen V, et al. Individual patient data meta-analysis of controlled attenuation parameter (CAP) technology for assessing steatosis. J Hepatol. 2017;66:1022–30. https://doi.org/10.1016/j.jhep.2016.12.022.

46. de Lédinghen V, Vergniol J, Capdepont M, Chermak F, Hiriart JB, Cassinotto C, et al. Controlled attenuation parameter (CAP) for the diagnosis of steatosis: a prospective study of 5323 examinations. J Hepatol. 2014;60:1026–31. https://doi.org/10.1016/j.jhep.2013.12.018.

47. Shi KQ, Tang JZ, Zhu XL, Ying L, Li DW, Gao J, et al. Controlled attenuation parameter for the detection of steatosis severity in chronic liver disease: a meta-analysis of diagnostic accuracy. J Gastroenterol Hepatol. 2014;29:1149–58. https://doi.org/10.1111/jgh.12519.

48. Winters AC, Mittal R, Schiano TD. A review of the use of transient elastography in the assessment of fibrosis and steatosis in the post-liver transplant patient. Clin Transpl. 2019;33:e13700. https://doi.org/10.1111/ctr.13700.

49. Mancia C, Loustaud-Ratti V, Carrier P, Naudet F, Bellissant E, Labrousse F, et al. Controlled attenuation parameter and liver stiffness measurements for steatosis assessment in the liver transplant of brain-dead donors. Transplantation. 2015;99:1619–24. https://doi.org/10.1097/TP.0000000000000652.

50. Hong YM, Yoon KT, Cho M, Chu CW, Rhu JH, Yang KH, et al. Clinical usefulness of controlled attenuation parameter to screen hepatic steatosis for potential donor of living donor liver transplant. Eur J Gastroenterol Hepatol. 2017;29:805–10. https://doi.org/10.1097/MEG.0000000000000876.

51. Yen YH, Kuo FY, Lin CC, Chen CL, Chang KC, Tsai MC, et al. Predicting hepatic steatosis in living liver donors via controlled attenuation parameter. Transplant Proc. 2018;50:3533–8. https://doi.org/10.1016/j.transproceed.2018.06.039.

52. Pisano G, Fracanzani AL, Caccamo L, Donato MF, Fargion S. Cardiovascular risk after orthotopic liver transplantation, a review of the literature and preliminary results of a prospective study. World J Gastroenterol. 2016;22:8869–82. https://doi.org/10.3748/wjg.v22.i40.8869.

53. Seo S, Maganti K, Khehra M, Ramsamooj R, Tsodikov A, Bowluset C, et al. De-novo nonalcoholic fatty liver disease after liver transplantation. Liver Transpl. 2007;13:844–7. https://doi.org/10.1002/lt.20932.

54. Contos MJ, Cales W, Sterling RK, Luketic VA, Shiffman ML, Mills AS, et al. Development of nonalcoholic fatty liver disease after orthotopic liver transplantation for cryptogenic cirrhosis. Liver Transpl. 2001;7:363–73. https://doi.org/10.1053/jlts.2001.23011.

55. Karlas T, Kollmeier J, Böhm S, Müller J, Kovacs P, Tröltzsch M, et al. Noninvasive characterization of graft steatosis after liver transplantation. Scand J Gastroenterol. 2015;50:224–32. https://doi.org/10.3109/00365521.2014.983156.

56. Chayanupatkul M, Dasani DB, Sogaard K, Schiano TD. The utility of assessing liver allograft fibrosis and steatosis post-liver transplantation using transient elastography with controlled attenuation parameter. Transplant Proc. 2020;S0041-1345(19)31521-0. https://doi.org/10.1016/j.transproceed.2020.02.160.

57. Bhati C, Idowu MO, Sanyal AJ, Rivera M, Driscoll C, Stravitz RT, et al. Long-term outcomes in patients undergoing liver transplantation for nonalcoholic steatohepatitis-related cirrhosis. Transplantation. 2017;101:1867–74. https://doi.org/10.1097/TP.0000000000001709.

58. Vergniol J, Foucher J, Terrebonne E, et al. Noninvasive tests for fibrosis and liver stiffness predict 5-year outcomes of patients with chronic hepatitis C. Gastroenterology. 2011;140:1970–79. e1-3. https://doi.org/10.1053/j.gastro.2011.02.058.

59. Shili-Masmoudi S, Wong GL, Hiriart JB, Liu K, Chermak F, Shu SS, et al. Liver stiffness measurement predicts long-term survival and complications in non-alcoholic fatty liver disease. Liver Int. 2020;40:581–9. https://doi.org/10.1111/liv.14301.

60. Crespo G, Lens S, Gambato M, Carrión JA, Mariño Z, Londoño MC, et al. Liver stiffness 1 year after transplantation predicts clinical outcomes in patients with recurrent hepatitis C. Am J Transplant. 2014;14:375–83. https://doi.org/10.1111/ajt.12594.

61. Pfeiffenberger J, Hornuss D, Houben P, Wehling C, von Haken R, Loszanowski V, et al. Routine liver elastography could predict actuarial survival after liver transplantation. J Gastrointestin Liver Dis. 2019;28:271–7. https://doi.org/10.15403/jgld-218.

62. Chin JL, Chan G, Ryan JD, McCormick PA. Spleen stiffness can non-invasively assess resolution of portal hypertension after liver transplantation. Liver Int. 2015;35:518–23. https://doi.org/10.1111/liv.12647.

63. Bayramov N, Yilmaz S, Salahova S, Bashkiran A, Zeynalov N, Isazade E, Bayramova T, et al. Liver graft and spleen elastography after living liver transplantation: our first results. Transplant Proc. 2019;51:2446–50. https://doi.org/10.1016/j.transproceed.2019.01.184.

Elastography in Autoimmune Liver Diseases

Laura Cristoferi, Marco Carbone, and Pietro Invernizzi

7.1 Introduction

Surrogate markers of liver fibrosis are increasingly replacing liver biopsy (LB) in the management of the most prevalent chronic liver diseases including viral hepatitis, alcohol-related liver diseases and non-alcoholic fatty liver diseases. In autoimmune liver diseases (AILDs), however, the validity of non-invasive tests (NITs) of fibrosis has not been fully established and their use is, therefore, limited. The main reason for this is the low prevalence of AILDs, mostly managed in referral centres, and the high heterogeneity in diagnostic delay, in therapeutic management, with the lack of curative treatment and in disease course which create a major hurdle for biomarker discovery.

To date, vibration-controlled transient elastography (VCTE) by FibroScan® (Echosens, Paris, France) has been the most widely used physical method of fibrosis assessment and demonstrated to have good accuracy in discriminating patient with advanced fibrosis and cirrhosis in AILDs [1–4].

L. Cristoferi (✉)
Division of Gastroenterology, Center for Autoimmune Liver Diseases, Department of Medicine and Surgery, University of Milano-Bicocca, Monza, MB, Italy

European Reference Network on Hepatological Diseases (ERN RARE-LIVER), San Gerardo Hospital, Monza, Italy

Bicocca Bioinformatics Biostatistics and Bioimaging Centre - B4, School of Medicine and Surgery, University of Milano-Bicocca, Monza, Italy
e-mail: l.cristoferi@campus.unimib.it

M. Carbone · P. Invernizzi
Division of Gastroenterology, Center for Autoimmune Liver Diseases, Department of Medicine and Surgery, University of Milano-Bicocca, Monza, MB, Italy

European Reference Network on Hepatological Diseases (ERN RARE-LIVER), San Gerardo Hospital, Monza, Italy

© Springer Nature Switzerland AG 2021
M. Fraquelli (ed.), *Elastography of the Liver and Beyond*,
https://doi.org/10.1007/978-3-030-74132-7_7

VCTE is rapid, non-invasive and reproducible and is performed at the bedside by a provider, and it acquires information from a much larger portion of the tissue compared with LB significantly reducing the risk of sampling error. These characteristics make it one of the best candidates for fibrosis staging in AILDs especially because of their patchy distribution in the liver that could bias staging and grading with LB that is currently the gold standard for fibrosis staging in AILDs.

In this chapter, we review the evidence on the use of VCTE in AILDs focusing on strengths and limitations.

7.2 Primary Biliary Cholangitis

Primary biliary cholangitis (PBC) is an autoimmune liver disease characterised by destructive cholangitis affecting the small intrahepatic bile ducts, leading to chronic cholestasis and progressive fibrosis. Many patients eventually develop end-stage liver disease with attendant need for liver transplantation [5].

The introduction of ursodeoxycholic acid (UDCA) has dramatically changed the pattern and course of the disease. In fact, the response to UDCA is a major predictor of long-term outcome. The two most important parameters in evaluating response to UDCA are alkaline phosphatase (ALP) and serum bilirubin which have been included in several (biochemical) criteria of response to UDCA [6].

Along with treatment response based on the liver biochemistry, fibrosis stage has itself a prognostic value in PBC. In fact, advanced histologic stage is an independent predictive factor for transplant-free survival, conferring a 1.5-fold increased risk for liver transplantation or death [7, 8]. Recently, the GLOBAL PBC study group and the UK-PBC study group demonstrated the histological assessment of fibrosis grants' prognostic value beyond biochemical treatment response at 1 year. This highlighted the need to incorporate liver fibrosis stage to individual risk stratification at diagnosis in PBC patients [9, 10]. The accurate, early identification of patients' fibrotic stage allows to optimise the patients' clinical pathway; e.g. patients with no clinically relevant fibrosis at lower risk of complication of end-stage liver disease if adequately treated can be de-escalated in the intensity of care, e.g. discharged to primary care; on the other hand, the early identification of patients with clinically relevant fibrosis at baseline will enable to enhance their management through earlier (second-line) treatment escalation and hepatocellular carcinoma (HCC) surveillance [11].

Percutaneous LB is currently the reference standard for liver fibrosis staging; however, due to its invasiveness and potential complications, it is not recommended by international PBC guidelines for fibrosis staging at diagnosis [6, 12, 13]. Moreover, the patchy distribution of the disease through the liver and a significant rate of intra- and inter-observer agreement may reduce LB diagnostic accuracy [14].

To date, several reports have tested the usefulness of serum biomarkers to assess liver fibrosis (i.e. serum levels of hyaluronic acid, procollagen III aminoterminal propeptide, collagen IV and FibroTest®). However, none of them demonstrated the ability to differentiate between early and advanced fibrosis in PBC with acceptable grade of specificity and sensitivity [15, 16]. Along with these biomarkers, the most clinical widespread surrogate markers of fibrosis, such as platelet count, albumin and bilirubin, prevent discrimination of fibrosis in non-advanced stages.

Non-invasive evaluation of liver fibrosis with liver stiffness measurements (LSM) by VCTE is considered the best surrogate marker for the detection of severe fibrosis or cirrhosis in patients with PBC, and there is an increasing interesting understanding of clinically relevant cut-off values. LSM by VCTE is currently recommended by European guidelines for disease staging at diagnosis and follow-up [6].

This recommendation is supported by a French study in PBC by Corpechot et al. ($N = 103$) in which VCTE was found to be of high performance in the diagnosis of severe liver fibrosis ($\geq$F3 according to Metavir staging system) or cirrhosis (F4) with sensitivity and specificity >90%. However, on the other hand, it showed rather poor sensitivity (despite high positive predictive value (PPV) and specificity) for the detection of mild or significant fibrosis ($\geq$F1 and $\geq$F2) with only 45% of patients with F2 at LB correctly classified and 32% and 23% under- and over-staged, respectively [4]. The optimal stiffness thresholds for the diagnosis of fibrosis stage $\geq$F1, $\geq$F2, $\geq$F3 and =F4 were 7.1, 8.8, 10.7 and 16.9 kPa. In addition, aiming at evaluating the prognostic role of VCTE, they retrospectively tested LSM progression over 5 years of follow-up analysing a monitoring cohort ($N = 150$). An optimal threshold of LSM increasing per year of 2.1 kPa and LSM >9.6 kPa at baseline have been found to be associated with 8.4- and 5.1-fold times increased risk of adverse outcome, respectively.

This study, while important, had some methodological flaws: the cohort was cross-sectional with patients at different phases of the disease course with a mean time from diagnosis of 6.7 years and only 11% of patients assessed at diagnosis and naïve to therapy; 14% of patients had histologically proven overlap with autoimmune hepatitis (AIH), and 18% of patients were receiving additional corticosteroids and/or mycophenolate mofetil; more importantly, this was a single-centre study lacking an external validation cohort [4]. Thus, the use of cut-offs individuated in this clinically heterogeneous cohort for disease staging at baseline, as suggested by guidelines, is not precise. Furthermore, the presence of potential confounding factors on LSM lecture, i.e. body mass index, cholestasis or high level of transaminases, has not been evaluated.

Other studies evaluated the accuracy of VCTE in assessing liver fibrosis PBC and results are summarised in Table 7.1 [4, 17–19].

Floreani et al. performed a cross-sectional single-centre study ($n = 114$), which demonstrated a good performance of VCTE in discriminating advanced fibrosis with an area under the receiver operating curve (AUROC) of 0.92 (CI 0.85–0.99) [17]. Significant fibrosis (F $\geq$ 3 according to Metavir staging system) was predicted in patients whose LSM was higher than 7.6 kPa with a PPV of 0.90 and a positive likelihood ratio (LR+) of 11.25, and it was ruled out with a negative predictive value (NPV) of 0.92. In this study, VCTE discriminated better intermediate stage of fibrosis with a cut-off of 5.9 kPa (F $\geq$ 2 sec. Metavir); however, the low NPV (62%) showed a mild accuracy in identifying true negative patients. In this study, patients

Table 7.1 Comparison of most important studies on VCTE in PBC

	Histological staging system	n	Cut-off (kPa)	Se	Sp	PPV	NPV	LR+	LR-	AUROC
Corpechot et al. [4]										
≥F1	Metavir	92	7.1	0.64	1.0	1.0	0.25	64	0.36	0.80
≥F2		52	8.8	0.67	1.0	1.0	0.75	67	0.17	0.91
≥F3		30	10.7	0.90	0.93	0.84	0.96	13.14	0.11	0.95
=F4		15	16.9	0.93	0.99	0.93	0.99	82.13	0.07	0.99
Floreani et al. [17]										
≥F2	Metavir	114	5.9	0.82	0.92	0.97	0.59	10.25	0.08	0.89
≥F3			7.6	0.90	0.92	0.90	0.92	11.25	0.10	0.92
=F4			11.6	0.99	0.94	0.77	1.00	16.7	0.01	0.99
Dominguez et al. [18]										
≥F3	Metavir	55	14.7	0.56	1.00	1.00	0.83	56	0.44	0.86
=F4			15.6	0.88	0.98	0.98	0.98	44	0.12	0.96
Cristoferi et al. [19]										
≥LS3	Ludwig	126	>11.0		0.99	0.94		91	0.08	0.89
≤LS2			≤6.5	0.91			0.96			

Se sensitivity, *Sp* specificity, *PPV* positive predictive value, *NPV* negative predictive value, *LR+* positive likelihood ratio, *AUROC* area under the receiver operating curves

with overlap with AIH were excluded and VCTE was performed within 6 months from liver biopsy.

Both studies evaluated the VCTE performance in identifying and excluding fibrosis against the other NITs (e.g. AST to platelet index (APRI), fibrosis-4 (FIB-4) score, hyaluronic acid (HA) levels, Mayo score and AST to ALT ratio). In the French study, the AUROCs from LSM by VCTE were significantly greater than those of the APRI, FIB-4, HA, AST to ALT ratio and Mayo score for the prediction of mild (F ≥ 2) and advanced fibrosis (F ≥ 3), and, in addition, the combination between biochemical indexes and VCTE did not improve diagnostic accuracy in a multiple regression model. Similar results are shown by the Italian study which demonstrated that LSM by VCTE alone outperformed both other NIT alone (i.e. APRI, FIB-4, FibroIndex and AST/ALT ratio) and in combination with VCTE in predicting advanced fibrosis; at multivariate logistic regression analysis, VCTE was the only independent variable associated with advance fibrosis (odds ratio = 1.389, 1.142–1.689, 95% CI).

Despite these two important studies, there remain critical unmet needs in this field. The first is to evaluate whether potential confounding factors such as cholestasis and inflammation can influence LSM values and increase the potential number of false positive. More importantly, considering the importance of fibrosis in the setting of risk stratification at diagnosis, there is a need of clinically relevant cut-offs able to correctly stage the disease at its onset in more homogeneous cohorts.

Our group tried to respond to these questions performing a diagnostic multicentre study (n = 126) in which we have enrolled patients at disease onset, naïve to therapy and with VCTE performance within 3 months from liver biopsy [19]. In our cohort, VCTE identified patients with advanced fibrosis with AUROC of 0.89; however, despite good sensitivity and specificity of a single cut-off approach identified at 7 kPa, NPV was 0.95 and PPV was only 0.62 with 19 patients falsely classified in advanced stage. Thus, we explored the use of a dual cut-off approach with a lower and a higher threshold to define areas of accurate prediction and a grey area where VCTE may not provide reliable prediction of advanced fibrosis. LSM cut-offs $\leq$6.5 kPa and >11.0 kPa enabled to exclude and confirm, respectively, advanced fibrosis (NPV = 0.94, PPV = 0.89, error rate = 5.6%). These values were externally validated in an independent cohort PBC patients (n = 91) with NPV = 0.93, PPV = 0.89 and error rate = 8.6%. Finally, we evaluated with a multivariable analysis role of potential confounding factors influencing the LSM lecture, and we found the only parameter affecting LSM was fibrosis stage, and no association was found with body mass index (BMI) and liver biochemistry.

A multicentre, international effort within the Globe study group to test longitudinal data of LSM and development of adverse outcome is ongoing.

7.3   Primary Sclerosing Cholangitis

Primary sclerosing cholangitis (PSC) is a chronic cholestatic autoimmune biliary disease characterised by a chronic inflammation of intra- and/or extra-hepatic bile ducts, leading to biliary strictures and eventually biliary cirrhosis. Usually, PSC progresses to end-stage liver disease within 10–20 years [20]. To date, no medical treatment has proven to effectively alter the course of disease. PSC patients are at greatly increased risk to develop hepatobiliary carcinoma, mainly cholangiocarcinoma, which is associated with a dismal prognosis [21]. However, for many patients, morbidity and mortality are mainly related to fibrosis progression to liver cirrhosis and its complications. The highly variable natural history of PSC, with possible intercurrent clinical events (e.g. cholangitis, biliary lithiasis) that could be dissociated from the severity of underlying liver disease with consequent fluctuant clinical symptoms and serum cholestasis marker, makes the prognostic assessment of these patients challenging. Indeed, reliable and solid prognostic tools able to estimate prognosis at individual level are still not available in PSC.

Limitations on the use of liver biopsy in PSC mainly relate to the patchy disease distribution [22], which increased the interest of developing disease-specific NITs.

To date, VCTE is the most explored and easy accessible tool for non-invasive fibrosis assessment in PSC (even if it is not recommended by the most recent guidelines [23, 24]). Although PSC mainly involves the large intra- and extra-hepatic bile ducts, advanced liver fibrosis impacts on adverse outcomes.

Corpechot et al. made an important effort to define the role of VCTE in PSC staging and predicting its outcomes. In a prospective, single-centre longitudinal study (n = 66), VCTE demonstrated to have a good accuracy in discriminating patients with advanced fibrosis ($\geq$F3 sec. Metavir) against liver histology with AUROC of 0.93, a sensitivity and specificity of 0.93 and 0.83, respectively, a PPV of 0.61 and

Table 7.2 Comparison of the most important studies on VCTE in PSC

	Histological staging system	n	Cut-off (kPa)	Se	Sp	PPV	NPV	LR+	LR−	AUROC
Corpechot et al. [3]	Metavir	66								
≥F1		60	7.4	0.60	0.86	0.97	0.20	4.28	0.46	0.71
≥F2		32	8.6	0.72	0.89	0.85	0.78	4.41	0.30	0.84
≥F3		15	9.6	0.93	0.83	0.61	0.98	13.14	0.08	0.93
=F4		9	14.4	1.00	0.88	0.56	1.00	82.13	0.01	0.95
Ehlken et al. [25]	Metavir	62								
≥F1		57	6.6	0.65	0.60	0.95	0.13	1.63	0.75	0.63
≥F2		27	8.8	0.82	0.89	0.85	0.86	7.45	0.08	0.91
≥F3		20	9.6	0.90	0.91	0.82	0.95	10.00	0.10	0.95
=F4		16	14.4	0.69	0.97	0.92	0.90	23.00	0.41	0.98

Se sensitivity, *Sp* specificity, *PPV* positive predictive value, *NPV* negative predictive value, *LR+* positive likelihood ratio, *AUROC* area under the receiver operating curves

NPV of 0.98 using a cut-off of 9.6 kPa (Table 7.2). Their results have been confirmed after removing patients with overlap with AIH and after internal validation based on 100 random replications, simulating 6600 virtual patients. Furthermore, they followed up the whole cohort ($n = 162$) for a median follow-up of 3.6 ± 18 years, and they demonstrated a tenfold increased risk of adverse events (i.e. death liver transplantation and hepatic complications) with a LSM at baseline > of 11.1 kPa (sensitivity 67%; specificity 81%; PPV, 38%; NPV, 93%; accuracy 79%) and LSM progression/year >1.5 kPa.

However, this study has some limitations. In fact, the small number of patients in the intermediate stage of fibrosis ($n = 23$ with stage F2–F3) and the low PPV (0.61) for the prediction of ≥F3 stage increase the probability to have false-negative patients. Furthermore, as pointed out by Ehlken et al., approximately 25% of patients with PSC have a high level of bilirubin at disease presentation, and the exclusion of patients with dominant stricture could have introduced a bias in the analysis [25]. Indeed, cholestasis is a known factor that can influence LSM value, and the interpretation of VCTE results should be done after excluding the presence of dominant stricture.

The French results have been confirmed by the German group ($n = 62$ with liver histology), which individuated the same cut-off of 9.6 kPa able to discriminate patients with advanced fibrosis with a specificity and sensitivity of 0.91 and 0.90, respectively, and a NPV and PPV of 0.95 and 0.82, respectively (AUROC 0.95) (Table 7.2). However, the small number of patients in the intermediate stage of fibrosis (F2/F3 = 13) reduces the power of the analysis.

Recently, Cazzagon et al. demonstrated that combined use of radiological score based on magnetic resonance cholangiopancreatography (MRCP) (Anali score which includes intrahepatic biliary duct dilatation, portal hypertension, hepatic dysmorphy and parenchymal enhancement heterogeneity when gadolinium is administered) and VCTE permits easy risk stratification in PSC. In a cohort of 162 patients followed for 753 patient/year, the optimal prognostic thresholds individuated by this study were 10.5 kPa for LS and 2 for the Anali score without Gd. Hazard ratios (95% confidence interval) were 2.07 (1.06–4.06) and 3.78 (1.67–8.59), respectively [26, 27]. The use in combination of these two thresholds allowed us to separate patients into low-, medium- and high-risk groups with 5-year cumulative rates of adverse outcome of 8%, 16% and 38%, respectively.

Finally, the application of Baveno VI criteria (LSM <20 kPa and PLT >150,000/mm^3) in patients with compensated cirrhosis and cholestatic liver disease (both PBC and PSC, $n = 227$) has been recently explored and seems to save 30–40% of esophagogastroduodenoscopies with a false-negative rate of 0% [28].

Magnetic resonance elastography (MRE) has been strongly correlated with histological stage at liver biopsy and seems accurate in detecting advanced fibrosis in patients with PSC [29]. M. Tafur et al. showed that MRE had a higher ability to quantify liver stiffness compared to VCTE, mainly due to its capability of assessing a broader liver area [30].

An important limitation of the above-mentioned studies is that analysis includes mainly patients with advanced disease, such as high grades of intrahepatic biliary stricture (Grades 3c and 4) or caudate hypertrophy. Moreover, not only both techniques can only give a semi-quantitative evaluation of bile duct strictures, but also biliary stricture severity addressed by MRCP is weakly correlated with LS values on MRE and does not correlate with LS on VCTE. This may limit their use in the future research on PSC.

Further studies in larger cohorts are needed to validate this result in order to determine clinically relevant cut-offs and rate of LSM progression over time to add to the poor arsenal of risk stratifiers in PSC a valid alternative.

7.4 Autoimmune Hepatitis

Autoimmune hepatitis (AIH) is an immune-mediated chronic liver disease characterised by the presence of interface hepatitis and portal plasma cell infiltration on histologic examination, elevated transaminase levels, circulating non-organ-specific autoantibodies and increased levels of immunoglobulin G [31]. An acute onset of disease is common, but most patients have a fluctuating course which led to progression to liver fibrosis and cirrhosis, HCC and end-stage liver disease [32].

AIH requires continuous treatment and care in most patients. Over 80% of patients have a good response to immunosuppressive therapy, which usually results in a good prognosis [33]. In 3% of AIH-treated patients, fibrosis progresses, either due to insufficient response, intolerance or non-adherence to therapy [34]. In fact, according to the American and European guidelines [35, 36], the assessment of liver fibrosis and cirrhosis is essential to guide treatment strategies in patients with AIH. Fibrosis progression may be present also in patients with normal values of transaminases but with persistent histological activity or in patients in which histological activity may lag biochemical remission by several months. This makes biochemical activity an imperfect biomarker to monitor the disease if considered alone.

In this setting, the use of non-invasive biomarkers of liver fibrosis may be helpful not only for disease staging but also for the monitoring of disease progression under treatment. Currently, although not generally recommended by current guidelines and the potential severe complications, many experts perform follow-up liver biopsies to assess inflammatory activity and disease progression.

VCTE is currently the only validated non-invasive method to estimate liver fibrosis in AIH with a reliable accuracy and reproducibility. One of the major limitations in the interpretation of LSM results in AIH is the presence of hepatic inflammation that has been demonstrated to be a potential confounding factor, leading to higher number of false-positive patients [37]. Therefore, LSM in AIH, particularly in the acute onset on in case of relapse, may be not reliable.

The most important evidences demonstrating the accuracy of VCTE in assessing fibrosis in AIH come from Hartl et al. [2]. In their first study, they examined a cohort of 34 patients with AIH comparing LSM with VCTE and liver histology and found the thresholds that best predicted fibrosis stages, defined as the highest sum of sensitivity plus specificity, were 5.8 kPa (F $\geq$ 2), 10.5 kPa (F $\geq$ 3) and 16.0 kPa (F $\geq$ 4). The accuracy was higher in diagnosing cirrhosis (sensitivity 0.83, specificity 1.0 with an AUROC of 0.92); however, for the discrimination of intermediate stage of fibrosis (severe, F3 and F4 vs. non-severe, F0–F2), the VCTE showed a worse performance with sensibility of 0.73 and specificity of 0.91 and an AUROC of 0.82. These results have been validated in an external cohort of 60 patients and showed a better performance in discriminating early from advanced fibrosis with the same cut-off of 10.5 kPa (AUROC 0.96, sensitivity 0.89, specificity 1.00). The reason of a better performance of the cut-offs in the validation cohort was probably due to the higher proportion of patients biopsied at first presentation of AIH and therefore a larger proportion of patients without (or with only a short period of) immunosuppression at the time of TE. In fact, assuming a role of inflammation in the LSM values, they put together both the cohorts ($n = 94$), and they divided the patients in three groups based on time from the induction with immunosuppression. In patients treated for more than 6 months, there was a weak correlation between LSM and inflammation, and the accuracy in assessing fibrosis was higher with respect to the group treated for less than 6 months (Table 7.3). Furthermore, they assessed that after this time interval, VCTE were reliable regardless of the achievement of biochemical remission. These results confirm the necessity, already reported in 2008 by Romanque et al. [37], to avoid performance of VCTE in an acute setting in AIH because inflammation could interfere with the fibrosis estimate with a greater number of false-positive patients.

The same group demonstrated the utility of VCTE in evaluating disease progression over time along with biochemical markers [1]. In patients with biochemical remission, LSM decrease progressively over time. On the other hand, in patients with active inflammation, despite normal LFTs, fibrosis may progress and LSM increase over time. These results highlight the importance of repeated VCTE measurements during follow-up that, associated with biochemical response, may help to assure the lack of disease progression.

Table 7.3 Comparison of the most important studies on VCTE in AIH

	Histological staging system	n	Cut-off (kPa)	Se	Sp	PPV	NPV	LR+	LR−	AUROC
Hartl et al. [2]	Metavir									
Whole cohort		92								
≥F2		52	5.8	0.90	0.72	0.83	0.84	3.2	0.14	0.87
≥F3		30	10.4	0.83	0.98	0.92	0.91	41.5	0.17	0.93
=F4		15	16.0	0.88	1.00	1.00	0.98	88.0	0.12	0.96
<3 months from induction		34								
≥F2			5.8	0.71	0.66	0.65	0.58	2.1	0.43	0.68
≥F3			10.4	0.60	0.88	0.75	0.85	5.0	0.45	0.80
=F4			16.0	0.60	0.93	0.60	0.93	8.6	0.04	0.71
6–12 months from induction		25								
≥F2			5.8	0.94	0.88	0.94	0.88	7.8	0.06	0.97
≥F3			10.4	1.00	1.00	1.00	1.00	99.0	0.001	1.00
=F4			16.0	1.00	1.00	1.00	1.00	99	0.001	1.00
>4 years from induction		27								
≥F2			5.8	1.00	0.77	0.80	0.88	4.3	0.01	0.94
≥F3			10.4	0.95	0.94	0.80	0.94	15.8	0.05	0.96
=F4			16.0	1.00	1.00	1.00	1.00	99.0	0.001	1.00
Xu et al. [38]	Metavir	100								
≥F2			6.45	0.82	0.86	0.97	0.49	6.6	0.13	0.88
≥F3			8.75	0.90	0.84	0.84	0.81	5.0	0.11	0.88
=F4			12.50	0.87	0.90	0.71	0.96	8.4	0.14	0.91

(continued)

Table 7.3 (continued)

	Histological staging system	n	Cut-off (kPa)	Se	Sp	PPV	NPV	LR+	LR−	AUROC
Anastasiou et al. [39]	Metavir	53								
≥F2			10.05	0.61	0.89	0.96	0.32	5.5	0.55	0.78
≥F3			12.10	0.59	0.83	0.81	0.62	3.5	0.49	0.74
=F4			19.00	0.82	0.93	0.76	0.95	11.7	0.19	0.84
Wu et al. [40]	Metavir									
≥F2		329	5.80–7.00	0.82	0.79			3.8	0.22	
		100	9.10–10.05	0.70	0.98			14.6	0.30	
≥F3		208	8.18–8.75	0.80	0.85			5.2	0.23	
		174	10.40–12.10	0.74	0.93			7.7	0.27	
=F4		268	11.00–12.67	0.88	0.99			7.4	0.12	
		147	16.00–19.00	0.86	0.97			21.7	0.14	

Se sensitivity, *Sp* specificity, *PPV* positive predictive value, *NPV* negative predictive value, *LR+* positive likelihood ratio, *AUROC* area under the receiver operating curves

Other studies have been conducted aiming at defining clinically relevant cut-offs in AIH, but the heterogeneity of cohorts (e.g. different time from immunosuppressive induction) and the small sample make the results less relevant (Table 7.3) [38, 39].

Recently, a systematic review on NITs of fibrosis in AIH has been published. All the studies, including those already reported here, had heterogeneous cohorts of patients with 39% of patients not treated, 26% under treatment and 35% after treatment [40]. Despite this, authors demonstrated good overall diagnostic performance of VCTE in patients with AIH for detecting significant ($\geq$F2), advanced fibrosis ($\geq$F3) and cirrhosis, by evaluating ten studies and an overall cohort of 329 patients. The cut-off points are represented in Table 7.3. On the contrary, performance of biochemical NITs (i.e. APRI and FIB-4) showed a poor performance in detection of advanced fibrosis and cirrhosis in AIH. To overcome the potential bias due to high levels of transaminase, they conducted a subgroup analysis by treatment status (patients not treated and patients after treatment) in which the good performance of VCTE was confirmed. However, data were limited, and further studies are needed to confirm these results in larger and more homogeneous cohorts of patients.

In this setting, a possible solution to avoid inflammation bias in assessing fibrosis is MRE that has been demonstrated to have a good performance in fibrosis assessment despite the presence of liver inflammation [41]. However, the small number of patients studied and the limited access to this tool may limit its use in daily clinical practice.

7.5 Conclusions

Assessing fibrosis is a key step in the prognosis and monitoring of patients with AILDs. We have now several non-invasive methods to assess disease stage, with VCTE by FibroScan being the most performant in all AILDs. Further studies are needed, for each of these conditions, to explore potential confounders to confirm VCTE reproducibility and validate the role of baseline staging and longitudinal monitoring.

References

1. Hartl J, Ehlken H, Sebode M, Peiseler M, Krech T, Zenouzi R, von Felden J, Weiler-Normann C, Schramm C, Lohse AW. Usefulness of biochemical remission and transient elastography in monitoring disease course in autoimmune hepatitis. J Hepatol. 2018;68:754–63.
2. Hartl J, Denzer U, Ehlken H, et al. Transient elastography in autoimmune hepatitis: timing determines the impact of inflammation and fibrosis. J Hepatol. 2016;65:769–75.
3. Corpechot C, Gaouar F, El Naggar A, Kemgang A, Wendum D, Poupon R, Carrat F, Chazouillères O. Baseline values and changes in liver stiffness measured by transient elastography are associated with severity of fibrosis and outcomes of patients with primary sclerosing cholangitis. Gastroenterology. 2014;146:970.
4. Corpechot C, Carrat F, Poujol-Robert A, Gaouar F, Wendum D, Chazouillères O, Poupon R. Noninvasive elastography-based assessment of liver fibrosis progression and prognosis in primary biliary cirrhosis. Hepatology. 2012;56:198–208.

5. Carey EJ, Ali AH, Lindor KD. Primary biliary cirrhosis. Lancet. 2015;386:1565–75.
6. Hirschfield GM, Beuers U, Corpechot C, Invernizzi P, Jones D, Marzioni M, Schramm C. EASL Clinical Practice Guidelines: the diagnosis and management of patients with primary biliary cholangitis. J Hepatol. 2017;67:145–72.
7. Corpechot C, Abenavoli L, Rabahi N, Chrétien Y, Andréani T, Johanet C, Chazouillères O, Poupon R. Biochemical response to ursodeoxycholic acid and long-term prognosis in primary biliary cirrhosis. Hepatology. 2008;48:871–7.
8. Floreani A, Caroli D, Variola A, Rizzotto ER, Antoniazzi S, Chiaramonte M, Cazzagon N, Brombin C, Salmaso L, Baldo V. A 35-year follow-up of a large cohort of patients with primary biliary cirrhosis seen at a single centre. Liver Int. 2011;31:361–8.
9. Murillo Perez CF, Hirschfield GM, Corpechot C, et al. Fibrosis stage is an independent predictor of outcome in primary biliary cholangitis despite biochemical treatment response. Aliment Pharmacol Ther. 2019;50:1127–36.
10. Carbone M, D'Amato D, Hirschfield GM, Jones DEJ, Mells GF. Letter: histology is relevant for risk stratification in primary biliary cholangitis. Aliment Pharmacol Ther. 2020;51:192–3.
11. Carbone M, Nardi A, Flack S, et al. Pretreatment prediction of response to ursodeoxycholic acid in primary biliary cholangitis: development and validation of the UDCA Response Score. Lancet Gastroenterol Hepatol. 2018;3:626–34.
12. Lindor KD, Bowlus CL, Boyer J, Levy C, Mayo M. Primary biliary cholangitis: 2018 practice guidance from the American Association for the Study of Liver Diseases. Hepatology. 2019;69:394–419.
13. Hirschfield GM, Dyson JK, Alexander GJM, et al. The British Society of Gastroenterology/UK-PBC primary biliary cholangitis treatment and management guidelines. Gut. 2018;67:1568–94.
14. Garrido MC, Hubscher SG. Accuracy of staging in primary biliary cirrhosis. J Clin Pathol. 1996;49:556–9.
15. Corpechot C. Utility of noninvasive markers of fibrosis in cholestatic liver diseases. Clin Liv Dis. 2016;20:143–58.
16. Patel K, Sebastiani G. Limitations of non-invasive tests for assessment of liver fibrosis. J Hepatol. 2020;2:100067.
17. Floreani A, Cazzagon N, Martines D, Cavalletto L, Baldo V, Chemello L. Performance and utility of transient elastography and noninvasive markers of liver fibrosis in primary biliary cirrhosis. Dig Liver Dis. 2011;43:887–92.
18. Gómez-Dominguez E, Mendoza J, García-Buey L, Trapero M, Gisbert JP, Jones EA, Moreno-Otero R. Transient elastography to assess hepatic fibrosis in primary biliary cirrhosis. Aliment Pharmacol Ther. 2008;27:441–7.
19. Cristoferi L, Nardi A, Viganò M, Rigamonti C, Degasperi E, Cardinale V, et al. Accuracy of liver stiffness measurement in assessing liver fibrosis in naive patients with primary biliary cholangitis. J Hepatol. 2020;73:s401–652.
20. Boonstra K, Beuers U, Ponsioen CY. Epidemiology of primary sclerosing cholangitis and primary biliary cirrhosis: a systematic review. J Hepatol. 2012;56:1181–8.
21. Bonato G, Cristoferi L, Strazzabosco M, Fabris L. Malignancies in primary sclerosing cholangitis--a continuing threat. Dig Dis. 2015;33:140–8.
22. De Vries E, Beuers U. Management of cholestatic disease in 2017. Liver Int. 2017;37:123–9.
23. Lindor KD, Kowdley KV, Harrison ME, American College of Gastroenterology. ACG Clinical Guideline: primary sclerosing cholangitis. Am J Gastroenterol. 2015;110:646–59.
24. Chapman MH, Thorburn D, Hirschfield GM, et al. British Society of Gastroenterology and UK-PSC guidelines for the diagnosis and management of primary sclerosing cholangitis. Gut. 2019;68:1356–78.
25. Ehlken H, Lohse AW, Schramm C. Transient elastography in primary sclerosing cholangitis - the value as a prognostic factor and limitations. Gastroenterology. 2014;147:542–3.
26. Lemoinne S, Cazzagon N, El Mouhadi S, et al. Simple magnetic resonance scores associate with outcomes of patients with primary sclerosing cholangitis. Clin Gastroenterol Hepatol. 2019;17:2785–2792.e3.

27. Cazzagon N, Lemoinne S, El Mouhadi S, et al. The complementary value of magnetic resonance imaging and vibration-controlled transient elastography for risk stratification in primary sclerosing cholangitis. Am J Gastroenterol. 2019;114:1878–85.
28. Moctezuma-Velazquez C, Saffioti F, Tasayco-Huaman S, et al. Non-invasive prediction of high-risk varices in patients with primary biliary cholangitis and primary sclerosing cholangitis. Am J Gastroenterol. 2019;114:446–52.
29. Eaton JE, Dzyubak B, Venkatesh SK, Smyrk TC, Gores GJ, Ehman RL, LaRusso NF, Gossard AA, Lazaridis KN. Performance of magnetic resonance elastography in primary sclerosing cholangitis. J Gastroenterol Hepatol. 2016;31:1184–90.
30. Tafur M, Cheung A, Menezes RJ, Feld J, Janssen H, Hirschfield GM, Jhaveri KS. Risk stratification in primary sclerosing cholangitis: comparison of biliary stricture severity on MRCP versus liver stiffness by MR elastography and vibration-controlled transient elastography. Eur Radiol. 2020;30:3735–47.
31. Manns MP, Lohse AW, Vergani D. Autoimmune hepatitis - update 2015. J Hepatol. 2015;62:S100–11.
32. Lohse AW, Mieli-Vergani G. Autoimmune hepatitis. J Hepatol. 2011;55:171–82.
33. Czaja AJ. Rapidity of treatment response and outcome in type 1 autoimmune hepatitis. J Hepatol. 2009;51:161–7.
34. Dhaliwal HK, Hoeroldt BS, Dube AK, Mcfarlane E, Underwood JCE, Karajeh MA, Gleeson D. Long-term prognostic significance of persisting histological activity despite biochemical remission in autoimmune hepatitis. Am J Gastroenterol. 2015;110:993–9.
35. European Association for the Study of the Liver. EASL Clinical Practice Guidelines: autoimmune hepatitis. J Hepatol. 2015;63:971–1004.
36. Manns MP, Czaja AJ, Gorham JD, Krawitt EL, Mieli-Vergani G, Vergani D, Vierling JM. AASLD Practise Guidelines. Diagnosis and management of autoimmune hepatitis. Hepatology. 2010;51:2193.
37. Romanque P, Stickel F, Dufour JF. Disproportionally high results of transient elastography in patients with autoimmune hepatitis. Liver Int. 2008;28:1177–8.
38. Xu Q, Sheng L, Bao H, Chen X, Guo C, Li H, Ma X, Qiu D, Hua J. Evaluation of transient elastography in assessing liver fibrosis in patients with autoimmune hepatitis. J Gastroenterol Hepatol. 2017;32:639–44.
39. Anastasiou OE, Büchter M, Baba HA, Korth J, Canbay A, Gerken G, Kahraman A. Performance and utility of transient elastography and non-invasive markers of liver fibrosis in patients with autoimmune hepatitis: a single centre experience. Hepat Mon. 2016;16:40737.
40. Wu S, Yang Z, Zhou J, Zeng N, He Z, Zhan S, Jia J, You H. Systematic review: diagnostic accuracy of non-invasive tests for staging liver fibrosis in autoimmune hepatitis. Hepatol Int. 2019;13:91–101.
41. Wang J, Malik N, Yin M, Smyrk TC, Czaja AJ, Ehman RL, Venkatesh SK. Magnetic resonance elastography is accurate in detecting advanced fibrosis in autoimmune hepatitis. World J Gastroenterol. 2017;23:859–68.

Transient Elastography for the Diagnosis of Liver Fibrosis and Cirrhosis in People with Alcohol-Associated Liver Disease

8

Taisiia Turankova, Giovanni Casazza, and Chavdar S. Pavlov

8.1   Introduction

The use of alcohol resulted in about three million deaths (5.3% of all deaths) worldwide and 132.6 million disability-adjusted life years (DALYs)—i.e., 5.1% of all DALYs in 2016 [1]. Alcohol-associated liver disease (ALD) is a public health concern, being the cause of half of all cirrhosis-related deaths (Fig. 8.1) [1].

ALD represents a spectrum of liver injury attributed to alcohol abuse. Liver injury ranges from hepatic steatosis to more advanced forms which include alcoholic hepatitis, alcohol-associated fibrosis, alcohol-associated cirrhosis, and liver cancer [2, 3].

In chronic liver disease of different etiologies, fibrosis progression is a result of an imbalanced deposition of extracellular matrix and degradation. Repeated tissue injury represents the wound healing response to liver damaging factors, such as viruses, fat, alcohol, etc. Fibrosis stage is one of the most important prognostic factors in ALD. The progression of fibrosis depends on the alcohol consumption and leads to the destruction of the lobular architecture, i.e., cirrhosis. Early detection of cirrhosis and abstinence in people with ALD minimize the risk of complications and improve prognosis [4].

Liver biopsy is considered the reference standard for the assessment of hepatic fibrosis stage. It can be obtained by percutaneous needle techniques, transjugular method, ultrasound-guided fine-needle, or surgical specimens [5]. The usefulness of obtaining liver biopsy specimen would usually depend on the liver biopsy technique and the physician's experience and skills. However, liver biopsy is invasive, has

T. Turankova · C. S. Pavlov (✉)
Department of Therapy, I.M. Sechenov First Moscow State Medical University, Moscow, Russian Federation

G. Casazza
Dipartimento di Scienze Biomediche e Cliniche "L. Sacco", Università degli Studi di Milano, Milan, Italy

© Springer Nature Switzerland AG 2021
M. Fraquelli (ed.), *Elastography of the Liver and Beyond*,
https://doi.org/10.1007/978-3-030-74132-7_8

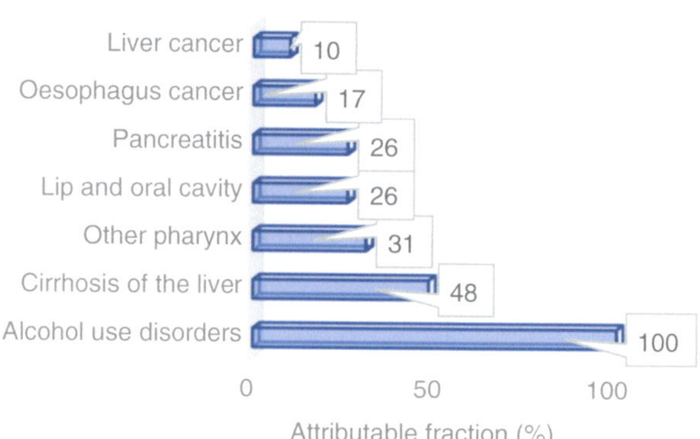

Fig. 8.1 Alcohol-attributable fractions for selected causes of death, disease type, and injury, 2016. (Adapted from [2])

drawbacks such as sampling error, and it is not completely free of risks and complications [6].

Several noninvasive tests (i.e., transient elastography, other ultrasound-based elastography techniques, or magnetic resonance elastography) for assessing the stage of liver fibrosis in people with ALD have been proposed as alternatives to the liver biopsy, but none has been sufficiently validated yet [7].

The 2018 EASL guideline recognizes liver biopsy as the most precise diagnostic method for staging liver fibrosis. However, there are no recommendations on what noninvasive methods should be used in the routine clinical practice for screening and defining liver fibrosis in people with ALD [8].

8.2   Liver Fibrosis and Staging Assessment

Fibrosis is defined by a detrimental process in progressive chronic liver disease. Many of the chronic liver diseases are asymptomatic, presenting with almost normal laboratory tests, and progress slowly to cirrhosis over the years, making the diagnosis of liver fibrosis difficult in routine clinical practice. Hagström et al. have identified an increased risk of development of severe liver disease in dose-response pattern (adjusted risk ratio (RR) for each gram/day increase of 1.02; 95% CI 1.01–1.02) associated with alcohol consumption [9]. Daily drinking, regardless of the alcohol amount consumed, appears to increase the risk of alcoholic cirrhosis, at least in men. The risk factor for developing alcoholic cirrhosis remains high, no matter at what age people start their alcohol consumption [10].

Alcohol liver injury is caused by ethanol metabolites (i.e., acetaldehyde and acetate) which increase redox state, steatosis, production of reactive oxygen species, and lipid peroxidation. These in turn cause production of proteins that alter normal liver functions, induce cell death, and/or liver inflammation. In addition, in ALD, lipopolysaccharide derived from a breakdown in the intestinal wall determines liver

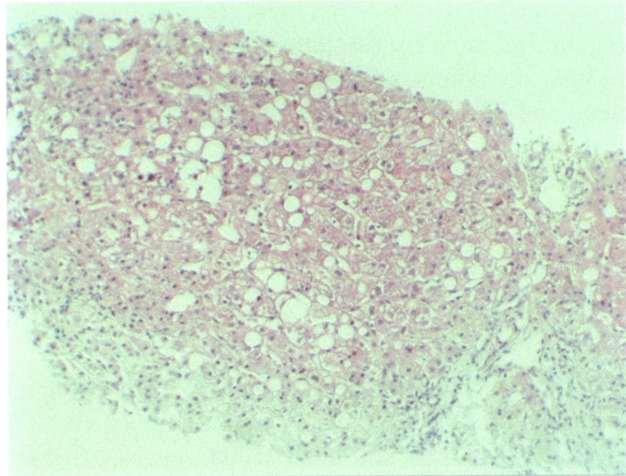

Fig. 8.2 Histopathologic image showing the morphology of alcohol-related liver disease

injury and fibrosis as a result of the induction of oxidative stress, the cytokine release, and subsequent infiltration of immune cells [11].

Cigarette smoking, obesity, sex, and the additional presence of chronic hepatitis B or hepatitis C virus infection are other factors which may also influence the risk of progression to cirrhosis [12].

With the advance of chronic liver disease, excessive deposition of Type I and III collagens is found not only in portal tracts, but also in the lobule, creating both fibrous septa and severe alterations to sinusoidal ultrastructure [13, 14].

Liver biopsy detects and measures liver fibrosis, and the amount of fibrosis measured defines the stages of liver fibrosis. Assessment is performed during a morphological investigation of a liver tissue, using semiqualitative scores defined with several variables. The most widely used scoring systems for assessment of fibrosis are the Knodell Histology Activity Index (HAI) [15], the Scheuer HAI [16], the Ishak HAI [17], and the Metavir scoring system [5]. According to these scoring systems, the histological changes characterizing the stages of fibrosis are defined as stage 0—no fibrosis; stage 1—perisinusoidal fibrosis; stage 2—perisinusoidal fibrosis with periportal fibrosis; stage 3—bridging fibrosis; and stage 4—fully developed cirrhosis. Cirrhosis is defined as hepatic bridging fibrosis and nodular regeneration (Fig. 8.2). At this stage of ALD, a successful treatment and abstinence from alcohol usually would result in improvement of parenchymal architecture and regression of fibrosis [8].

8.3 Noninvasive Laboratory Tests and Machine-Based Techniques for Assessment of Hepatic Fibrosis

Good alternatives to liver biopsy for assessment of fibrosis in people with ALD are some noninvasive technologies based on laboratory tests or imaging, or elastographic techniques.

Unlike the liver biopsy procedure, these tools are less operator-dependent and require less time for reaching the diagnosis. Some laboratory tests are FibroTest (α2-macroglobulin, apolipoprotein A1, haptoglobin, gamma glutamyl transpeptidase, and total bilirubin), aspartate transaminase-platelet ratio index (APRI), and FIB-4 (platelets, aspartate transaminase, alanine aminotransferase, and age), Hepa-Score (α2-macroglobulin, hyaluronic acid, and gamma glutamyl transpeptidase), ELF (hyaluronic acid, tissue inhibitor of metalloproteinase-1, and procollagen 3 peptide N-terminal), and FibroMeter (platelets, hyaluronic acid or gamma glutamyl transpeptidase, prothrombin index, aspartate transaminase, and α2-macroglobulin). All of these tests consist of combinations of various variables (validated and non-validated) [18].

Ultrasound (US) is the first noninvasive imaging method for diagnosis of focal lesions in the liver. However, although inexpensive, its accuracy in the diagnosis of alcoholic fibrosis is still unclear due to the lack of studies with liver biopsy as a comparator [19, 20]. Liver size, bluntness of the liver edge, coarseness of the liver parenchyma, nodularity of the liver surface, size of the lymph nodes around the hepatic artery, irregularity and narrowness of the inferior vena cava, portal vein velocity, and spleen size are among the ultrasound parameters for assessing fibrosis and cirrhosis in people with ALD. As liver fibrosis reduces tissue elasticity, measurement of liver stiffness is an attractive surrogate for severity of fibrosis. In addition to ultrasound and ultrasound-based liver elastography, there are other alternative approaches for fibrosis assessment such as Fibroscan (Echosens, Paris, France [21]); acoustic radiation force impulse imaging (ARFI; Siemens) [22]; shear wave elastography (SWE; Supersonic Imaging) [23], and magnetic resonance elastography (MRE) [24]. The diagnostic test accuracy of these techniques is presented in Table 8.1.

The use of noninvasive tests could be tailored to first tier screening of people at risk in order to diagnose early the people with progressive liver disease and offer targeted interventions for the prevention of decompensation [8]. Estimate of liver fibrosis progression in a person is considered an important surrogate end point that may facilitate treatment decisions by clarifying the vulnerability of an individual at risk of progression to cirrhosis [8].

8.4 Transient Elastography for Fibrosis Assessment in ALD

Fibroscan is the most studied and used technique among hepatologists and gastro-enterologists. In people with ALD, liver stiffness correlates with the degree of fibrosis and is measured in kPa by transient elastography [32–34]. This noninvasive method, used in portable devices, makes it possible to test large groups of people and improve the quality of screening.

During the transient elastography procedure, measurements are performed in the right lobe of the liver through intercostal spaces on fasting patients lying in dorsal decubitus with the right arm in maximal abduction.

Table 8.1 Study performance of machine-based techniques for the diagnosis of fibrosis and cirrhosis in patients with biopsy-proven ALD

Study	LSM type	Participants (n)	Cirrhotics (%)	Fibrosis stage	Cutoff value	Sensitivity	Specificity	LR+	LR−	AUROC (95% CI)
Nguyen-Khac et al. (2008) [25]	TE	103	32	F ≥ 2	7.8 kPa	0.8	0.9	8.00	0.22	0.91
				F ≥ 3	11 kPa	0.86	0.8	4.30	0.18	0.90
				F = 4	15.5 kPa	0.85	0.84	5.31	0.18	0.92
Nahon et al. (2008) [26]	TE	147	53.7	F ≥ 3	11.6 kPa	0.87	0.89	7.91	0.15	0.4
				F = 4	22.7 kPa	0.84	0.83	4.94	0.19	0.87
Thiele et al. (2015) [27]	SWE	199	18.1	F ≥ 3	10.2 kPa	0.82	0.93	11.7	0.19	0.94
				F = 4	16.4 kPa	0.94	0.91	10.4	0.07	0.95
Zhang et al. (2015) [28]	ARFI	99	9.09	F ≥ 2	1.27 m/s	0.77	0.85	5.13	0.27	0.84
				F ≥ 3	1.40 m/s	0.84	0.82	4.67	0.20	0.87
				F = 4	1.65 m/s	0.89	0.84	5.56	0.13	0.89
Kiani et al. (2016) [29]	ARFI	82	15.85	F ≥ 2	1.63 m/s	0.82	0.83	4.82	0.22	0.87
				F ≥ 3	1.84 m/s	0.82	0.78	3.73	0.23	0.86
				F = 4	1.94 m/s	0.92	0.81	4.84	0.10	0.89
Bensamoun et al. (2013) [30]	MRE	90	14.44	F ≥ 2	2.57 kPa	0.78	0.78	3.55	0.28	0.85
				F ≥ 3	3.31 kPa	0.96	0.95	19.2	0.04	0.97
				F = 4	4.00 kPa	1	0.92	12.5	0.00	0.98
Singh et al. (2015) [31]	MRE	697 (21 ALD)	N/A	F ≥ 2	3.66 kPa	0.7	0.77	3.04	0.39	0.81
				F ≥ 3	4.11 kPa	0.92	0.81	4.84	0.10	0.93

LSM liver stiffness measurement, *LR* likelihood ratio, *AUROC* area under the receiver operating characteristics, *TE* transient elastography, *SWE* shear wave elastography, *ARFI* acoustic radiation force impulse imaging, *MRE* magnetic resonance elastography

Liver stiffness values in the general population are influenced independently by sex, body mass index, and metabolic syndrome, mean of 'normal' liver stiffness values which lie between 3.3 and 7.0 kPa, using the 5th and 95th percentiles [35, 36].

Detection of fibrosis F0 or F1 is of no clinical relevance as these initial hepatic fibrosis stages do not influence prognosis, and if the individual abstains from alcohol consumption, the fibrosis will reverse [37].

Results of liver stiffness measurements by transient elastography were compared with histological staging of hepatic fibrosis by liver biopsy in publications. The cutoff values, proposed by study authors, for diagnosis of the stages of fibrosis in people with ALD varied. For example, the study by Nguyen-Khac et al., with 103 patients analyzed, showed that liver stiffness was correlated with fibrosis ($r = 0.72$, $p < 0.014$) [median for F1 at 6.3 kPa, area under the ROC (receiver operating characteristics) curve (AUROC) 0.84 (95% CI 0.73–0.95); F2 at 8.4 kPa, AUROC 0.91 (95% CI 0.85–0.98); F3 at 15 kPa, AUROC 0.91 (95% CI 0.82–0.97); and F4 at 47.3 kPa, 0.92 AUROC 0.91 (95% CI 0.87–0.98)] [25]. The study by Foucher et al. reported similar results in 711 patients, among whom 12.5% were with ALD [38]. With a cutoff value of 17.6 kPa, the negative predictive value for the diagnosis of cirrhosis was 92% and the positive predictive value was 91% [39].

The study by Cassinotto et al. analyzing a cohort of 145 patients with alcoholic disorders showed liver stiffness median of 7.9 kPa for F1 [AUROC 0.84 (95% CI: 0.77–0.89)]; of 9.93 kPa for F2 [AUROC 0.83 (95% CI: 0.78–0.87)]; of 11.3 kPa for F3 [AUROC 0.86 (95% CI: 0.81–0.89)]; and of 26.2 kPa for F4 [AUROC 0.90 (95% CI: 0.86–0.93)] [39].

A study by Mueller et al., conducted in 50 people with ALD, showed that the activity of glutamic oxaloacetic transaminase (aspartate transaminase) reduced to <100 u/mL significantly improved the diagnostic accuracy of transient elastography in the diagnosis of cirrhosis. The activity of steatohepatitis increased liver stiffness in the patients, regardless of the stage of fibrosis [40]. A later study by Mueller showed that the inflammation-adapted liver stiffness cutoff values, calculated for ALD, improved the diagnostic accuracy and the agreement with histological fibrosis stages (See adapted Table 8.2) [41].

The study by Bardou-Jacquet et al. showed that transient elastography decreased significantly after alcohol cessation over a long period of follow-up (median follow-up of 32.5 weeks) in 85% of abstinent patients [median (range): −4.9 (−6.1 to −1.9)], leading to a modification of the putative fibrosis stage in 28–71% of patients according to different cutoff values [42].

Table 8.2 Cutoff values and AUROCs in patients with and without elevated aspartate aminotransferase (AST) levels both for ALD. Table with adapted results from [41]

Fibrosis stage	F0 vs. F1/2		F1/2 vs. F3		F3 vs. F4	
	Cutoff (kPa)	AUROC	Cutoff (kPa)	AUROC	Cutoff (kPa)	AUROC
All	6.1	0.744	8.1	0.684	17.1	0.864
AST <40 U/L	4.9	0.700	6.8	0.705	10.5	0.868
AST >40 U/L	6.1	0.713	8.1	0.673	16.9	0.873

To use transient elastography in clinical practice, the cutoff values need to be confirmed both in people who continue to abuse alcohol and in abstinent people. In 2015, a Cochrane systematic review meta-analyzed available data from 14 studies with 834 patients diagnosed with ALD (Table 8.3) [37].

Although the cutoff values for stiffness varied among the studies and were not defined a priori, the most commonly used cutoff value for the detection of advanced fibrosis (F3 or worse) was 9.5 and 12.5 kPa for cirrhosis (Table 8.4) [37].

The Forest plot (Fig. 8.3) summarizes diagnostic accuracy main results in terms of sensitivity and specificity for the diagnosis of liver cirrhosis.

Table 8.3 Studies included in the review [37]

Study	Year	Country	No of included patients with ALD/n of enrolled patients	Study design	Time interval between TE and LB
Anastasiou et al. (2010) [43]	n/a	Greece	14/65	Prospective cohort study	3 days
Boursier et al. (2009) [44]	From September 2003 to June 2007	France, Morocco	106/390	Prospective cohort study	1 week
Carl et al. (2012) [45]	From 1 May 2008 to 31 July 2011	UK	4/266	Retrospective cohort study	n/a
de Ledinghen et al. (2012) [46]	From September 2009 to March 2011	France, China	34/286	Prospective cohort study	Within 1 week
Dolman et al. (2013) [47]	From 2008 to 2011	Netherlands, UK	20/130	Retrospective study using data from a consecutive cohort of participants	2 months
Kim et al. (2009) [48]	n/a	Korea	45/45	Prospective cohort study	With the interval of 11.2 ± 22 days (0 to about 92 days)
Lannerstedt et al. (2013) [49]	From 2007 to 2010	Norway	16/418	Retrospective cohort study	8 participants had TE at <2 months, and 8 had TE at >1.9–8.6 years

(continued)

Table 8.3 (continued)

Study	Year	Country	No of included patients with ALD/*n* of enrolled patients	Study design	Time interval between TE and LB
Nguyen-Khac et al. (2008) [25]	From April 2005 to January 2007	France	103/160	Prospective cohort study	TE and LB performed on the same day
Fernandez et al. (2012) [50]	n/a	Belgium	139	Retrospective cohort study	Within 6 months
Mueller et al. (2010) [41]	From June 2007 to March 2009	Germany	101/101	Prospective cohort study	A mean observation interval of 5.3 days. Range 3–10 days.
Lemoine et al. (2008) [51]	From January 2004 to September 2006	France	48/92	Prospective cohort study	TE and LB were performed on the same day
Janssens et al. (2010) [52]	From January 2006 to February 2008	Belgium	49/255	Prospective cohort study	1 week
Nahon et al. (2008) [26]	From November 2005 to November 2006	France	147/174	Prospective cohort study	TE and LB performed on the same day
Bardou-Jacquet et al. (2013) [42]	From June 2005 to November 2010	France	8/572 participants with ALD had liver biopsy during follow-up	Retrospective cohort study	2 LB within 4 weeks, and 6 LB within the median of follow-up 32.5 weeks (15–85 weeks)

TE transient elastography, *LB* liver biopsy, *ALD* alcohol liver disease, *UK* United Kingdom of Great Britain and Northern Ireland

Only 3 of the 14 studies were judged to be at low risk of bias. No serious concerns regarding the applicability of the studies in answering the main study question of the review were identified, i.e., the diagnostic test accuracy of transient elastography compared with liver biopsy. Due to the small number of studies reporting data on common cutoff values, the optimal cutoff values for the fibrosis stages could not be identified. However, transient elastography seems to be a good diagnostic method

Table 8.4 The results of the Cochrane systematic review [37]

Fibrosis stage	No. of studies	No. of participants	Cutoff value, kPa	Summary sensitivity	Summary specificity	LR−	LR+
F2	8	342	7.5	0.94 (95% CI 0.86–0.97)	0.89 (95% CI 0.76–0.95)	0.07	8.2
F3	8	564	9.5	0.92 (95% CI 0.89–0.96)	0.70 (95% CI 0.61–0.79)	0.11	3.1
F4	7	330	12.5	0.95 (95% CI 0.87–0.98)	0.71 (95% CI 0.56–0.82)	0.07	3.3

Study	TP	FP	FN	TN	Cut-off for >=F2	Sensitivity (95% CI)	Specificity (95% CI)
Boursier 2009	94	1	5	6	7.0	0.95 [0.89, 0.98]	0.86 [0.42, 1.00]
Lannerstedt 2013	14	0	0	2	7.0	1.00 [0.77, 1.00]	1.00 [0.16, 1.00]
anastasiou 2010	3	2	1	8	7.15	0.75 [0.19, 0.99]	0.80 [0.44, 0.97]
de Ledinghen 2013	32	0	1	1	7.2	0.97 [0.84, 1.00]	1.00 [0.03, 1.00]
Kim 2009	39	0	1	5	7.5	0.97 [0.87, 1.00]	1.00 [0.48, 1.00]
Dolman 2013	7	2	1	10	7.65	0.88 [0.47, 1.00]	0.83 [0.52, 0.98]
Nguyen-Khac 2008	62	2	15	24	7.8	0.81 [0.70, 0.89]	0.92 [0.75, 0.99]
Thiele 2015	69	10	14	105	9.6	0.83 [0.73, 0.90]	0.91 [0.85, 0.96]
Carl 2012	3	0	0	1	13.5	1.00 [0.29, 1.00]	1.00 [0.03, 1.00]

Study	TP	FP	FN	TN	Cut-off for >=F3	Sensitivity (95% CI)	Specificity (95% CI)
Mueller 2010	41	14	4	42	8.0	0.91 [0.79, 0.98]	0.75 [0.62, 0.86]
Boursier 2009	77	7	12	10	9.5	0.87 [0.78, 0.93]	1.59 [0.33, 0.82]
Kim 2009	35	2	1	7	9.5	0.97 [0.85, 1.00]	0.78 [0.40, 0.97]
Dolman 2013	4	4	1	11	9.5	0.80 [0.28, 0.99]	0.73 [0.45, 0.92]
Lannersted 2013	13	1	0	2	9.5	1.00 [0.75, 1.00]	0.67 [0.09, 0.99]
Femandez 2012	67	21	7	44	10.5	0.91 [0.81, 0.96]	0.68 [0.55, 0.79]
Nguyen-Khac 2008	46	10	7	40	11.0	0.87 [0.75, 0.95]	0.80 [0.66, 0.90]
Nahon 2008	96	4	14	33	11.6	0.87 [0.80, 0.93]	0.89 [0.75, 0.97]
de Ledinghen 2013	26	1	4	3	9.5	0.87 [0.69, 0.96]	0.75 [0.19, 0.99]
janssens 2010	23	4	9	13	17.0	0.72 [0.53, 0.86]	0.78 [0.50, 0.93]

Study	TP	FP	FN	TN	Cut-off for >=F4	Sensitivity (95% CI)	Specificity (95% CI)
Anastasiou 2010	3	2	1	8	7.15	0.75 [0.19, 0.99]	0.80 [0.44, 0.97]
Boutsier 2009	62	10	7	27	12.5	0.90 [0.80, 0.96]	0.73 [0.56, 0.86]
Kim 2009	29	8	0	8	12.5	1.00 [0.88, 1.00]	0.50 [0.25, 0.75]
Mueller 2010	25	15	1	60	12.5	0.96 [0.80, 1.00]	0.80 [0.69, 0.88]
Bardou-Jacquet 2013	5	2	0	1	12.5	1.00 [0.48, 1.00]	0.33 [0.01, 0.91]
de Ledinghen 2013	25	2	2	5	12.5	0.93 [0.76, 0.99]	0.71 [0.29, 0.96]
Dolman 2013	3	1	0	16	12.5	1.00 [0.29, 1.00]	0.94 [0.71, 1.00]
Lannerstedt 2013	8	4	0	4	12.5	1.00 [0.63, 1.00]	0.50 [0.16, 0.84]
Carl 2012	1	1	0	2	15.1	1.00 [0.03, 1.00]	0.67 [0.09, 0.99]
Femandez 2012	51	11	6	71	15.7	0.89 [0.78, 0.96]	0.87 [0.77, 0.93]
Nguyen-Khac 2008	28	11	5	59	19.5	0.85 [0.68, 0.95]	0.84 [0.74, 0.92]
Janssens 2010	16	7	4	22	19.6	0.80 [0.56, 0.94]	0.76 [0.56, 0.90]
Thiele 2015	35	16	1	147	19.7	0.97 [0.85, 1.00]	0.90 [0.85, 0.94]
Nahon 2008	66	12	13	56	22.7	0.84 [0.74, 0.91]	0.82 [0.71, 0.91]
Lemoine 2008	36	1	4	7	34.9	0.90 [0.76, 0.97]	0.88 [0.47, 1.00]

Fig. 8.3 Forest plot SR 2015

to rule out liver cirrhosis (F4) in people with alcoholic liver disease. Transient elastography may also help in ruling out severe fibrosis (F3 or worse). Liver biopsy investigation remains an option if the certainty to rule in or rule out the stage of hepatic fibrosis or cirrhosis remains insufficient after a clinical follow-up or any other noninvasive test considered useful by the clinician.

In a 2018 individual patient data meta-analysis with 1026 patients, Nguyen-Khac et al. showed liver stiffness cutoff values of 7.0 kPa [AUROC 0.83 (95% CI 0.79–0.87) for F ≥ 1 fibrosis], of 9.0 kPa [AUROC 0.86 (95% CI 0.82–0.90) for F ≥ 2], of 12.1 kPa [AUROC 0.90 (95% CI 0.86–0.94) for F ≥ 3], and of 18.6 kPa [AUROC 0.91 (95% CI 0.83–0.99) for F = 4] [53]. The study concludes that liver stiffness cutoff values are influenced by the increased AST concentrations, bilirubin concentrations, or both.

8.5   Discussion

Fibrosis stage is one of the most important prognostic factors in alcohol-associated liver disease and useful for patient stratification. Early staging of hepatic fibrosis in people with alcoholic liver diseases could motivate patients and physicians in finding an optimal strategy for achieving abstinence.

There are several factors that can influence the results of noninvasive methods of liver fibrosis evaluation. It is important to remember that liver stiffness can arise not only from fibrosis, but from edema or inflammation.

Thus, interpretation of the results in a proper clinical context is essential; for example, acute hepatitis can yield stiffness values comparable to cirrhosis, or the applicability of a test in obese people can be a problem. Improvement of current and new technologies may avoid the influence of systematic bias on the diagnostic accuracy assessments.

The currently cutoff values proposed by Pavlov et al. [37] for the different stages of hepatic fibrosis by transient elastography may be used in clinical practice, but caution is needed because the reported values are only the most common cutoff values used by the study authors.

The major issue is that there are only few studies properly designed to assess TE in people with ALD. Most of the studies enrolled people with a mixed etiology of the liver disease, and people with ALD are only a small proportion of the overall number of included patients. This might be a potential source of bias. Moreover, there are no studies that are properly designed in order to find and validate the optimal cutoff value in people with alcoholic liver disease. To correctly diagnose the stage of hepatic fibrosis in people with alcoholic liver disease using transient elastography assessment, prospective studies should consider a single aetiology as the best cutoff values for hepatic fibrosis in people with alcoholic liver disease remain to be validated.

Hepatic fibrosis should be diagnosed with both transient elastography and liver biopsy, and in this sequence. Transient elastography cutoff values should be pre-specified and validated. The time interval between the two investigations should not exceed 3 months, which is the interval, mainly required for people without cirrhosis. Assessment of results should be properly blinded. Only studies with low risk of bias, fulfilling the Standards for Reporting of Diagnostic Accuracy may answer the review question.

8.6   Conclusion

In ALD patients, when chronic liver disease is suspected, liver biopsy remains the reference standard for the diagnosing and staging of liver fibrosis. However, it is an invasive procedure with risk of adverse events. There is a great need for reliable high-quality comparative studies in people with alcohol-associated liver disease and the use of noninvasive imaging techniques that can correctly assess the stage of liver fibrosis. Most of the data available in the literature are derived from studies in which people with ALD are only a minority among the studied population. However, even with these methodological limitations, regarding the identification of advanced fibrosis, transient elastography seems to be one of the most accurate and validated modalities so far. Thus, liver stiffness measurement by transient elastography is an appropriate for first-line investigation in primary care since it has been shown to be cost-effective, and it is well-suited for second-line investigation in referral centers in order to select patients who might require liver biopsy or need follow-up in the liver clinic [54]. The cutoff values and the required parameters to diagnose liver fibrosis by transient elastography in ALD patients should also be further validated.

Acknowledgment *Authorship*: All authors approved the final version of the manuscript.
Declaration of Personal Interests: TT: none known; GC: none known; CS Pavlov: none known.

References

1. World Health Organization, Management of Substance Abuse Team. Global status report on alcohol and health 2018. Geneva: WHO; 2018.
2. Asrani SK, Devarbhavi H, Eaton J, Kamath PS. Burden of liver diseases in the world. J Hepatol. 2019;70:151–71. https://doi.org/10.1016/j.jhep.2018.09.014.
3. Crabb DW, Im GY, Szabo G, Mellinger JL, Lucey MR. Diagnosis and treatment of alcohol-associated liver diseases: 2019 practice guidance from the American Association for the Study of Liver Diseases. Hepatology. 2020;71:306–33. https://doi.org/10.1002/hep.30866.
4. Lackner C, Tiniakos D. Fibrosis and alcohol-related liver disease. J Hepatol. 2019;70:294–304. https://doi.org/10.1016/j.jhep.2018.12.003.
5. Bedossa P, Poynard T. An algorithm for the grading of activity in chronic hepatitis C. The METAVIR Cooperative Study Group. Hepatology. 1996;24:289–93. https://doi.org/10.1002/hep.510240201.
6. Seeff LB, Everson GT, Morgan TR, Curto TM, Lee WM, Ghany MG, et al. Complication rate of percutaneous liver biopsies among persons with advanced chronic liver disease in the HALT-C trial. Clin Gastroenterol Hepatol. 2010;8:877–83. https://doi.org/10.1016/j.cgh.2010.03.025.
7. Poynard T, Munteanu M, Deckmyn O, Ngo Y, Drane F, Castille JM, et al. Validation of liver fibrosis biomarker (FibroTest) for assessing liver fibrosis progression: proof of concept and first application in a large population. J Hepatol. 2012;57:541–8. https://doi.org/10.1016/j.jhep.2012.04.025.
8. Thursz M, Gual A, Lackner C, Mathurin P, Moreno C, Spahr L, et al. EASL Clinical Practice Guidelines: management of alcohol-related liver disease. J Hepatol. 2018;69:154–81. https://doi.org/10.1016/j.jhep.2018.03.018.
9. Hagström H, Hemmingsson T, Discacciati A, Andreasson A. Alcohol consumption in late adolescence is associated with an increased risk of severe liver disease later in life. J Hepatol. 2018;68:505–10. https://doi.org/10.1016/j.jhep.2017.11.019.
10. Askgaard G, Grønbæk M, Kjær MS, Tjønneland A, Tolstrup JS. Alcohol drinking pattern and risk of alcoholic liver cirrhosis: a prospective cohort study. J Hepatol. 2015;62:1061–7. https://doi.org/10.1016/j.jhep.2014.12.005.
11. Schaffert CS, Duryee MJ, Hunter CD, Hamilton BC III, DeVeney AL, Huerter MM, et al. Alcohol metabolites and lipopolysaccharide: roles in the development and/or progression of alcoholic liver disease. World J Gastroenterol. 2009;15:1209–18. https://doi.org/10.3748/wjg.15.1209.

12. Schwartz JM, Reinus JF. Prevalence and natural history of alcoholic liver disease. Clini Liv Dis. 2012;16:659–66. https://doi.org/10.1016/j.cld.2012.08.001.
13. Gressner AM. Hepatic fibrogenesis: the puzzle of interacting cells, fibrogenic cytokines, regulatory loops, and extracellular matrix molecules. Z Gastroenterol. 1992;30(Suppl 1):5–16.
14. Crawford JM, Bioulac-Sage P, Hytiroglou P. Structure, function, and, responses to injury. In: MacSween's pathology of the liver. 7th ed. Amsterdam: Elsevier; 2018. https://www.elsevier.com/books/macsweens-pathology-of-the-liver/burt/978-0-7020-6697-9. Accessed 23 Jun 2020.
15. Knodell RG, Ishak KG, Black WC, Chen TS, Craig R, Kaplowitz N, Kiernan TW, Wollman J. Formulation and application of a numerical scoring system for assessing histological activity in asymptomatic chronic active hepatitis. J Hepatol. 2003;38:382–6. https://doi.org/10.1016/s0168-8278(03)00005-9.
16. Scheuer PJ. Classification of chronic viral hepatitis: a need for reassessment. J Hepatol. 1991;13:372–4. https://doi.org/10.1016/0168-8278(91)90084-O.
17. Ishak K, Baptista A, Bianchi L, Callea F, De Groote J, Gudat F, et al. Histological grading and staging of chronic hepatitis. J Hepatol. 1995;22:696–9. https://doi.org/10.1016/0168-8278(95)80226-6.
18. Poynard T, Ngo Y, Perazzo H, Munteanu M, Lebray P, Moussalli J, et al. Prognostic value of liver fibrosis biomarkers. Gastroenterol Hepatol (N Y). 2011;7:445–54.
19. Aubé C, Oberti F, Korali N, Namour M-A, Loisel D, Tanguy J-Y, et al. Ultrasonographic diagnosis of hepatic fibrosis or cirrhosis. J Hepatol. 1999;30:472–8. https://doi.org/10.1016/S0168-8278(99)80107-X.
20. Pavlov CS, Casazza G, Semenistaia M, Nikolova D, Tsochatzis E, Liusina E, et al. Ultrasonography for diagnosis of alcoholic cirrhosis in people with alcoholic liver disease. Cochrane Database Syst Rev. 2016;3:CD011602. https://doi.org/10.1002/14651858.CD011602.pub2.
21. FibroScan® Accurate for Assessment of Fibrosis & Steatosis. n.d. https://www.fibroscan.com/en/products. Accessed 26 Jun 2020.
22. Rifai K, Cornberg J, Mederacke I, Bahr MJ, Wedemeyer H, Malinski P, et al. Clinical feasibility of liver elastography by acoustic radiation force impulse imaging (ARFI). Dig Liver Dis. 2011;43:491–7. https://doi.org/10.1016/j.dld.2011.02.011.
23. Ferraioli G, Tinelli C, Dal Bello B, Zicchetti M, Filice G, Filice C, et al. Accuracy of real-time shear wave elastography for assessing liver fibrosis in chronic hepatitis C: a pilot study. Hepatology. 2012;56:2125–33. https://doi.org/10.1002/hep.25936.
24. Yin M, Talwalkar JA, Glaser KJ, Manduca A, Grimm RC, Rossman PJ, et al. Assessment of hepatic fibrosis with magnetic resonance elastography. Clin Gastroenterol Hepatol. 2007;5:1207–1213.e2. https://doi.org/10.1016/j.cgh.2007.06.012.
25. Nguyen-Khac E, Chatelain D, Tramier B, Decrombecque C, Robert B, Joly J-P, et al. Assessment of asymptomatic liver fibrosis in alcoholic patients using fibroscan: prospective comparison with seven non-invasive laboratory tests. Aliment Pharmacol Ther. 2008;28:1188–98. https://doi.org/10.1111/j.1365-2036.2008.03831.x.
26. Nahon P, Kettaneh A, Tengher-Barna I, Ziol M, de Lédinghen V, Douvin C, et al. Assessment of liver fibrosis using transient elastography in patients with alcoholic liver disease. J Hepatol. 2008;49:1062–8. https://doi.org/10.1016/j.jhep.2008.08.011.
27. Thiele M, Detlefsen S, Sevelsted Møller L, Madsen BS, Fuglsang Hansen J, Fialla AD, et al. Transient and 2-dimensional shear-wave elastography provide comparable assessment of alcoholic liver fibrosis and cirrhosis. Gastroenterology. 2016;150:123–33. https://doi.org/10.1053/j.gastro.2015.09.040.
28. Zhang D, Li P, Chen M, Liu L, Liu Y, Zhao Y, et al. Non-invasive assessment of liver fibrosis in patients with alcoholic liver disease using acoustic radiation force impulse elastography. Abdom Imaging. 2015;40:723–9. https://doi.org/10.1007/s00261-014-0154-5.
29. Kiani A, Brun V, Lainé F, Turlin B, Morcet J, Michalak S, et al. Acoustic radiation force impulse imaging for assessing liver fibrosis in alcoholic liver disease. World J Gastroenterol. 2016;22:4926–35. https://doi.org/10.3748/wjg.v22.i20.4926.

30. Bensamoun SF, Leclerc GE, Debernard L, Cheng X, Robert L, Charleux F, et al. Cutoff values for alcoholic liver fibrosis using magnetic resonance elastography technique. Alcohol Clin Exp Res. 2013;37:811–7. https://doi.org/10.1111/acer.12025.

31. Singh S, Venkatesh SK, Wang Z, Miller FH, Motosugi U, Low RN, et al. Diagnostic performance of magnetic resonance elastography in staging liver fibrosis: a systematic review and meta-analysis of individual participant data. Clin Gastroenterol Hepatol. 2015;13:440–451.e6. https://doi.org/10.1016/j.cgh.2014.09.046.

32. Sandrin L, Fourquet B, Hasquenoph J-M, Yon S, Fournier C, Mal F, et al. Transient elastography: a new noninvasive method for assessment of hepatic fibrosis. Ultrasound Med Biol. 2003;29:1705–13. https://doi.org/10.1016/j.ultrasmedbio.2003.07.001.

33. Afdhal NH. Fibroscan (transient elastography) for the measurement of liver fibrosis. Gastroenterol Hepatol (N Y). 2012;8:605–7.

34. de Lédinghen V, Vergniol J. Transient elastography for the diagnosis of liver fibrosis. Expert Rev Med Dev. 2010;7:811–23. https://doi.org/10.1586/erd.10.46.

35. Basnet BK, Kc S, Sharma D, Shrestha D. Transient elastographic values of healthy volunteers in a tertiary care hospital. J Nepal Med Assoc. 2014;52:661–7.

36. Roulot D, Czernichow S, Le Clésiau H, Costes J-L, Vergnaud A-C, Beaugrand M. Liver stiffness values in apparently healthy subjects: influence of gender and metabolic syndrome. J Hepatol. 2008;48:606–13. https://doi.org/10.1016/j.jhep.2007.11.020.

37. Pavlov CS, Casazza G, Nikolova D, Tsochatzis E, Burroughs AK, Ivashkin VT, et al. Transient elastography for diagnosis of stages of hepatic fibrosis and cirrhosis in people with alcoholic liver disease. Cochrane Database Syst Rev. 2015;1:CD010542. https://doi.org/10.1002/14651858.CD010542.pub2.

38. Foucher J, Chanteloup E, Vergniol J, Castéra L, Le Bail B, Adhoute X, et al. Diagnosis of cirrhosis by transient elastography (FibroScan): a prospective study. Gut. 2006;55:403–8. https://doi.org/10.1136/gut.2005.069153.

39. Cassinotto C, Lapuyade B, Mouries A, Hiriart J-B, Vergniol J, Gaye D, et al. Non-invasive assessment of liver fibrosis with impulse elastography: comparison of Supersonic Shear Imaging with ARFI and FibroScan®. J Hepatol. 2014;61:550–7. https://doi.org/10.1016/j.jhep.2014.04.044.

40. Mueller S, Millonig G, Sarovska L, Friedrich S, Reimann FM, Pritsch M, et al. Increased liver stiffness in alcoholic liver disease: differentiating fibrosis from steatohepatitis. World J Gastroenterol. 2010;16:966–72. https://doi.org/10.3748/wjg.v16.i8.966.

41. Mueller S, Englert S, Seitz HK, Badea RI, Erhardt A, Bozaari B, et al. Inflammation-adapted liver stiffness values for improved fibrosis staging in patients with hepatitis C virus and alcoholic liver disease. Liver Int. 2015;35:2514–21. https://doi.org/10.1111/liv.12904.

42. Bardou-Jacquet E, Legros L, Soro D, Latournerie M, Guillygomarc'h A, Le Lan C, et al. Effect of alcohol consumption on liver stiffness measured by transient elastography. World J Gastroenterol. 2013;19:516–22. https://doi.org/10.3748/wjg.v19.i4.516.

43. Anastasiou J, Alisa A, Virtue S, Portmann B, Murray-Lyon I, Williams R. Noninvasive markers of fibrosis and inflammation in clinical practice: prospective comparison with liver biopsy. Eur J Gastroenterol Hepatol. 2010;22:474–80. https://doi.org/10.1097/MEG.0b013e328332dd0a.

44. Boursier J, Vergniol J, Sawadogo A, Dakka T, Michalak S, Gallois Y, et al. The combination of a blood test and Fibroscan improves the non-invasive diagnosis of liver fibrosis. Liver Int. 2009;29:1507–15. https://doi.org/10.1111/j.1478-3231.2009.02101.x.

45. Carl I, Addley J, McDougall NI, Cash WJ. Transient hepatic elastography reliably excludes cirrhosis in an unselected liver disease population. J Hepatol. 2012;56(Suppl 2):S409–10. https://doi.org/10.1016/S0168-8278(12)61059-9.

46. de Lédinghen W, et al. Diagnosis of liver fibrosis and cirrhosis using liver stiffness measurement: comparison between M and XL probe of FibroScan®. J Hepatol. 2012;56:833. https://doi.org/10.1016/j.jhep.2011.10.017.

47. Dolman GE, Nieboer D, Steyerberg EW, Harris S, Ferguson A, Zaitoun AM, et al. The performance of transient elastography compared to clinical acumen and routine tests - what is the incremental diagnostic value? Liver Int. 2013;33:172–9. https://doi.org/10.1111/liv.12017.

48. Kim SG, Kim YS, Jung SW, Kim HK, Jang JY, Moon JH, et al. The usefulness of transient elastography to diagnose cirrhosis in patients with alcoholic liver disease. Korean J Hepatol. 2009;15:42–51. https://doi.org/10.3350/kjhep.2009.15.1.42.
49. Lannerstedt H, Konopski Z, Sandvik L, Haaland T, Løberg EM, Haukeland JW. Combining transient elastography with FIB4 enhances sensitivity in detecting advanced fibrosis of the liver. Scand J Gastroenterol. 2013;48:93–100. https://doi.org/10.3109/00365521.2012.746389.
50. Fernández M, Trepo E, Gustot T, Degré D, Verset L, Demetter P, et al. Fibroscan (transient elastography) is the most reliable non-invasive method for the assessment of severe fibrosis and cirrhosis in alcoholic liver disease. 2012.
51. Lemoine M, Katsahian S, Ziol M, Nahon P, Ganne-Carrie N, Kazemi F, et al. Liver stiffness measurement as a predictive tool of clinically significant portal hypertension in patients with compensated hepatitis C virus or alcohol-related cirrhosis. Aliment Pharmacol Ther. 2008;28:1102–10. https://doi.org/10.1111/j.1365-2036.2008.03825.x.
52. Janssens F, de Suray N, Piessevaux H, Horsmans Y, de Timary P, Stärkel P. Can transient elastography replace liver histology for determination of advanced fibrosis in alcoholic patients: a real-life study. J Clin Gastroenterol. 2010;44:575–82. https://doi.org/10.1097/MCG.0b013e3181cb4216.
53. Nguyen-Khac E, Thiele M, Voican C, Nahon P, Moreno C, Boursier J, et al. Non-invasive diagnosis of liver fibrosis in patients with alcohol-related liver disease by transient elastography: an individual patient data meta-analysis. Lancet Gastroenterol Hepatol. 2018;3:614–25. https://doi.org/10.1016/S2468-1253(18)30124-9.
54. Hadefi A, Degré D, Trépo E, Moreno C. Noninvasive diagnosis in alcohol-related liver disease. Health Sci Rep. 2020;3:e146. https://doi.org/10.1002/hsr2.146.

Elastography After Treatment and During Follow-Up

9

Mirella Fraquelli, Ilaria Fanetti, and Andrea Costantino

9.1 Introduction

Liver fibrosis is the prognostic hallmark of chronic liver diseases (CLD), independently of their etiology [1], since it significantly correlates with relevant outcomes, such as cirrhosis development, liver-related complications, and mortality. For such reasons, the assessment of liver fibrosis has always been considered of strategic importance.

Until the early 2000s, liver fibrosis used to be evaluated by histological examination of the liver obtained through liver biopsy. However, liver biopsy has several disadvantages, including poor patient compliance, sampling errors, a minor but still consistent risk of complications, and limited usefulness for dynamic follow-up [2, 3]. Together, these drawbacks of liver biopsy have boosted the search for noninvasive methods of fibrosis progression assessment that could simplify the management of patients with CLD.

Since 2004, the severity of liver fibrosis in CLD patients has been assessed through liver stiffness measurement (LS) by vibration-controlled transient elastography (VCTE, also commonly known as transient elastography, TE, FibroScan®) and, thereafter, also by US elastography techniques implemented on regular ultrasound machines [4–9]. TE is the most frequently used technique in clinical practice: the EASL guidelines currently recommend it for the evaluation of patients with CLD [10].

After the evidence of the tight correlation between fibrosis regression after treatment (by IFN or more recently direct-acting agents, DAA) and the improvement of primary relevant outcomes [11–13], the longitudinal assessment of liver stiffness after antiviral therapy has also become crucial. Mallet et al. have firstly

M. Fraquelli (✉) · I. Fanetti · A. Costantino
Gastrointestinal and Endoscopy Unit, Fondazione IRCCS Ca' Granda Ospedale Maggiore Policlinico, Milan, Italy
e-mail: mirella.fraquelli@policlinico.mi.it

© Springer Nature Switzerland AG 2021
M. Fraquelli (ed.), *Elastography of the Liver and Beyond*,
https://doi.org/10.1007/978-3-030-74132-7_9

demonstrated that cirrhosis regression in CHC patients significantly improved clinically relevant outcomes, such as all-cause mortality [11]. In this study, in fact, 96 patients with histologically proven HCV-related cirrhosis were treated with an IFN-based regimen and underwent at least one post-treatment biopsy. In a median follow-up of 118 months (range 86–138), cirrhosis regression was observed in 18 patients (19%), who, interestingly, also showed decreased disease-related morbidity and improved survival.

Since then, many studies investigating the use of elastographic techniques to monitor treatment response have been published with the common aim of understanding how fibrosis changes during and after antiviral treatment.

However, the shared lack of histological post-treatment assessment mainly for ethical reasons can represent a methodological flaw in most of such studies.

In addition, as already reported by Prati et al. in a previous chapter of this book, besides hepatic fibrosis, LSM can be influenced by several confounders: interpreting the results of these studies should be done with caution.

In fact, earlier studies using liver biopsy as the reference standard have demonstrated that LS measurement is a sum of fibrosis and inflammation and that it might be influenced by liver steatosis [14–16]. The influence of inflammation can be supported in CHC patients following HCV clearance [17–19] and by the decrease of LSM following alcohol withdrawal [20]. It has also been suggested in CHB patients whose liver stiffness dynamic profiles paralleled those of ALT as occurred during ALT flares in patients with hepatitis exacerbation [21, 22]. Other possible confounding factors that have been described are sinusoidal pressure [20], extrahepatic cholestasis [23], and liver congestion due to heart failure [24, 25].

Thus, post-treatment LS reduction has to be interpreted with caution, taking into account all the available information. Also, it is still unclear at which moment to perform LS assessment best, whether early or later during post-treatment follow-up.

9.2 Chronic HCV Infection

Over the last 20–30 years, HCV infection has been the major cause of liver fibrosis and cirrhosis worldwide, because of its high global prevalence and the lack of any effective treatment to achieve viral clearance in most cases. Indeed, the natural history of the HCV disease shows fibrosis progression over time, both in untreated patients and in nonresponders [26].

More recently, thanks to the widespread application of a highly effective short-duration treatment regimen based on direct-acting agents (DAA), most HCV patients have been successfully treated to rapid virus elimination. Thus, fibrosis reversal and cirrhosis regression have become the main issues of hepatologic studies, wondering how much fibrosis reversal should be expected and, in case of cirrhosis, if the disease would revert to a less severe form of CLD.

In the next paragraphs, we shall summarize the main results of the studies that have assessed LS modifications in CHC patients after antiviral therapy (IFN- or DAA-based regimens) using either liver histology as the reference standard or without histological confirmation.

9.3   Liver Stiffness Changes Following IFN-Based Regimens

9.3.1   Studies with Histological Confirmation

Some studies, primarily performed on patients receiving IFN-based therapy with or without ribavirin, have adopted liver histology as the reference standard and demonstrated that cirrhosis reversed in a substantial proportion of patients [27–33].

D'Ambrosio et al. [28] have assessed the long-term histological benefits of SVR in 38 HCV patients with cirrhosis who underwent paired pre- and post-treatment liver biopsies taken 61 months after SVR. For 33 of them, post-treatment TE measurement was also available at the time of the second biopsy. For these patients, TE accuracy in assessing the stage of liver fibrosis was evaluated. In all patients, the median area of fibrosis was significantly reduced from baseline (2.3% after treatment, $p < 0.0001$), and cirrhosis regression was seen in 20 (61%) of the cases. For what concerns TE accuracy, a significant correlation was found between TE and both fibrosis stage ($r = 0.56$; $p = 0.001$) and morphometry ($r = 0.56$, $p = 0.001$) as well as between fibrosis stage and area of fibrosis ($r = 0.72$, $p = 0.001$).

The median TE value was 9.8 kPa, lower in regressed than not regressed patients (9.1 kPa vs. 12.9 kPa, $p = 0.01$). In detail, TE was <12 kPa in 5 (38%) F4 patients and in 19 (95%) F3 patients ($p = 0.0007$) with 61% sensitivity and 95% specificity in the diagnosis of F4 after treatment.

Interestingly, this study showed for the first time a low predictive power of the viremic cutoff value of 12 kPa in the setting of cirrhotics with eradicated HCV, probably as a consequence of liver remodeling and fibrosis reabsorption, suggesting that liver biopsy still remains the only reliable approach for staging liver fibrosis following SVR.

Chen et al. [32] studied a series of HCV patients who had undergone a baseline liver biopsy before 2004 and performed, either by liver biopsy or LSM using TE, a follow-up liver fibrosis assessment over a time length of more than 10 years. The patients who had undergone a baseline liver biopsy but had no follow-up fibrosis assessment were recalled to perform LS assessment. Fibrosis was categorized as mild-moderate (METAVIR F0–F2, LS ≤9.5 kPa) or advanced (F3–F4, LS >9.5 kPa). One hundred thirty-one patients were included in the analysis, 83% of whom received interferon-based antiviral therapy and 40% achieving SVR. At follow-up (the median period between fibrosis assessments being 14 years), liver fibrosis assessment was performed by LS in 86% and liver biopsy in 14%. The results of this study showed fibrosis progression in only 7% of patients who achieved SVR in comparison to 30% of the patients not responding to antiviral therapy, over a decade. Interestingly, the three participants who developed fibrosis progression despite SVR showed additional cofactors, such as concomitant alcohol abuse and diabetes. At multivariate analysis, SVR was independently associated with prevention from liver fibrosis progression.

In their prospective study, Tachi et al. [34] enrolled 336 HCV patients, of whom 121 with SVR. LS measurement was performed by ARFI elastography on all patients the same day as liver biopsy. LS significantly correlated with the histological fibrosis score, both in viremic and SVR patients. However, in accordance with the same fibrosis stage, LS resulted significantly lower in SVR as compared to non-SVR subjects. In addition, the LS values were affected by necroinflammatory activity, their being higher in HCV patients with Grades 2 or 3 as compared with patients with Grades 0 or 1. In accordance with D'Ambrosio et al. [28], in this study too, the viremic cutoff values were not the most accurate ones for diagnosing liver cirrhosis in SVR patients.

9.3.2 Studies Without Histological Confirmation

These studies (their characteristics are summarized in Table 9.1) have assessed the longitudinal changes of LS determination after SVR as an indirect marker of hepatic fibrosis [18, 19, 26, 35–43]. Overall, SVR has always been associated with the post-treatment reduction of liver stiffness, although most of the studies are heterogeneous as there are differences related to different study design formats, prevalence of cirrhosis, the different elastography techniques used, and the follow-up time points.

Frequently, these studies are limited by a short follow-up period of around 24 weeks.

Ogawa et al. [19] studied 145 Japanese HCV patients who underwent a PEG-IFN plus ribavirin combination therapy to assess any association between LS measured by TE and treatment efficacy. LS values significantly decreased in SVR patients in comparison with non-SVR patients at the end of treatment (EOT), and up to 96 weeks after EOT. Among the non-SVR patients, TE values were significantly diminished for patients with biochemical response in comparison with those without, at EOT, and up to 96 weeks after EOT.

In a French study, Vergniol et al. [35] looked at 416 treatment-naive patients, 112 of whom started treatment after enrollment. In the treatment group, the TE values were significantly higher before and after treatment than among untreated patients at baseline and after 1 year. However, there was no significant difference between treated and untreated patients at the end of follow-up. TE values fell in all treated patients, independently of their virological response, without any significant difference between treated and untreated patients at the end of follow-up. At multivariate analysis, treatment was the only factor independently associated with TE values reduction.

Another French study [18] involved 91 patients with CHC and significant fibrosis (LS >7.0 kPa) at baseline. Liver stiffness significantly decreased during therapy (PEG-IFN and ribavirin) and continued to diminish after treatment only in patients who achieved SVR. At multivariate analysis, only SVR was associated with long-term liver stiffness improvement.

Wang et al. [33] reported similar results in SVR patients while showing a progressive increase in the LS values of nonresponders during follow-up.

In the paper by Calvaruso et al. [42], long-term responders to IFN-based therapies revealed lower LS values than those untreated and still viremic, whereas Arima et al. [35] observed a significant LS reduction after SVR and in relapsers. An

Table 9.1 Main characteristics of the studies involving CHC patients who were treated by IFN-based antiviral regimens and underwent paired liver stiffness assessment by elastography

Study	Treated Patients (n)	Cirrhotics	Tx	SVR	LSM type	Pre-Tx LSM values (kPa or m/s) in SVR	Post-Tx LSM values (kPa or m/s) in SVR	Time LSM after EOT (max available)
Ogawa et al. (2009) [19]	126	13%	IFN + RBV	45%	TE	10.3 ± 4.8	5.4 (median)	96 W
Vergniol et al. (2009) [35]	112	21%	IFN	63%	TE	10.65 ± 9.55	7.30 ± 8.45	24 W
Arima et al. (2010) [36]	145	64%	IFN ± RBV	100%	TE	8 (5–11.9)	5.3 (4.1–6.3)	104 W
Macías et al. (2010) [37]	143 (68% HCV-HIV)	18%	IFN ± RBV	56%	TE	7.7 (6.0–10.8)	6.0 (4.7–8.1)	24 W
Wang et al. (2010) [38]	144	32%	IFN + RBV	66%	TE	6.1 (3.0–70.6)	5.5 (2.7–33.8)	24 W
Hezode et al. (2011) [18]	91	36%	IFN + RBV	65%	TE	10 (8.2–14.1)	Δ −3.4 (−4.7–1.1)	24 W
Martinez et al. (2012) [39]	323	17%	IFN + RBV	63%	TE	9.3 ± 5.9	7.4 ± 4.4	24 W
Poynard et al. (2013) [26]	595	NA	IFN ± RBV	29%	TE	NA	NA	>24 W
Osakabe et al. (2015) [40]	87	NA	IFN ± RBV	47%	ARFI	1.27 (1.11–1.49)[a]	1.05 (0.95–1.16)[a]	104 W
Soliman et al. (2020) [41]	150	50%	IFN	90%	TE	F4: 21.3 (17.3–28)	F4: 13.4 (10.9–19.7)	48 W
						F2/3: 10.4 (9–11)	F2/3: 6 (5.6–6.6)	

CHC chronic hepatitis C viral infection, *SVR* sustained virological response, *LSM* liver stiffness measurement, *Tx* therapy, *EOT* end of treatment, *NA* not available, *W* week

[a]m/s

interesting aspect of the Calvaruso et al. paper is that at multivariate logistic analysis, γ-GT and histological steatosis were independently associated with the persistence of higher LS values, again pointing out the importance of confounders in LS results interpretation.

9.4 Liver Stiffness Changes Following DAA Regimens

9.4.1 Studies with Histological Confirmation

Significant improvement of fibrosis noninvasive markers has been documented also after successful treatment with DAA characterized by short-duration schedules (12 weeks) and high sustained virological response (SVR) rates (>90%).

The main characteristics of the studies [44–46] that used liver histology as the reference standard and performed paired liver biopsy before treatment and after SVR are summarized in Table 9.2.

Pan et al. [44] included 84 HCV patients with advanced fibrosis or cirrhosis who underwent DAA treatment and achieved SVR. Overall, 62% of them showed improved liver stiffness as assessed by TE, which was consistent with the regression of at least one stage of fibrosis. Fifteen patients with liver biopsies prior to SVR underwent biopsy after SVR, and 13 of these patients had a concordant improvement of liver stiffness. The post-SVR liver biopsies of only four patients showed F1–F2, while 11 patients showed F3–F4; however, the morphometry of the first 11 biopsied patients revealed that ten patients had a 46% average decrease in collagen content.

In the study by Enomoto et al. [45] among 691 patients with CHC who achieved SVR after DAA, 51 underwent liver biopsy 41 ± 20 weeks after EOT despite normal transaminases. Of them, 20 patients also had liver biopsy specimens obtained at a median of 1.2 years before their treatment start, and the comparison revealed a significant regression of the inflammation grade but not of the fibrosis stage.

In their retrospective analysis of 43 patients with paired liver biopsy specimens after SVR with DAA therapy, Huang et al. [46] observed that inflammation improvement and fibrosis regression were achieved in 83% and 38% of patients, respectively. Interestingly, LS measured by TE could predict post-SVR fibrosis, and pre-SVR LS values were significantly lower in patients with fibrosis regression.

9.4.2 Studies Without Histological Confirmation

Several studies have observed a significant decrease of LS values by measurement with different elastographic techniques after successful DAA treatment [47–81]. These studies too are heterogeneous in terms of study design formats, prevalence of cirrhosis, and length of follow-up. The main results of these studies are summarized in Table 9.3.

Table 9.2 Main characteristics of the studies involving CHC patients who were treated with DAA antiviral regimens and underwent paired liver biopsy and/or liver stiffness assessment by transient elastography

Study	Patients (n)	Cirrhotics	SVR	Patients with paired TE	Pre-Tx LSM values (kPa) in SVR	Post-Tx LSM values (kPa) in SVR	Time LSM after EOT (max available)	Patients with paired LB	Fibrosis improvement	Δ Time paired LB
Pan et al. (2018) [44]	84	24%	100%	28	NA	6.5[a]	1.2–1.9 Y	15	73%	2.3–3.9 Y
Enomoto et al. (2018) [45]	141	5%	100%	20	11.5 ± 6.4	7.7 ± 5.4	48 W	20	65%	41 SD (±20) W
Huang et al. (2020) [46]	40	35%	100%	40	9.5[a]	7.6[a]	12 W	40	83%	36 W

CHC chronic hepatitis C viral infection, *SVR* sustained virological response, *EOT* end of treatment, *DAA* direct-acting agents, *LB* liver biopsy, *LSM* liver stiffness measurement, *NA* not available, *W* week, *Y* year

[a]Median

Table 9.3 Main characteristics of the studies involving CHC patients who were mainly treated with DAA antiviral regimen and underwent liver stiffness assessment by transient elastography

Study	Treated patients (n)	Cirrhotics	Tx	SVR	LSM type	Pre-Tx LSM values (kPa)	Post-Tx LSM values (kPa)	Time LSM after EOT (max available)
Knop et al. (2016) [47]	54	100%	DAA	100%	TE	32.5 (9.1–75)	21.2 (5.4–70)	24 W
					ARFI	2.7 (1.2–4.1)	2.4 (1.2–3.9)	
Chekuri et al. (2016) [48]	100	42%	IFN (52) DAA (48)	100%	TE	12.70 (8.3–21.1)	7.70 (5.3–11.6)	48 W
Pons et al. (2017) [49]	41	100%	DAA	98%	TE	20.8 (16.3–29.5)	14.3 (10.8–22.9)	48 W
Elsharawy et al. (2017) [50]	337	45%	DAA	92%	TE	14.63 ± 10.68	11.8 ± 8.8	12 W
Dolmazashvilia et al. (2017) [51]	304	57%	DAA (152) IFN + SOF + RBV (152)	85%	TE	16.9 (11.8–27.7)	11.9 (8.2–20.9)	24 W
Bachofner et al. (2017) [52]	392	13%	DAA	93%	TE	14.3 (10.2–21.5)	9.1 (6.1–13.9)	40 W (143 pts)
Sporea et al. (2017) [53]	211	100%	DAA	100%	TE	27.4 ± 11.9	21.3 ± 11	12 W
Tada et al. (2017) [55]	210	NA	DAA	100%	SWE	10.2 (7.7–14.7)	7.6 (6.3–10.3)	24 W
Tada et al. (2018) [54]	198	NA	DAA	100%	MRI	3.10 (2.7–4.1)	2.80 (2.4–3.7)	24 W
Hamada et al. (2018) [56]	196	NA	DAA (107) IFN (89)	100%	SWE	8.3 (3.4 ± 36.2)	5.9 (2.7 ± 31.3)	24 W
Ohya et al. (2018) [57]	302	NA	DAA	96%	TE	NA	NA	48 W
Ravaioli et al. (2018) [58]	139	100%	DAA	100%	TE	18.6 (15–26)	13.8 (10.4–20.4)	EOT
Noureddin et al. (2018) [59]	101	0	DAA	100%	TE	7.4 ± 1.9	6.1 ± 3.6	48 W
Omar et al. (2018) [60]	52 POST OLT	46% F3–F4	DAA	100%	TE	F2: 9 (8.8–9.25) F34: 15.35 (12–24.15)	F2: 5.5 (4.5–6.7) F34: 9.2 (6.3–15.6)	72 W
Chan et al. (2018) [61]	70	24%	DAA IFN + DAA (4)	96%	TE	8.0 (5.4, 12.4)	NA	48 W

Persico et al. (2018) [62]	749	70%	DAA	98%	TE	19.3 (±11.2)	14.2 (±11.7)	12 W
Facciorusso et al. (2018) [63]	112	32%	DAA (82) IFN (30)	100%	TE	12.3 (9–17.8)	6.6 (5.3–7.4)	5 Y (62 pts)
Akuta et al. (2018) [64]	217	21%	192 (88% Tx COMPLETE)	96%	TE	F4: 23.9 (17.6–31.6) F0–3: 6.05 (4.4–7.7)	F4: 17.6 (12–22.3) F0–3: 5.1 (3.9–6.4)	24 W
Ogasawara et al. (2018) [65]	214	52%	DAA	91%	TE	11.25 (2.4–51.4)	5.45	72 W
Kobayashi et al. (2018) [66]	57	NA	DAA	100%	TE	8.3 (5.0–14.8)	5.4 (4.0–13.4)	48 W
Flisiak et al. (2018) [67]	200	58%	DAA	100%	TE	EOT: 16.6 ± 11.8	12.7 ± 9.1	48 W (120 pts)
Lee et al. (2019) [68]	270	31%	DAA	93%	TE	13.2 ± 12.6	10.5	12 W
Rout et al. (2019) [69]	372	26%	DAA	100%	TE	6.9 (5.1–12.7)	6.1 (4.8–9.4)	48 W (265 pts)
Hsu et al. (2019) [70]	388	34%	DAA	98%	ARFI	1.78 (1.25–2.3)	1.38 (1.14–1.8)	12 W (199 pts)
Giannini et al. (2019) [71]	52	52%	DAA	100%	TE	15.2 (12.0–20.0)	9.3 (7.5–12.0)	60 W
Soliman et al. (2020) [41]	150	50%	DAA	90%	TE	F4: 21.8 (17.3–31.8) F23: 10.2 (9.2–11.2)	F4: 14.9 (11–19) F23: 6.2 (5.6–7.1)	48 W
Kohla et al. (2020) [72]	165	9%	DAA	100%	SWE	8.49 ± 0.83	5.74 ± 3.21	36 W
Kawagishi et al. (2020) [73]	116	20%	DAA	100%	TE	NA	NA	24 W
Stasi et al. (2020) [74]	294	48%	DAA	100%	NA	13.4 ± 9.97	NA	96 W

CHC chronic hepatitis C viral infection, *SVR* sustained virological response, *EOT* end of treatment, *DAA* direct-acting agents, *LSM* liver stiffness measurement, *NA* not available, *W* week, *Y* year

A finding that is common to most of the published studies is the very rapid decrease of LS values shortly after starting DAA treatment paralleling the transaminases decrease: it is likely to be related to necroinflammation decrease.

For example, in the study by Pons et al. [49] concerning 41 patients treated with DAA therapy, LS was assessed before, during, and after treatment, up to 48 weeks using TE. LS decreased very rapidly in CLD patients during DAA treatment, with a higher decrease observed in patients with baseline ALT values higher than twice the upper limit of normality than in those with ALT lower than twice the upper limit of normal.

In the paper by Kobayashi et al. [66] covering 57 patients who received DDA therapy and achieved SVR, there is an interesting finding: ALT levels decreased overall with significant difference among baseline, EOT, and SVR24 and thereafter remained stable. The median LS values as measured by TE decreased significantly at each timepoint between baseline and SVR24. Therefore, LS at SVR24 might reflect the actual stage of liver fibrosis in patients achieving SVR after DAA.

9.5 HBV Infection

Similar to CHC patients, fibrosis represents also as the major determinant of prognosis for CHB patients [82], and its longitudinal assessment during antiviral therapy is very important for establishing treatment strategies. Indeed, HBV inhibition can lead to fibrosis and even cirrhosis reversion leading to improved clinically relevant outcomes [83–85].

Three studies [83–85] (see Table 9.4) with paired liver biopsy before and after treatment documented the regression of liver fibrosis after antiviral therapy.

Dienstag et al. [83] enrolled 63 patients (17% cirrhotic) who underwent three sets of liver biopsies: before and after 1 year on lamivudine treatment and after 2 years on further open-label treatment. At the end of the first year, 57% of the patients showed a >2 point improvement in necroinflammatory activity; after two additional years on lamivudine, 19% of patients continued to improve. As to fibrosis, bridging fibrosis improved by >1 degree in 63% of the cases, while cirrhosis improved in 73%. Only 2% showed progression to cirrhosis and 9% showed progression to bridging fibrosis.

Chang et al. [84] followed 69 patients (7% cirrhotic) treated with entecavir therapy who underwent paired liver biopsy after a median time of 6 years. At the time of their long-term biopsy, all the patients presented with a hepatitis B virus DNA level <300 copies/mL, and 86% had a normalized ALT level. Histological improvement ($\geq$2-point decrease in the Knodell necroinflammatory score and no worsening of the Knodell fibrosis score) was observed in 96% of patients, and a $\geq$1-point improvement in the Ishak fibrosis score was found in 88% of patients.

In a randomized controlled trial, Marcellin et al. [85] studied 585 patients who entered a 7-year study of open-label tenofovir DF treatment, with a pre-specified repeat liver biopsy at Week 240. Three hundred forty-eight patients (54% of the whole study population) had their baseline and Year 5 liver biopsy results showing

Table 9.4 Main characteristics of the studies involving CHB patients who were treated with antiviral regimens and underwent paired liver biopsy

Study	Patients (n)	Cirrhotics (%)	Tx	LSM	Patients with paired LB	Δ Time paired LB	LB cirrhosis reversal	LB fibrosis reversal	LB grade improvement
Dienstag et al. (2003) [83]	63	17%	LMV	No	63	3 Y	73%	NA	56%
Chang et al. (2010) [84]	57	7%	ETV ± LMV	No	57	6 (3–7) Y	100%	88%	75%
Marcellin et al. (2013) [85]	641	28%	TDF	No	348	5 Y	74%	51%	90%

CHB chronic hepatitis B, *Tx* treatment, *LMV* lamivudine, *NUCs* nucleos(t)ide analogue, *ETV* entecavir, *ADV* adefovir, *CLV* clevudine, *IFN* interferon, *LB* liver biopsy, *TEL* telbivudine, *NA* not available, *Y* Years

an histological improvement in 87% of the cases; in particular, 51% had fibrosis regression at Week 240, and out of 96 (28%) patients with cirrhosis at baseline, 74% no longer had cirrhosis (≥1 unit decrease in score), whereas only 3 out of 252 patients without cirrhosis at baseline progressed to cirrhosis at Year 5.

In addition, in a Chinese study by Wu et al. [88], LS was sequentially performed by TE every 26 weeks on 120 treatment-naive CHB patients receiving entecavir. The TE results were compared to the results of paired liver biopsy performed at baseline and at Week 78 on antiviral therapy. Interestingly, LS values presented a rapid-to-slow decline pattern and decreased more rapidly in patients with histological fibrosis regression than in those without fibrosis improvement at Week 78. At multivariate analysis, the LS percent decline at Weeks 52 and 78 was an independent predictive factor for histological fibrosis regression at Week 78 on antiviral therapy.

Several studies (their main characteristics are summarized in Table 9.5) have investigated the longitudinal changes in liver stiffness before, during, and after antiviral therapy using elastography techniques [19, 83–109] and have documented a significant reduction of LS values after antiviral treatment as compared to basal determination. However, the majority of these studies are limited by short periods of observation and lack of paired histological assessment.

Several interesting results can be inferred from the studies with relatively longer periods (≥3 years) of treatment with NUCs.

In the study by Osakabe et al. [97], LS was measured by TE in 212 CHB patients who underwent NUC treatment. Liver biopsies were performed in 51 patients. Changes of LS were assessed in 29 patients treated with NUCs and 52 patients without antiviral therapy. LS measured at an interval of 512 days was significantly reduced by antiviral therapy, from 12.9 (range 6.2–17.9) to 6.6 kPa (4.4–10.3). Eleven out of 19 (58%) patients with baseline fibrosis stages of F3–F4 deduced from LS had a ≥2-point reduction of the deduced stage at the last LS measurement.

Andersen et al. [98] studied 66 patients (53 cirrhotics and 13 with advanced fibrosis) prior to treatment. Among the patients with cirrhosis before treatment, 49% had liver stiffness below 11.0 kPa at follow-up, suggesting cirrhosis regression. Among the patients with advanced fibrosis (F3) prior to treatment, 77% had liver stiffness below 8.1 kPa after treatment, suggesting improvement of fibrosis. However, histological assessment was not available in this study.

Fung et al. [99] examined longitudinally liver stiffness changes as measured by TE in a cohort of 426 CHB patients, 110 of whom received oral antiviral therapy. There was a significant decline of LS at follow-up measurement compared to baseline in treated patients with elevated ALT at baseline and subsequent normalization after 3 years (6.1 kPa vs. 7.8 kPa, respectively) and in untreated patients who had persistently normal ALT. Antiviral therapy ALT levels during follow-up were independent significant factors associated with LSM decline.

A recent meta-analysis [109] identified 24 studies in adults with hepatitis B who underwent TE before and at least 6 months after their start on NUC therapy.

Table 9.5 Main characteristics of the studies involving CHB patients who underwent antiviral regimens and underwent paired liver biopsy and/or paired liver stiffness assessment by transient elastography

Study	Patients (*n*)	Cirrhotics (%)	Tx	Virological response	LB	Paired LB	Paired TE	TE values (kPa) Pre-Tx	TE values (kPa) Post-Tx	Δ Time paired TE
Enomoto et al. (2010) [89]	56	23%	ETV	95%	Yes	0	20	11.2 (7.0–15.2)	7.8 (5.1–11.9)	1 Y
Kim et al. (2010) [90]	41	56%	LMV, ADV, ETV	96%	Yes	4	41	11.7 (4.1–36.3)	11.8 (3.8–20.9)	1 Y
Lim et al. (2011) [91]	62	39%	ETV	82%	Yes	15	62	15.1 (5.6–75.0)	8.8 (3.0–33.8)	1 Y
Wong et al. (2011) [87]	71	11%	CLV, ADV	70%	Yes	71	71	8.8 (3.1–26.3)	6.6 (3.3–18.8)	1 Y
Ogawa et al. (2011) [19]	44	9%	LMV ± ADV	86%	Yes	0	22	8.2 (10.5 ± 6.5)	5.3 (6.8 ± 4.0)	3 Y
Zeng et al. (2016) [92]	175	NA	NUCs / IFN	54% / 34%	Yes	67	175	8.9 ± 3.3	5.3 ± 1.3	2 Y
Sun et al. (2017) [93]	71	72%	ETV	NA	Yes	71	0	12.0 (8.4, 15.2)	NA	NA

(continued)

Table 9.5 (continued)

Study	Patients (n)	Cirrhotics (%)	Tx	Virological response	LB	Paired LB	Paired TE	TE values (kPa) Pre-Tx	TE values (kPa) Post-Tx	Δ Time paired TE
Jeon et al. (2017) [94]	540	100%	NA	NA	Yes	0	0	14.5 (9.6–21.3)	NA	NA
Liang et al. (2017) [86]	534	NA	TEL ± ADV	73%	Yes	164	534	8.6 (2.6–49.5)	5.3 (2.7–36.8)	2 Y
Stasi et al. (2017) [95]	50	NA	NUCs	100%	Yes	0	20	12.60 ± 6.31	7.28 ± 3.17	2 Y
Oliveri et al. (2008) [96]	87	NA	NUCs, IFN	NA	No	0	9	12.3 ± 3.3	5.6 ± 1.1	1 Y
Andersen et al. (2011) [98]	66	80%	NUCs	NA	No	0	66	53 F4	27 F4	4 Y
Osakabe et al. (2011) [97]	29	NA	LMV, ETV	NA	No	0	27	12.9 (6.2–17.9)	4.7 (3.1–7.9)	3 Y
Fung et al. (2011) [99]	426	NA	26% treated: LMV, ETV, ADV, TEL, TDF	NA	No	0	426	6.0 (1.5–28.0)	5.6 (3.0–46.4)	3 Y
Kim et al. (2013) [100]	121	52%	ETV	92%	No	0	121	14.3 (9.0–23.5)	7.3 (5.3–11.8)	3 Y

Yan et al. (2013) [101]	58	7%	NA	NA	No	0	58	8.8 (3.2–47.3)	5.5 (2.8–21.5)	1 Y
Jang et al. (2014) [102]	76	NA	NUCs	70%	No	0	76	6.5 (4.7–9.2)	5.3 (3.9–6.7)	1.5 Y
Kuo et al. (2014) [103]	233	43%	ETV	NA	No	0	233	12.5 (5.2–63.9)	10.1 (4.4–67.8)	1.3 Y
Wang et al. (2015) [104]	236	39%	TDF	98%	No	0	80	10.2 ± 6.2	7.3 ± 5.7	1 Y
Tenggara et al. (2017) [105]	41	41%	ETV, TBV	NA	No	0	41	10.8 (4.1–61.5)	5.9 (NA)	1 Y
Chon et al. (2017) [106]	120	86%	LMV, ETV	NA	No	0	NA	14.5 ± 7.2	NA	NA
Rinaldi et al. (2018) [107]	200	10%	ETV, TDF	NA	No	0	189	12.4 (±9.3)	8.22 (±4.9)	2 Y
Wu et al. (2018) [88]	120	54%	ETV	NA	Yes	0	120	13.8 (9.6–20.3)	7.7 (5.7–12.0)	78 W

CHB chronic hepatitis B, *Tx* treatment, *LMV* lamivudine, *NUCs* nucleos(t)ide analogue, *ETV* entecavir, *ADV* adefovir, *CLV* clevudine, *IFN* interferon, *LB* liver biopsy, *TEL* telbivudine, *NA* not available, *W* week, *Y* year

Antiviral therapy was associated with a progressive decline in liver stiffness in patients with hepatitis B; in particular, in patients with high baseline ALT and viral load, LSM significantly declined by 2.2 kPa, 2.53 kPa, 3.73 kPa, 4.15 kPa, and 5.19 kPa at 6 months, 1 year, 2 years, 3 years, and 5 years from the start of therapy, respectively.

Overall, TE seems to be a useful tool to monitor fibrosis changes in CHB patients undergoing antiviral treatment with NUC. However, without histological confirmation with paired liver biopsies, it is unclear whether the decrease in LS values is associated with improvement in necroinflammation, regression of liver fibrosis, or both. Actually, some studies have observed a significant LS reduction during NUC treatment even in the presence of limited or no improvement of histological fibrosis [86, 87, 91].

Finally, in CHB patients, the optimal threshold values to identify residual severe fibrosis or cirrhosis after NUC treatment are likely to be lower than those identified in treatment-naive patients, but such values need definition in further studies.

9.6 Conclusions

In the literature, there is consistent evidence indicating that LS values significantly decrease during and after antiviral therapy in both CHC and HBV patients.

Some studies with paired liver biopsy, before and after antiviral treatment, have documented a significant reduction of necroinflammatory activity and fibrosis score in both the conditions.

On the other hand, the major limitation of most of the studies is that they were performed without the availability of paired histological results, and thus it remains unclear whether the reduction of TE values is closely correlated with the regression of liver fibrosis or simply related to the improvement in necroinflammatory scores.

Another relevant issue that should to be considered is about the time at which the determination of liver stiffness is performed. Actually, on the basis of the present knowledge, the rapid decrease in liver stiffness after viral clearance is likely to be related to the reduction of necroinflammation, while the *true* reduction of liver fibrosis related to an architectural remodeling of the liver parenchyma is likely to occur later on, when a further slow decrease in liver stiffness is possibly observed. Unfortunately, the majority of the studies in the literature have follow-up periods usually around 12 months long too short to discriminate between the two phases.

Given that the first and rapid reduction of LS is mainly attributable to the disappearance of inflammation paralleling, as in some studies, the decrease in transaminase levels [61, 86, 87, 91], LS monitoring during antiviral treatment does not appear clinically relevant.

Then, in the next period, there is a gradual LS reduction that is compatible with an improvement in fibrosis. However, as the cutoff values currently used for elastography techniques have been defined and tested on patients with active chronic hepatitis, it is not reliable to interpret TE evaluation in long-term HCV responders or in patients on a NUC regimen with these same cutoff values. Indeed, liver remodeling occurring after treatment could decrease TE ability to rule the presence of cirrhosis out and the routine use of noninvasive tests after antiviral treatment has a high false-negative rate. Thus, as indicated by the guidelines of many scientific societies [8–10, 110], screening for hepatocellular carcinoma and other main complications of liver cirrhosis should be continued despite the decrease in liver stiffness in both CHC and CHB patients.

In addition, when considering the literature results, the possible presence of such confounding factors as obesity, steatosis, diabetes, or concomitant alcohol abuse should be accounted for, because the liver elasticity in such subsets of patients might be affected and, sometimes, might worsen in spite of antiviral therapy.

In summary, according to the results in the literature, liver biopsy still remains the only reliable approach in CHC patients to stage liver fibrosis after SVR.

In non-cirrhotic CHC patients, for whom clinical surveillance is not indicated, routine LS measurement during treatment or after SVR does not add to their clinical disease management.

In this setting, a periodical clinical assessment including LS measurement might be indicated only in the presence of cofactors (such as alcohol abuse or metabolic syndrome, diabetes, etc.) [110].

In CHC patients with severe fibrosis/cirrhosis prior to treatment, the progressive decrease of LS observed after 6–12 months of follow-up is likely to be related to fibrosis regression. However, LS monitoring after SVR, having a high false-negative rate, cannot be used to diagnose residual cirrhosis or to stop HCC surveillance.

On the other hand, a sudden LS increase during follow-up after SVR should always be considered as a warning signal for the presence of cofactors or the development of such relevant complications as HCC or clinical decompensation.

In CHB patients, a significant reduction of fibrosis or reversal of liver cirrhosis is reported after prolonged treatment with NUCs. In this case, serial LS measurements a few months after treatment and normalization of ALT can be useful to define a reliable baseline value to monitor the changes in liver fibrosis.

As concerns both CHC and CHB patients with severe fibrosis or cirrhosis, the prognostic value of LS determination (before and after antiviral treatment) to stratify patients according to major clinical outcomes (survival, OLT, etc.) and the risk of developing major complications, such as HCC, is addressed in other chapters of this book.

References

1. Bravo AA, Sheth SG, Chopra S. Liver biopsy. N Engl J Med. 2001;344:495–500.
2. Piccinino F, Sagnelli E, Pasquale G, Giusti G. Complications following percutaneous liver biopsy. A multicentre retrospective study on 68,276 biopsies. J Hepatol. 1986;2:165–73.
3. Bedossa P, Dargere D, Paradis V. Sampling variability of liver fibrosis in chronic hepatitis C. Hepatology. 2003;38:1449–57.
4. Sandrin L, Fourquet B, Hasquenoph JM, Yon S, Fournier C, Mal F, et al. Transient elastography: a new noninvasive method for assessment of hepatic fibrosis. Ultrasound Med Biol. 2003;29:1705–13.

5. Ziol M, Handra-Luca A, Kettaneh A, Christidis C, Mal F, Kazemi F, et al. Noninvasive assessment of liver fibrosis by measurement of stiffness in patients with chronic hepatitis C. Hepatology. 2005;41:48–54.
6. Castera L, Vergniol J, Foucher J, Le Bail B, Chanteloup E, Haaser M, et al. Prospective comparison of transient elastography, Fibrotest, APRI, and liver biopsy for the assessment of fibrosis in chronic hepatitis C. Gastroenterology. 2005;128:343–50.
7. Foucher J, Chanteloup E, Vergniol J, Castéra L, Le Bail B, Adhoute X, et al. Diagnosis of cirrhosis by transient elastography (Fibroscan): a prospective study. Gut. 2006; 55:403–8.
8. Dietrich CF, Bamber J, Berzigotti A, Bota S, Cantisani V, Castera L, et al. EFSUMB guidelines and recommendations on the clinical use of liver ultrasound elastography, Update 2017. Ultraschall Med. 2017;38(4):e48. https://doi.org/10.1055/a-0641-0076.
9. Ferraioli G, Wong VW-S, Castera L, Berzigotti A, Sporea I, Dietrich C, et al. Liver ultrasound elastography: an update to the world federation for ultrasound in medicine and biology guidelines and recommendations. Ultrasound Med Biol. 2018;44(12):2419–40.
10. European Association for the Study of the Liver. EASL recommendations on treatment of hepatitis C 2016. J Hepatol. 2017;66:153–94. https://doi.org/10.1016/j.jhep.2016.09.001.
11. Mallet V, Gilgenkrantz H, Serpaggi J, Verkarre V, Vallet-Pichard A, Fontaine H, Pol S. Brief communication: the relationship of regression of cirrhosis to outcome in chronic hepatitis C. Ann Intern Med. 2008;149(6):399–403.
12. George SL, Bacon BR, Brunt EM, Mihindukulasuriya KL, Hoffmann J, Di Bisceglie AM. Clinical, virologic, histologic, and biochemical outcomes after successful HCV therapy: a 5-year follow-up of 150 patients. Hepatology. 2009;49:729–38. https://doi.org/10.1002/hep.22694.
13. Veldt BJ, Heathcote EJ, Wedemeyer H, Reichen J, Hofmann WP, Zeuzem S, et al. Sustained virologic response and clinical outcomes in patients with chronic hepatitis C and advanced fibrosis. Ann Intern Med. 2007;147:677–84.
14. Lupşor M, Badea R, Stefănescu H, Grigorescu M, Sparchez Z, Serban A, et al. Analysis of histopathological changes that influence liver stiffness in chronic hepatitis C. Results from a cohort of 324 patients. J Gastrointestin Liver Dis. 2008;17:155–63.
15. Arena U, Vizzutti F, Abraldes JG, Corti G, Stasi C, Moscarella S, et al. Reliability of transient elastography for the diagnosis of advanced fibrosis in chronic hepatitis C. Gut. 2008;57:1288–93.
16. Fraquelli M, Rigamonti C, Casazza G, Donato MF, Ronchi G, Conte D, et al. Etiology-related determinants of liver stiffness values in chronic viral hepatitis B or C. J Hepatol. 2011 Apr;54(4):621–8.
17. Andersen ES, Moessner BK, Christensen PB, Kjær M, Krarup H, Lillevanget S, et al. Lower liver stiffness in patients with sustained virological response 4 years after treatment for chronic hepatitis C. Eur J Gastroenterol Hepatol. 2011;23:41–4.
18. Hezode C, Castera L, Roudot-Thoraval F, Bouvier-Alias M, Rosa I, Roulot D, et al. Liver stiffness diminishes with antiviral response in chronic hepatitis C. Aliment Pharmacol Ther. 2011;34:656–63.
19. Ogawa E, Furusyo N, Toyoda K, Takeoka H, Maeda S, Hayashi J. The longitudinal quantitative assessment by transient elastography of chronic hepatitis C patients treated with pegylated interferon alpha-2b and ribavirin. Antivir Res. 2009;83(2):127.
20. Mueller S, Millonig G, Sarovska L, Friedrich S, Reimann FM, Pritsch M, et al. Increased liver stiffness in alcoholic liver disease: differentiating fibrosis from steatohepatitis. World J Gastroenterol. 2010;16:966–72.
21. Coco B, Oliveri F, Maina AM, Ciccorossi P, Sacco R, Colombatto P, et al. Transient elastography: a new surrogate marker of liver fibrosis influenced by major changes of transaminases. J Viral Hepat. 2007;14(5):360–9.
22. Viganò M, Massironi S, Lampertico P, Iavarone M, Paggi S, Pozzi R, et al. Transient elastography assessment of the liver stiffness dynamics during acute hepatitis B. Eur J Gastroenterol Hepatol. 2010;22:180–4.

23. Millonig G, Reimann FM, Friedrich S, Fonouni H, Mehrabi A, Buchler MW, et al. Extrahepatic cholestasis increases liver stiffness (FibroScan) irrespective of fibrosis. Hepatology. 2008;48:1718–23.

24. Millonig G, Friedrich S, Adolf S, Fonouni H, Golriz M, Mehrabi A, et al. Liver stiffness is directly influenced by central venous pressure. J Hepatol. 2010;52:206–10.

25. Colli A, Pozzoni P, Berzuini A, Gerosa A, Canovi C, Molteni EE, et al. Decompensated chronic heart failure: increased liver stiffness measured by means of transient elastography. Radiology. 2010;257(3):872–8.

26. Poynard T, Moussalli J, Munteanu M, Thabut D, Lebray P, Rudler M, et al. Slow regression of liver fibrosis presumed by repeated biomarkers after virological cure in patients with chronic hepatitis C. J Hepatol. 2013;59:675–83. https://doi.org/10.1016/j.jhep.2013.05.015.

27. D'Ambrosio R, Aghemo A, Rumi MG, Ronchi G, Donato MF, Paradis V, et al. A morphometric and immunohistochemical study to assess the benefit of a sustained virological response in hepatitis C virus patients with cirrhosis. Hepatology. 2012;56(2):532–43.

28. D'Ambrosio R, Aghemo A, Fraquelli M, Rumi MG, Donato MF, Paradis V, et al. The diagnostic accuracy of Fibroscan for cirrhosis is influenced by liver morphometry in HCV in patients with a sustained virological response. J Hepatol. 2013;59:251–6. https://doi.org/10.1016/j.jhep.2013.03.013.

29. Patel K, Friedrich-Rust M, Lurie Y, Grigorescu M, Stanciu C, Lee C-M, et al. FibroSURE and FibroScan in relation to treatment response in chronic hepatitis C virus. World J Gastroenterol. 2011;17(41):4581–9.

30. El Saadany S, Soliman H, Ziada DH, Hamisa M, Hefeda M, Selim A, et al. Fibroscan versus liver biopsy in the evaluation of response among the Egyptian HCV infected patients to treatment. Egypt J Radiol Nucl Med. 2016;47(1):1–7.

31. Stasi C, Arena U, Zignego AL, Corti G, Monti M, Triboli E, et al. Longitudinal assessment of liver stiffness in patients undergoing antiviral treatment for hepatitis C. Dig Liver Dis. 2013;45:840–3. https://doi.org/10.1016/j.dld.2013.03.023.

32. Chen Yi Mei SLG, Thompson AJ, Christensen B, Cunningham G, McDonald L, Bell S, et al. Sustained virological response halts fibrosis progression: a long-term follow-up study of people with chronic hepatitis C infection. PLoS One. 2017;12(10):e0185609.

33. Chen SH, Lai HC, Chiang IP, Su WP, Lin CH, Kao JT, et al. Changes in liver stiffness measurement using acoustic radiation force impulse elastography after antiviral therapy in patients with chronic hepatitis C. PLoS One. 2018;13(1):e0190455.

34. Tachi Y, Hirai T, Kojima Y, Miyata A, Ohara K, Ishizu Y, et al. Liver stiffness measurement using acoustic radiation force impulse elastography in hepatitis C virus-infected patients with a sustained virological response. Aliment Pharmacol Ther. 2016;44:346–55.

35. Vergniol J, Foucher J, Castéra L, Bernard PH, Tournan R, Terrebonne E, et al. Changes of non-invasive markers and fibroScan values during HCV treatment. J Viral Hepat. 2009;16(2):132–40.

36. Arima Y, Kawabe N, Hashimoto S, Harata M, Nitta Y, Murao M, et al. Reduction of liver stiffness by interferon treatment in the patients with chronic hepatitis C. Hepatol Res. 2010;40:383–92.

37. Macìas J, del Valle J, Rivero A, Mira JA, Camacho A, Merchante N, et al. Changes in liver stiffness in patients with chronic hepatitis C with and without HIV co-infection treated with pegylated interferon plus ribavirin. J Antimicrob Chemoter. 2010;65(10):2204–11.

38. Wang JH, Yen YH, Yao CC, Hung CH, Chen CH, Hu TH, et al. Liver stiffness-based score in hepatoma risk assessment for chronic hepatitis C patients after successful antiviral therapy. Liver Int. 2016;36(12):1793–9.

39. Martinez SM, Foucher J, Combis J-M, Metivier S, Brunetto M, Capron D, et al. Longitudinal liver stiffness assessment in patients with chronic hepatitis C undergoing antiviral therapy. PLoS One. 2012;7(10):e47715.

40. Osakabe K, Ichino N, Nishikawa T, Sugiyama H, Kato M, Shibata A, et al. Changes of shear-wave velocity by interferon-based therapy in chronic hepatitis C. World J Gastroenterol. 2015;21(35):10215–23.

41. Soliman H, Ziada D, Salama M, Hamisa M, Badawi R, Hawash N, et al. Predictors for fibrosis regression in chronic HCV patients after the treatment with DAAS: results of a real-world color study. Endocr Metab Immune Disord Drug Targets. 2020;20(1):104–11.

42. Calvaruso V, Di Marco V, Ferraro D, Petta S, Calì A, Bavetta MG, et al. Fibrosis evaluation by transient elastography in patients with long-term sustained HCV clearance. Hepat Mon. 2013;13:e7176.

43. Poynard T, Ngo Y, Munteanu M, Tabut D, Massard J, Moussali J, et al. Biomarkers of liver injury for hepatitis clinical trials: a meta-analysis of longitudinal studies. Antivir Ther. 2010;15(4):617–31.

44. Pan JJ, Bao F, Du E, Skillin C, Frenette C, Waalen J, et al. Morphometry confirms fibrosis regression from sustained virologic response to direct-acting antivirals for hepatitis C. Hepatol Commun. 2018;2(11):1320–30.

45. Enomoto M, Ikura Y, Tamori A, Kozuka R, Motoyama H, Kawamura E, et al. Short-term histological evaluations after achieving a sustained virologic response to direct-acting antiviral treatment for chronic hepatitis C. United European Gastroenterol J. 2018;6:1391–400.

46. Huang R, Rao H, Yang M, Gao Y, Wang J, Jin Q, et al. Noninvasive measurements predict liver fibrosis well in hepatitis C virus patients after direct-acting antiviral therapy. Dig Dis Sci. 2020;65(5):1491–500.

47. Knop V, Hoppe D, Welzel T, Vermehren J, Herrmann E, Vermehren A, et al. Regression of fibrosis and portal hypertension in HCV-associated cirrhosis and sustained virologic response after interferon-free antiviral therapy. J Viral Hepat. 2016;23:994–1002.

48. Chekuri S, Nickerson J, Bichoupan K, Sefcik R, Doobay K, Chang S, et al. Liver stiffness decreases rapidly in response to successful hepatitis C treatment and then plateaus. PLoS One. 2016;11(7):e0159413.

49. Pons M, Santos B, Simón-Talero M, Ventura-Cots M, Riveiro-Barciela M, Esteban R, et al. Rapid liver and spleen stiffness improvement in compensated advanced chronic liver disease patients treated with oral antivirals. Ther Adv Gastroenterol. 2017;10(8):619–29.

50. Elsharkawy A, Abdel Alem S, Fouad R, El Raziky M, El Akel W, Abdo M, et al. Changes in liver stiffness measurements and fibrosis scores following sofosbuvir based treatment regimens without interferon. J Gastroenterol Hepatol. 2017;32:1624–30.

51. Dolmazashvili E, Abutidze A, Chkhartishvili N, Karchava M, Sharvadze L, Tsertsvadze T. Regression of liver fibrosis over a 24-week period after completing direct-acting antiviral therapy in patients with chronic hepatitis C receiving care within the national hepatitis C elimination program in Georgia: results of hepatology clinic HEPA experience. Eur J Gastroenterol Hepatol. 2017;29(11):1223–30.

52. Bachofner JA, Valli PV, Kroger A, Bergamin I, Kunzler P, Baserga A, et al. Direct antiviral agent treatment of chronic hepatitis C results in rapid regression of transient elastography and fibrosis markers fibrosis-4 score and aspartate aminotransferase platelet ratio index. Liver Int. 2017;37:369–76. https://doi.org/10.1111/liv.13256.

53. Sporea I, Lupușoru R, Mare R, Popescu A, Gheorghe L, Iacob S, et al. Dynamics of liver stiffness values by means of transient elastography in patients with HCV liver cirrhosis undergoing interferon free treatment. Gastrointest Liver Dis. 2017;26:145–50.

54. Tada T, Kumada T, Toyoda H, Sone Y, Takeshima K, Ogawa S, et al. Viral eradication reduces both liver stiffness and steatosis in patients with chronic hepatitis C virus infection who received direct-acting anti-viral therapy. Aliment Pharmacol Ther. 2018;47(7):1012–22.

55. Tada T, Kumada T, Toyoda H, Mizuno K, Sone Y, Kataoka S, et al. Improvement of liver stiffness in patients with hepatitis C virus infection who received direct-acting antiviral therapy and achieved sustained virological response. J Gastroenterol Hepatol. 2017;32(12):1982–8.

56. Hamada K, Saitoh S, Nishino N, Fukushima D, Horikawa Y, Nishida S, et al. Shear wave elastography predicts hepatocellular carcinoma risk in hepatitis C patients after sustained virological response. PLoS One. 2018;13(4):e0195173.

57. Ohya K, Akuta N, Suzuki F, Fujiyama S, Kawamura Y, Kominami Y, et al. Predictors of treatment efficacy and liver stiffness changes following therapy with Sofosbuvir plus Ribavirin in patients infected with HCV genotype 2. J Med Virol. 2018;90(5):919–25.

58. Ravaioli F, Conti F, Brillanti S, Andreone P, Mazzella G, Buonfiglioli F, et al. Hepatocellular carcinoma risk assessment by the measurement of liver stiffness variations in HCV cirrhotics treated with direct acting antivirals. Dig Liver Dis. 2018;50(6):573–9.

59. Noureddin M, Wong MM, Todo T, Lu SC, Sanyal AJ, Mena EA. Fatty liver in hepatitis C patients post-sustained virological response with direct-acting antivirals. World J Gastroenterol. 2018;24(11):1269–77.

60. Omar H, Said M, Eletreby R, Mehrez M, Bassam M, Abdellatif Z, et al. Longitudinal assessment of hepatic fibrosis in responders to direct-acting antivirals for recurrent hepatitis C after liver transplantation using noninvasive methods. Clin Transpl. 2018;32(8):e13334.

61. Chan J, Gogela N, Zheng H, Lammert S, Ajayi T, Fricker Z, et al. Direct-acting antiviral therapy for chronic HCV infection results in liver stiffness regression over 12 months post-treatment. Dig Dis Sci. 2018;63(2):486–92.

62. Persico M, Rosato V, Aglitti A, Precone D, Corrado M, De Luna A, et al. Sustained virological response by direct antiviral agents in HCV leads to an early and significant improvement of liver fibrosis. Antivir Ther. 2018;23(2):129–38.

63. Facciorusso A, Del Prete V, Turco A, Buccino RV, Nacchiero MC, Muscatiello N. Long-term liver stiffness assessment in hepatitis C virus patients undergoing antiviral therapy: results from a 5-year color study. J Gastroenterol Hepatol. 2018;33(4):942–9.

64. Akuta N, Toyota J, Karino Y, Ikeda F, Ido A, Tanaka K, et al. Potent viral suppression and improvements in alpha-fetoprotein and measures of fibrosis in Japanese patients receiving a daclatasvir/asunaprevir/beclabuvir fixed-dose combination for the treatment of HCV genotype-1 infection. J Gastroenterol. 2018;53(9):1089–97.

65. Ogasawara N, Kobayashi M, Akuta N, Kominami Y, Fujiyama S, Kawamura Y, et al. Serial changes in liver stiffness and controlled attenuation parameter following direct-acting antiviral therapy against hepatitis C virus genotype 1b. J Med Virol. 2018;90(2):313–9.

66. Kobayashi N, Iijima H, Tada T, Kumada T, Yoshida M, Aoki T, et al. Changes in liver stiffness and steatosis among patients with hepatitis C virus infection who received direct-acting antiviral therapy and achieved sustained virological response. Eur J Gastroenterol Hepatol. 2018;30(5):546–51.

67. Flisiak R, Janczewska E, Lucejko M, Karpinska E, Zerebska-Michaluk D, Nazzal K, et al. Durability of virologic response, risk of de novo hepatocellular carcinoma, liver function and stiffness 2 years after treatment with ombitasvir/paritaprevir/ritonavir±dasabuvir ±ribavirin in the AMBER, real-world experience study. J Viral Hepat. 2018;25(11):1298–305.

68. Lee Y-C, Hu T-H, Hung C-H, Lu S-N, Chen C-H, Wang J-H. The change in liver stiffness, controlled attenuation parameter and fibrosis-4 index for chronic hepatitis C patients with direct-acting antivirals. PLoS One. 2019;14(4):e0214323.

69. Rout G, Nayak B, Patel AH, Gunjan D, Singh V, Kedia S, et al. Therapy with oral directly acting agents in hepatitis C infection is associated with reduction in fibrosis and increase in hepatic steatosis on transient elastography. J Clin Exp Hepatol. 2019;9(2):207–14.

70. Hsu W-F, Lai H-C, Su W-P, Lin C-H, Chuang P-H, Chen S-H, et al. Rapid decline of noninvasive fibrosis index values in patients with hepatitis C receiving treatment with direct-acting antiviral agents. BMC Gastroenterol. 2019;19:63.

71. Giannini E, Crespi M, Demarzo M, Bodini G, Furnari M, Marabotto E, et al. Improvement in hepatitis C virus patients with advanced, compensated liver disease after sustained virological response to direct acting antivirals. Eur J Clin Investig. 2019;49(3):e13056.

72. Kohla MAS, El Fayoumi A, Akl M, Abdelkareem M, Elsakhawy M, Waheed S, et al. Early fibrosis regression by shear wave elastography after successful direct-acting anti-HCV therapy. Clin Exp Med. 2020;20(1):143–8.

73. Kawagishi N, Suda G, Kimura M, Maehara O, Shimazaki T, Yamada R, et al. High serum angiopoietin-2 level predicts non-regression of liver stiffness measurement-based liver fibrosis stage after direct-acting antiviral therapy for hepatitis C. Hepatol Res. 2020;50(6):671–81.

74. Stasi C, Sadalla S, Carradori E, Monti M, Petraccia L, Madia F, et al. Longitudinal evaluation of liver stiffness and outcomes in patients with chronic hepatitis C before and after short- and long-term IFN-free antiviral treatment. Curr Med Res Opin. 2020;36(2):245–9.

75. Bernuth S, Yagmur E, Schuppan D, Sprinzl MF, Zimmermann A, Schad A, et al. Early changes in dynamic biomarkers of liver fibrosis in hepatitis C virus-infected patients treated with sofosbuvir. Dig Liver Dis. 2016;48:291–7.
76. Yada N, Sakurai T, Minami T, Arizumi T, Takita M, Inoue T, et al. Ultrasound elastography correlates treatment response by antiviral therapy in patients with chronic hepatitis C. Oncology. 2014;87(Suppl1):118–23.
77. Suda T, Okawa O, Masaoka R, Gyotoku Y, Tokutomi N, Katayama Y, et al. Shear wave elastography in hepatitis C patients before and after antiviral therapy. World J Hepatol. 2017;9(1):64–8.
78. Lu M, Li J, Zhang T, Rupp LB, Trudeau S, Holmberg SD, et al. Serum biomarkers Indicate long-term reduction in liver fibrosis in patients with sustained virological response to treatment for HCV infection. Clin Gastroenterol Hepatol. 2016;14(7):1044–55.
79. Elsharkawy A, Abdel Alem S, Fouad R, El Raziky M, El Akel W, Abdo M, et al. Changes in liver stiffness measurements and fibrosis scores following sofosbuvir based treatment regimens without Interferon. J Gastroenterol Hepatol. 2017;32(9):1624–30. https://doi.org/10.1111/jgh.13758.
80. Nascimbeni F, Lebray P, Fedchuk L, Oliveira CP, Alvares-da-Silva MR, Varault A, et al. Significant variations in elastometry measurements made within short-term in patients with chronic liver diseases. Clin Gastroenterol Hepatol. 2015;13:763–71.e1-e6. https://doi.org/10.1016/j.cgh.2014.07.037.
81. Sáez-Royuela F, Linares P, Cervera LA, Almohalla C, Jorquera F, Lorenzo S, et al. Evaluation of advanced fibrosis measured by transient elastography after hepatitis C virus protease inhibitor-based triple therapy. Eur J Gastroenterol Hepatol. 2016;28(3):305–12.
82. Fattovich G, Brollo L, Giustina G, Noventa F, Pontisso P, Alberti A, et al. Natural history and prognostic factors for chronic hepatitis type B. Gut. 1991;32:294–8.
83. Dienstag JL, Goldin RD, Heathcote EJ, Hann HWL, Woessner M, Stephenson SL, et al. Histological outcome during long-term lamivudine therapy. Gastroenterology. 2003;124:105–17. https://doi.org/10.1053/gast.2003.50013.
84. Chang T-T, Liaw Y-F, Wu S-S, Schiff E, Han K-H, Lai C-L, et al. Long-term entecavir therapy results in the reversal of fibrosis/cirrhosis and continued histological improvement in patients with chronic hepatitis B. Hepatology. 2010;52:886–93. https://doi.org/10.1002/hep.2378.
85. Marcellin P, Gane E, Buti M, Afdhal N, Sievert W, Jacobson IM, et al. Regression of cirrhosis during treatment with tenofovir disoproxil fumarate for chronic hepatitis B: a 5-year open-label follow-up study. Lancet. 2013;381(9865):468–75.
86. Liang X, Xie Q, Tan D, Ning Q, Niu J, Bai X, et al. Interpretation of liver stiffness measurement-based approach for the monitoring of hepatitis B patients with antiviral therapy: a 2-year prospective study. J Viral Hepat. 2017;25(3):296–305.
87. Wong GL-H, Wong VW-S, Choi PC-L, Chan AW-H, Chim AM-L, Yiu KK-L, et al. On-treatment monitoring of liver fibrosis with transient elastography in chronic hepatitis B patients. Antiv Ther. 2011;16:165–72.
88. Wu SD, Liu LL, Cheng JL, Liu Y, Cheng LS, Wang SQ, et al. Longitudinal monitoring of liver fibrosis status by transient elastography in chronic hepatitis B patients during long-term entecavir treatment. Clin Exp Med. 2018;18(3):433–43.
89. Enomoto M, Mori M, Ogawa T, Fujii H, Kobayashi S, Iwai S, et al. Usefulness of transient elastography for assessment of liver fibrosis in chronic hepatitis B: regression of liver stiffness during entecavir therapy. Hepatol Res. 2010;40(9):853–61.
90. Kim SU, Park JY, Kim DY, Ahn SH, Choi EH, Seok JY, et al. Non-invasive assessment of changes in liver fibrosis via liver stiffness measurement in patients with chronic hepatitis B: impact of antiviral treatment on fibrosis regression. Hepatol Int. 2010;4(4):673–80.
91. Lim SG, Cho SW, Lee YC, Jeon SJ, Lee MH, Cho YJ, et al. Changes in liver stiffness measurement during antiviral therapy in patients with chronic hepatitis B. Hepato-Gastroenterol. 2011;58(106):539–45.
92. Zeng D-W, Dong J, Liu Y-R, Jiang J-J, Zhu Y-Y. Noninvasive models for assessment of liver fibrosis in patients with chronic hepatitis B virus infection. World J Gastroenterol. 2016;22(29):6663–72.

93. Sun Y, Zhou J, Wang L, Wu X, Chen Y, Piao H, et al. New classification of liver biopsy assessment for fibrosis in chronic hepatitis B patients before and after treatment. Viral Hepat. 2017;65(5):1438–50.
94. Jeon MY, Lee HW, Kim SU, Heo JY, Han S, Kim BK, et al. Subcirrhotic liver stiffness by FibroScan correlates with lower risk of hepatocellular carcinoma in patients with HBV-related cirrhosis. Hepatol Int. 2017;11(3):268–76.
95. Stasi C, Salomoni E, Arena U, Corti G, Montalto P, Bartalesi F, et al. Non-invasive assessment of liver fibrosis in patients with HBV-related chronic liver disease undergoing antiviral treatment: a preliminary study. Eur J Pharmacol. 2017;5(806):105–9.
96. Olivieri F, Coco B, Ciccorossi P, Colombatto P, Romagnoli V, Cherubini B, et al. Liver stiffness in the hepatitis B virus carrier: a non-invasive marker of liver disease influenced by the pattern of transaminases. World J Gastroenterol. 2008;14(40):6154–62.
97. Osakabe K, Ichino N, Nishikawa T, Sugiyama H, Kato M, Kitahara S, et al. Reduction of liver stiffness by antiviral therapy in chronic hepatitis B. J Gastroenterol. 2011;46(11):1324–34.
98. Andersen ES, Weiland O, Leutscher P, Krarup H, Westin J, Moessner B, et al. Low liver stiffness among cirrhotic patients with hepatitis B after prolonged treatment with nucleoside analogs. Scand J Gastroenterol. 2011;46:760–6.
99. Fung J, Lai CL, Wong DK, Seto WK, Hung I, Yuen MF. Significant changes in liver stiffness measurements in patients with chronic hepatitis B: 3-year follow-up study. J Viral Hepat. 2011;18:e200–5.
100. Kim BK, Oh HJ, Park JY, Kim DY, Ahn SH, Han KH, et al. Early on-treatment change in liver-related events in chronic hepatitis B patients receiving antiviral therapy. Liver Int. 2013;33(2):180–9.
101. Yan L-B, Zhu X, Bai L, Liang L-B, Chen E-Q, Du L-Y, et al. Impact of mild to moderate elevations of alanine aminotransferase on liver stiffness measurement in chronic hepatitis B patients during antiviral therapy. Hepatol Res. 2013;43(2):185–91.
102. Jang W, Yu SI, Sinn DH, Park SH, Park H, Park JY, et al. Longitudinal change of liver stiffness by transient elastography in chronic hepatitis B patients treated with nucleos(t)ide analogue. Clin Res Hepatol Gastroenterol. 2014;38:195–200.
103. Kuo Y-H, Lu S-N, Chen C-H, Chang K-C, Hung C-H, Tai W-C, et al. The changes of liver stiffness and its associated chronic hepatitis B patients with entecavir therapy. PLoS One. 2014;9(3):e93160.
104. Wang H-M, Hung C-H, Lee C-M, Lu S-N, Wang J-H, Yen Y-H, et al. Three-year efficacy and safety of tenofovir in nucleos(t)ide analog-naïve and nucleos(t)ide analog-experienced chronic hepatitis B patients. J Gastroenterol Hepatol. 2016;31:1307–14.
105. Tengaara IR, Lesmana CR, Gani RA. Treatment response monitoring of chronic hepatitis B patients using transient elastography and aspartate aminotransferase-to-pleatelet ratio index (APRI). Acta Med Indones. 2017;49(3):220–6.
106. Chon YE, Park JY, Myoung S-M, Jung KS, Kim BK, Kim SU, et al. Improvement of liver fibrosis after long-term antiviral therapy assessed by fibrosa in chronic hepatitis B patients with advanced fibrosis. Am J Gastroenterol. 2017;112(6):882–91.
107. Rinaldi L, Ascione A, Messina V, Rosato V, Valente G, Sangiovanni V, et al. Influence of antiviral therapy on the liver stiffness in chronic HBV hepatitis. Infection. 2018;46(2):31–238.
108. Lai CL, Chien RN, Leung NW, Chang TT, Guan R, Tai DI, et al. A one-year trial of lamivudine for chronic hepatitis B. Asia Hepatitis Lamivudine Study Group. N Engl J Med. 1998;339(2):61–8.
109. Facciorusso A, Garcia Perdomo HA, Muscatiello N, Buccino RV, Wong VW, Singh S. Systematic review with meta-analysis: change in liver stiffness during anti-viral therapy in patients with hepatitis B. Dig Liver Dis. 2018;50(8):787–94.
110. Lim JK, et al. American Gastroenterological Association Institute guidelines on the role of elastography in the evaluation of liver fibrosis. Gastroenterology. 2017;152:15436–1543.

Laurent Castera

10.1 Available Elastography Methods

10.1.1 Principle and Characteristics

They are two different kinds of elastography methods: ultrasound (US)- and magnetic resonance (MR)-based. The former uses ultrasound to detect the velocity of the microdisplacements (shear waves) induced in the liver tissue, whereas the latter uses the magnetic resonance scanner [1]. The shear wave's velocity is then converted into a liver stiffness measurement, expressed in kilopascals (kPa) or in meter/second (m/s). US-based elastography methods include transient elastography (TE); point shear wave elastography (pSWE), also known as Acoustic Radiation Force Impulse Imaging (ARFI); and two-dimensional shear wave elastography (2D-SWE).

Transient elastography (TE) was the first commercially available elastography system (FibroScan, Echosens, Paris, France), introduced in Europe in 2003 and FDA approved in the United States in 2013 [2]. VCTE delivers a 50 Hz mechanical impulse to the skin surface and then measures the velocity of the generated shear wave (Fig. 10.1). There are several probes available, with the M probe used for standard examinations and the XL probe introduced to increase the reliability of TE measurements in high BMI patients [3].

pSWE/ARFI techniques, integrated in conventional ultrasound systems, use focused US "push" pulses to deform internal tissue and generate shear waves [4]. Originally available in Siemens systems (Virtual Touch Quantification™ Acuson 2000, Siemens Healthineers, Erlangen, Germany), ARFI methods are now integrated into their clinical ultrasound systems by most vendors [1]. Region of interest (ROI) localization can be chosen under B-mode visualization. A single acoustic

L. Castera (✉)
Service d'Hépatologie, Hôpital Beaujon, Assistance Publique-Hôpitaux de Paris, INSERM
UMR 1149-CRI, Université de Paris, Clichy, France
e-mail: laurent.castera@bjn.aphp.fr

© Springer Nature Switzerland AG 2021
M. Fraquelli (ed.), *Elastography of the Liver and Beyond*,
https://doi.org/10.1007/978-3-030-74132-7_10

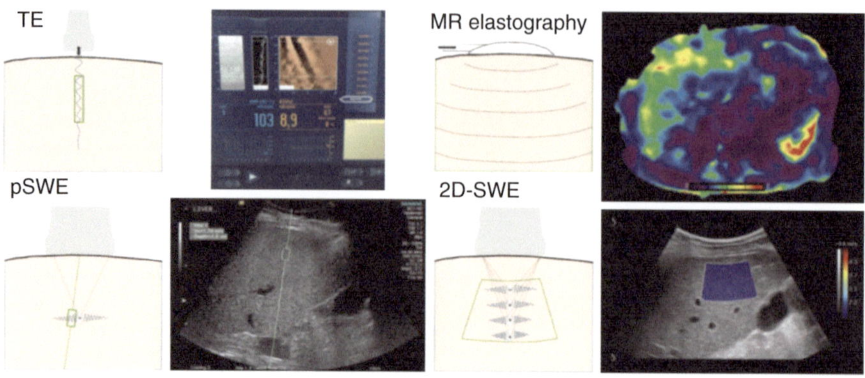

Fig. 10.1 This figure illustrates the four elastography methods available: US elastography, including TE (FibroScan, Echosens), pSWE/ARFI (Virtual Touch Quantification, Siemens Acuson S2000), 2D-SWE (Aixplorer, Supersonic Imagine), and MR elastography. Region of interest (ROI) for each method is depicted by enclosed green area. (Adapted from ref. [1])

impulse is used to induce a shear wave within a small ROI (approximately 1.0×0.5 cm), and the velocity of shear waves is measured in meter/second or kPa. The technique for shear wave induction, the frequencies used, as well as the size of ROI differ between companies and need be taken into account when interpreting the results [5–7]. Measurement should be performed 1–3 cm below the liver capsule. The median of ten measurements should be used for clinical interpretation. Improved quality is obtained by pSWE estimation algorithms, which warn the user if measurement is not adequate. In addition, quality criteria such as an IQR/median $\leq 30\%$ and standard deviation $\leq 30\%$ have been reported to improve accuracy [6].

2D-SWE, like ARFI, is integrated in conventional ultrasonography systems, enabling the additional performance of elastography with the same probes as abdominal ultrasound (Fig. 10.1). Originally available clinically in Supersonic Imagine system (Aixplorer™, Supersonic Imagine, Aix-en-Provence, France), 2D-SWE are now integrated in their systems by several vendors [1]. Multiple shear waves are induced using acoustic impulses. The size of the ROI can be increased to approximately 2×2 cm and shown as either single image or in real-time. Velocity of stiffness can then be measured at varying locations within this ROI, and statistical quantities such as the mean, standard deviation, minimum and maximum values of the 2D-SWE, or Young's modulus in kPa are calculated and displayed. The measurement box should be placed at least 10 mm below the liver capsule. At least three measurements should be obtained, and the report should include median and IQR. The technique for shear wave induction, as well as the frequencies used, differs between companies and should be taken into account when interpreting the results. All 2D-SWE systems have some kind of quality indicators of the shear wave speed estimate. However, quality criteria for clinical interpretation remain poorly evaluated [5–7].

In contrast to US elastography systems, MR elastography (MRE) quantifies mechanical properties through "direct inversion" of the visualized "wave field" into a map of the mechanical parameter of interest without the intermediate step of measuring shear wave speed. MRE requires a special adaptation and proprietary hardware and software installment (Resoundant Inc., Rochester, MN, USA) over conventional MRI scanners and reports the shear stiffness of tissue, which is the magnitude of the complex shear modulus, $|G^*|$. MRE was FDA approved in 2009 and initially introduced on GE systems, but has since become available on Siemens and Philips MR systems. Magnetic resonance elastography (MRE) enables the measurement of liver stiffness with a 2D gradient echo using a 1.5 or 3 T magnetic resonance systems [1].

Care must be taken when comparing results between US and MR elastography due to the different parameters reported. An obstacle to direct comparison between techniques is the frequency dependence of biological tissue. Higher frequency shear waves produce higher stress and strain rates, resulting in higher stiffness measurements. This can be problematic when comparing US elastography techniques, as TE operates at 50 Hz, whereas ARFI and 2D-SWE operate at frequencies of 100–500 Hz [8]. The frequency dependence, method of measurement, and parameter reported (wave speed, E, or G^*) should be considered when comparing elastography techniques.

10.1.2 Reliability, Failure Rates, and Applicability of Elastography Methods

In the largest series to date, on more than 13,000 examinations in 7261 European patients with chronic liver disease seen over a 5-year period, failure to obtain any measurement was observed in 3% of cases and unreliable results (not meeting manufacturer's recommendations) in 16% [9], mostly due to patient obesity or limited operator experience. As a result, TE applicability was 81%. The introduction of the XL probe has improved the applicability of TE to more than 95% in patients with NAFLD [10, 11]. Excellent interobserver reproducibility has been reported for TE, with intraclass correlation coefficient (ICC) of 0.98 in a cohort of 200 patients with various chronic liver diseases in whom 800 TE examinations were performed by two operators [12]. However, reproducibility was significantly reduced in patients with steatosis, increased BMI, and mild degrees of liver fibrosis.

The reliability of both pSWE/ARFI and 2D-SWE was compared in 79 patients with measurements performed by three radiologists [13]. Failure rate was low for both methods (5% for 2D-SWE and 1% for pSWE/ARFI), and intraobserver agreement was significantly better for pSWE/ARFI than 2D-SWE (0.915 vs. 0.829). Shear wave speeds measured with 2D-SWE were higher than pSWE/ARFI suggesting that care should be taken when comparing methods. Scan-rescan repeatability of 2D-SWE measurements performed on the same day by the same operator has been shown to be excellent with ICC of 0.95 and 0.93 for an expert and novice operator, respectively [14]. However, intraobserver reproducibility between measurements performed in the same subject on different days revealed ICC values of 0.84 and 0.65 for an expert and novice operator, respectively. There is further evidence to suggest that operator experience has an effect on pSWE/ARFI measurements [15], so operators are recommended to be suitably trained. With the introduction of pSWE/ARFI and 2D-SWE into commercial US systems by many manufacturers, interplatform variability may be an issue.

As for MRE, the failure rate is low (5.6%) in the largest series to date [16]. The majority of these failures (71%) were attributed to iron deposition and the use of the 2D-GRE sequence. The test-retest repeatability of MRE is high [17–20], with reported ICC of 0.95 [18]. In order to become a widely accepted method for diagnosis and staging of fibrosis, MRE must produce consistent results regardless of the MR system used. Good interplatform reproducibility when using a 2D-GRE sequence at 1.5 T has been reported, with ICC between 0.82 and 0.99 [21–23].

In summary, MRE and 2D-SWE appear to produce the highest rate of successful measurements; however, the introduction of the XL probe has improved the applicability of TE in overweight patients. Reproducibility is good to excellent among all elastography techniques.

10.1.3 Limitations of Liver Stiffness Measurement with Different Methods

Though each elastography method has its own limitations, some drawbacks apply to all techniques. For example, liver stiffness values increase after meal intake [24–30]; therefore, elastography examinations should be performed after fasting for at least 2 h [5], though fasting for 4–6 h prior to measurement has also been recommended [8]. Similarly, cholestasis has been shown to cause increased liver stiffness with TE [31], pSWE/ARFI [32], and MRE [33].

2D-SWE and pSWE/ARFI can be performed with one probe in all patients, independent of body weight, as the ROI can be positioned manually at different depths in the liver. As compared to TE, ascites is not a limitation for 2D-SWE and pSWE/ARFI enabling their performance in decompensated liver cirrhosis for prognostic reasons. The risk of overestimating liver stiffness values has been reported with other confounding factors including ALT flares [34–36], congestive heart failure [37], excessive alcohol intake [38–40], and acute viral hepatitis [34, 41]. The influence of steatosis is still a matter of debate with conflicting results, some studies suggesting a detrimental effect [42, 43], whereas others do not [44–46].

In summary, US elastography techniques need to be performed using a standardized protocol and with critically interpreted results, taking confounding factors into account [5].

Although considered a highly accurate technique, MRE has several limitations. The primary drawback with liver MRE is the sensitivity of 2D gradient recalled echo (GRE) sequence to iron deposition. There is conflicting evidence on the effect of BMI on MRE measurements: a recent study found that BMI was not a contributing factor in failure [47], but found waist circumference to be a significant factor of failure. In contrast, a recent large retrospective study investigating the cause of MRE failure using a 2D-GRE sequence [48] found that BMI, iron deposition, massive ascites, and the use of 3 T were significantly associated with MRE failure. The overall failure rate was low at 1.5 T (3.5%) though it increased to 15.3% at 3 T, likely due to increased $T_2{}^*$ relaxation at higher field strength.

10.1.4 Respective Advantages and Inconveniences of the Different Methods

Advantages and inconvenience of the different elastography methods are summarized in Table 10.1. Advantages of TE are that it is a widely available point-of-care technique, with a short procedure time (<5 min) and immediate results, that can be performed in the outpatient clinic by a nurse after a short learning curve. Quality criteria are well defined, based on at least ten validated measurements and an interquartile range (IQR, reflects variations among measurements) of less than 30% of the median value (IQR/LSM ≤30%). It is the most validated technique with the highest level of evidence in most diseases. The main limitations of TE in clinical practice are that it requires a dedicated device and that its applicability is limited (80%) in case of obesity and limited operator experience, when using the M probe. However, the use of XL probe in patients with BMI higher than 30 kg/m² increases applicability above 95%.

Advantages of pSWE/ARFI and 2D-SWE are that they can be easily implemented on commercial ultrasound machines, enabling hepatocellular carcinoma surveillance with the same machine in patients with cirrhosis, for instance. The larger ROI used in pSWE/ARFI and 2D-SWE possibly has an advantage over TE; however, these techniques also require more operator training and expertise. Quality criteria for the performance and interpretation of pSWE/ARFI and 2D-SWE are not well defined by the manufacturers.

Advantages of MRE include its ability to analyze almost the entire liver and its applicability to patients with obesity or ascites. However, MRE has limited availability and is too costly and time-consuming to be used in routine practice and thus more suited for research.

10.2 Performance of Elastography Techniques for Diagnosing Cirrhosis

Early detection of compensated cirrhosis is critical in the management and surveillance of patients with chronic liver disease as these patients are the most at risk of developing complications related to portal hypertension or liver insufficiency and hepatocellular carcinoma [49].

The diagnostic accuracy of TE for cirrhosis is based on large meta-analyses including several thousands of patients in viral hepatitis B [50] and C [51], NAFLD [52] and ALD [53], and considered excellent (AUROCs 0.93–0.96) with sensitivities and specificities of 84–91% and 85–89%, respectively (Table 10.2). However, a meta-analysis based on individual data is still awaited. Actually, TE is better at

Table 10.1 Comparison of elastography methods for liver fibrosis staging (Adapted from ref. [10])

Techniques	Units (range)	Quality criteria	Failure (%)	Confounders Inflammation obesity others	Level of evidence	Availability	Cost		
TE	kPa (2–75)	Well-defined IQR/M <30%	#3 XL	++	++ XL probe	Congestion Steatosis?	High	+++	$
pSWE/ARFI	m/s (0.5–4.4)	Not well defined	2	+? Limited data	+? limited data	Similar to TE? Limited data	Intermediate	++	$$
2D-SWE	kPa (2–150)	Not well defined	13	+? Limited data	+? limited data	Similar to TE? Limited data	Intermediate	++	$$
MRE	kPa[a] (2–11)	Emerging QIBA consensus statement	<5	+	–	Congestion Iron overload	Low	+	$$$

[a]MR elastography is reported as shear modulus, while US elastography techniques are reported in Young's modulus. Young's modulus is three times the shear modulus

Table 10.2 Diagnostic performances (meta-analyses) for cirrhosis of different elastography methods, taking liver biopsy as reference

	Etiology	Studies (*N*)	Patients (*N*)	AUC	Cutoff (kPa)	Se	Sp
US elastography							
TE							
Li et al. [50]	HBV	27	4386	0.93	9.0–16.9	86	87
Friedrich-Rust et al. [51]	CLD (HCV)	50	8206	0.94	13.0	91	89
Xiao et al. [52]	NAFLD	13	1780	0.94	10.3–11.3	88	86
Nguyen-Khac et al. [53]	ALD	10	1026	0.91	18.6	84	85
pSWE/ARFI							
Hu et al. [58]	HBV/HCV	21	2691	0.91	2.4 m/s	86	84
2D-SWE							
Hermann et al. [59]	HBV	1	400	0.95	11.5	80	93
	HCV	1	379	0.93	13.0	86	88
	NAFLD	1	156	0.92	13.0	75	88
MR elastography							
MRE							
Singh et al. [61]	CLD	12	697	0.92	4.7	91	81
Xiao et al. [60]	HBV	9	1470	0.97	4.6	89	92
Xiao et al. [52]	NAFLD	3	384	0.97	4.1–6.7	87	93

ruling out, rather than ruling in, liver cirrhosis (with negative predictive value higher than 90%). Different cutoffs have been proposed for different causes of liver diseases (HCV, HBV, NAFLD, and ALD), but no consensus has been reached. As shown in Table 10.2, cutoffs for cirrhosis ranged from 9.0 kPa in HBV to 18.6 kPa in ALD. This may be related to the so-called spectrum bias, depending on the uneven distribution of different fibrosis stages in different cohorts [54, 55]. For instance, in ALD cohorts, prevalence of cirrhosis is usually higher (40–50%) than in HBV (10–20%). Also, cutoffs in ALD should be adjusted according to transaminase levels and ongoing alcohol intake. In that respect, the Baveno VI consensus workshop recommended a diagnosis of compensated liver cirrhosis in asymptomatic patients using TE, if liver stiffness values are repeatedly (two different days, fasting) $\geq$15 kPa [49]. Recently, it has been shown that in NAFLD patients, the same cutoffs of <10 kPa and $\geq$15 kPa could be used to rule out and rule in compensated cirrhosis, respectively, when using M probe in patients with BMI <30 kg/m^2 and XL probe in those with BMI >30 kg/m^2 [46]. Finally, when compared head-to-head with serum markers, TE outperforms all of them [56, 57].

pSWE/ARFI performance for diagnosing cirrhosis has been evaluated mainly in viral hepatitis with high accuracy (AUROC 0.91) and cutoff of 2.4 m/s [58]. 2D-SWE has been evaluated in a meta-analysis [59], based on individual data in 1340 patients with chronic liver diseases, reporting high accuracies (AUROCs 0.93–0.95) for cirrhosis with an optimal cutoff of 13.5 kPa.

As for MRE, evidence is based on a few hundreds of patients [52, 60, 61], but with excellent accuracy (97%) for diagnosing cirrhosis. However, widespread use of this method will depend on cost and availability. Finally, it should be kept in mind that cutoffs for cirrhosis are system specific.

10.3 Comparison of Elastography Methods and Other Noninvasive Tests

All elastography methods have higher accuracy for diagnosing advanced fibrosis and cirrhosis than lower fibrosis stages. When evaluating US elastography methods alone, a meta-analysis of 13 studies including 1163 patients found that pSWE/ARFI had similar diagnostic performance than TE for advanced fibrosis and cirrhosis [62]. Studies comparing TE to pSWE/ARFI [63] and 2D-SWE [64, 65] have found ARFI methods to provide similar or superior diagnostic performance to TE. In comparisons of all three methods, pSWE, 2D-SWE, and TE [66–68], 2D-SWE was the slightly superior method for staging fibrosis [66] with variable reliability compared to pSWE/ARFI [67, 68].

A few comparative studies investigating the diagnostic accuracy of MR and US elastography methods have been published. Though MRE was generally found to be superior to TE in diagnosing fibrosis in mixed cohorts [69–71] and NAFLD patients [72, 73], other studies have found both techniques to perform similarly [47, 74]. Less literature on the comparison of MRE to pSWE/ARFI and 2D-SWE is available, though a meta-analysis assessing the diagnostic accuracy of pSWE/ARFI (15 studies, 2128 patients) and MRE (11 studies, 982 patients) for staging fibrosis found that MRE is more accurate than pSWE/ARFI, particularly in diagnosing early stages of fibrosis [75]. MRE has also been compared to 2D-SWE in a mixed etiology cohort [76] which found comparable diagnostic accuracy for both techniques in staging fibrosis. MRE has also been shown to outperform serum markers [69, 77–81], morphologic features [82], and diffusion measurements [69, 83–87].

10.4 New Technical Developments

10.4.1 Controlled Attenuation Parameter (CAP)

A more recent application of TE is the controlled attenuation parameter (CAP) [88]. CAP, which is available on both M and XL probes, estimates the attenuation of the US signal decibels per meter (dB/m) and (range from 100 to 400 dB/m) and is used as a method to grade steatosis. A meta-analysis (19 studies including 2736 patients with chronic liver disease), using the M probe, reported excellent accuracy for detecting steatosis based on histopathology [89]. Recently, two large multicenter studies using the XL probe in NAFLD patients reported high applicability (>95%) and good performance for steatosis detection, but poor performance for quantification [90, 91]. Although there are no consensual cutoffs, a CAP value >275 dB/m had a positive predictive value >90% for detecting steatosis. When compared to proton density fat fraction (PDFF) MR spectroscopy, using liver biopsy as reference, CAP was outperformed by MRI-PDFF for grading steatosis [72, 73, 92].

In summary, CAP is a promising point-of-care technique for rapid and standardized steatosis detection in patients with NAFLD. CAP needs to be compared to US that, despite its limitations, remains the most widely used tool for first-line steatosis assessment.

10.4.2 3D MRE

Though the acquisition of all three directions of motion is not a new development [93], advances in inversion algorithms and the increasing availability of research 3D MRE imaging sequences have made the technique more accessible. 3D MRE enables the determination of additional parameters compared to 2D owing to the acquisition of the full wave field and fewer assumptions about the material model during inversion. These parameters, such as volumetric strain, which has been shown to be sensitive to pressure-related changes [94] and may have applications in the diagnosis of portal hypertension, are still being evaluated to establish clinical benefit. The acquisition of all three motion directions also addresses the issue of artificially increased wavelengths due to oblique 2D waves violating the planar wave assumption [95]. In a head-to-head comparison between 3D MRE and 2D MRE, 3D MRE at 40 Hz was superior to 2D MRE at 60 Hz with an AUROC for the detection for advanced fibrosis of 0.98 (3D MRE) versus 0.92 (2D MRE) [96]. However, processing of 3D MRE takes a much longer time and has yet not been applied in multicenter studies. 3D MRE appears to be an extremely promising tool for longitudinal changes in fibrosis assessment. Further studies are needed to determine its role in fibrosis assessment in routine clinical practice. Spleen stiffness has also been assessed with 3D MR elastography [97], with liver stiffness and spleen stiffness significantly associated with the presence of esophageal varices.

10.4.3 Multifrequency MRE

Generally, MRE examinations are performed by imaging shear waves at a single frequency (typically at 60 Hz). The stiffness of tissue is dependent on the frequency of the imaged waves, so examinations at a frequency other than 60 Hz will result in a different stiffness measurement. The use of multifrequency MRE, where acquisitions acquired at multiple frequencies are performed, may lead to the development of parameters that are independent of frequency through viscoelastic modeling [98–100] or via analysis of the regression line of stiffness and frequency [101]. Another application of multifrequency data is combining the wave fields from each frequency to improve the resulting elastogram. This is achieved by accounting for areas of low displacement and wave nodes that are present in each wave field, but the location of which varies depending on frequency. A downside of the acquisition of multiple frequencies is the increased scan time, as each additional frequency incrementally increases the scan time limiting clinical adoption, and the associated challenges with increased wave attenuation at higher frequencies. Thus, the diagnostic benefit of multifrequency over single-frequency MRE must be established.

10.5 Conclusions

US and MR elastography techniques have developed into accurate methods for quantitative, noninvasive diagnosis of liver fibrosis in a wide range of etiologies. Interpretation of results should take into account potential confounding factors of liver stiffness measurements, pitfalls, and technical limitations. MR elastography has equivalent, or slightly better, diagnostic accuracy to TE, pSWE/ARFI, and 2D-SWE while providing stiffness measurement over a larger area of the liver. However, MRE requires further validation, and the higher cost and limited availability will likely limit adoption worldwide. In liver referral centers performing a large number of MR imaging examinations, it is feasible to incorporate MRE into the standard imaging protocols to provide a fibrosis staging tool. The weight of published data on TE has allowed the establishment of cutoffs for staging liver fibrosis and diagnosing cirrhosis in clinical practice for most etiologies. pSWE/ARFI and 2D-SWE have shown similar diagnostic accuracy than TE, and it is reasonable to assume that once sufficient data has been acquired to fully validate these methods, they will also become a recommended noninvasive measurement tool for staging of liver fibrosis. The emergence of advanced techniques like 3D MRE and CAP may increase the accuracy of fibrosis and steatosis staging in liver disease, although more data is needed.

References

1. Kennedy P, Wagner M, Castera L, Hong CW, Johnson CL, Sirlin CB, et al. Quantitative elastography methods in liver disease: current evidence and future directions. Radiology. 2018;286(3):738–63.
2. Sandrin L, Fourquet B, Hasquenoph JM, Yon S, Fournier C, Mal F, et al. Transient elastography: a new noninvasive method for assessment of hepatic fibrosis. Ultrasound Med Biol. 2003;29(12):1705–13.
3. Myers RP, Pomier-Layrargues G, Kirsch R, Pollett A, Duarte-Rojo A, Wong D, et al. Feasibility and diagnostic performance of the FibroScan XL probe for liver stiffness measurement in overweight and obese patients. Hepatology. 2012;55(1):199–208.
4. Friedrich-Rust M, Poynard T, Castera L. Critical comparison of elastography methods to assess chronic liver disease. Nat Rev Gastroenterol Hepatol. 2016;13(7):402–11.
5. Castera L, et al. EASL-ALEH Clinical Practice Guidelines: non-invasive tests for evaluation of liver disease severity and prognosis. J Hepatol. 2015;63(1):237–64.
6. Dietrich C, Bamber J, Berzigotti A, Bota S, Cantisani V, Castera L, et al. EFSUMB Guidelines and recommendations on the clinical use of liver ultrasound elastography, update 2017 (long version). Ultraschall in der Medizin. 2017;38(04):e16–47.

7. Ferraioli G, Filice C, Castera L, Choi BI, Sporea I, Wilson SR, et al. WFUMB guidelines and recommendations for clinical use of ultrasound elastography: Part 3: liver. Ultrasound Med Biol. 2015;41(5):1161–79.

8. Barr RG, Ferraioli G, Palmeri ML, Goodman ZD, Garcia-Tsao G, Rubin J, et al. Elastography assessment of liver fibrosis: society of radiologists in ultrasound consensus conference statement. Radiology. 2015;276(3):845–61.

9. Castera L, Foucher J, Bernard PH, Carvalho F, Allaix D, Merrouche W, et al. Pitfalls of liver stiffness measurement: a 5-year prospective study of 13,369 examinations. Hepatology. 2010;51(3):828–35.

10. Castera L, Friedrich-Rust M, Loomba R. Noninvasive assessment of liver disease in patients with nonalcoholic fatty liver disease. Gastroenterology. 2019;156(5):1264–81.e4.

11. Vuppalanchi R, Siddiqui MS, Van Natta ML, Hallinan E, Brandman D, Kowdley K, et al. Performance characteristics of vibration-controlled transient elastography for evaluation of nonalcoholic fatty liver disease. Hepatology. 2018;67(1):134–44.

12. Fraquelli M, Rigamonti C, Casazza G, Conte D, Donato MF, Ronchi G, et al. Reproducibility of transient elastography in the evaluation of liver fibrosis in patients with chronic liver disease. Gut. 2007;56(7):968–73.

13. Woo H, Lee JY, Yoon JH, Kim W, Cho B, Choi BI. Comparison of the reliability of acoustic radiation force impulse imaging and supersonic shear imaging in measurement of liver stiffness. Radiology. 2015;277(3):881–6.

14. Ferraioli G, Tinelli C, Zicchetti M, Above E, Poma G, Di Gregorio M, et al. Reproducibility of real-time shear wave elastography in the evaluation of liver elasticity. Eur J Radiol. 2012;81(11):3102–6.

15. Ferraioli G, Tinelli C, Lissandrin R, Zicchetti M, Bernuzzi S, Salvaneschi L, et al. Ultrasound point shear wave elastography assessment of liver and spleen stiffness: effect of training on repeatability of measurements. Eur Radiol. 2014;24(6):1283–9.

16. Yin M, Glaser KJ, Talwalkar JA, Chen J, Manduca A, Ehman RL. Hepatic MR Elastography: clinical performance in a series of 1377 consecutive examinations. Radiology. 2016;278(1):114–24.

17. Hines CDG, Bley TA, Lindstrom MJ, Reeder SB. Repeatability of magnetic resonance elastography for quantification of hepatic stiffness. J Magn Reson Imaging. 2010;31(3):725–31.

18. Lee YJ, Lee JM, Lee JE, Lee KB, Lee ES, Yoon J-H, et al. MR elastography for noninvasive assessment of hepatic fibrosis: reproducibility of the examination and reproducibility and repeatability of the liver stiffness value measurement. J Magn Reson Imaging. 2014;39(2):326–31.

19. Shi Y, Guo Q, Xia F, Sun J, Gao Y. Short- and midterm repeatability of magnetic resonance elastography in healthy volunteers at 3.0 T. Magn Reson Imaging. 2014;32(6):665–70.

20. Shire NJ, Yin M, Chen J, Railkar RA, Fox-Bosetti S, Johnson SM, et al. Test-retest repeatability of MR elastography for noninvasive liver fibrosis assessment in hepatitis C. J Magn Reson Imaging. 2011;34(4):947–55.

21. Serai SD, Yin M, Wang H, Ehman RL, Podbreesky DJ. Cross-vendor validation of liver magnetic resonance elastography. Abdom Imaging. 2015;40(4):789–94.

22. Trout AT, Serai S, Mahley AD, Wang H, Zhang Y, Zhang B, et al. Liver Stiffness measurements with MR elastography: agreement and repeatability across imaging systems, Field Strengths, and Pulse Sequences. Radiology. 2016;281(3):793–804.

23. Yasar TK, Wagner M, Bane O, Besa C, Babb JS, Kannengiesser S, et al. Interplatform reproducibility of liver and spleen stiffness measured with MR elastography. J Magn Reson Imaging. 2016;43(5):1064–72.

24. Arena U, Lupsor Platon M, Stasi C, Moscarella S, Assarat A, Bedogni G, et al. Liver stiffness is influenced by a standardized meal in patients with chronic hepatitis C virus at different stages of fibrotic evolution. Hepatology. 2013;58(1):65–72.

25. Berzigotti A, Gottardi AD, Vukotic R, Siramolpiwat S, Abraldes JG, García-Pagan JC, et al. Effect of meal ingestion on liver stiffness in patients with cirrhosis and portal hypertension. PLoS One. 2013;8(3):e58742.

26. Hines CDG, Lindstrom MJ, Varma AK, Reeder SB. Effects of postprandial state and mesenteric blood flow on the repeatability of MR elastography in asymptomatic subjects. J Magn Reson Imaging. 2011;33(1):239–44.
27. Jajamovich GH, Dyvorne H, Donnerhack C, Taouli B. Quantitative liver MRI combining phase contrast imaging, elastography, and DWI: assessment of reproducibility and postprandial effect at 3.0 T. PLoS One. 2014;9(5):e97355.
28. Mederacke I, Wursthorn K, Kirschner J, Rifai K, Manns MP, Wedemeyer H, et al. Food intake increases liver stiffness in patients with chronic or resolved hepatitis C virus infection. Liver Int. 2009;29(10):1500–6.
29. Popescu A, Bota S, Sporea I, Sirli R, Danila M, Racean S, et al. The influence of food intake on liver stiffness values assessed by acoustic radiation force impulse elastography—preliminary results. Ultrasound Med Biol. 2013;39(4):579–84.
30. Yin M, Talwalkar JA, Glaser KJ, Venkatesh SK, Chen J, Manduca A, et al. Dynamic postprandial hepatic stiffness augmentation assessed with MR elastography in patients with chronic liver disease. Am J Roentgenol. 2011;197(1):64–70.
31. Millonig G, Reimann FM, Friedrich S, Fonouni H, Mehrabi A, Büchler MW, et al. Extrahepatic cholestasis increases liver stiffness (FibroScan) irrespective of fibrosis. Hepatology. 2008;48(5):1718–23.
32. Pfeifer L, Strobel D, Neurath MF, Wildner D. Liver stiffness assessed by acoustic radiation force impulse (ARFI) technology is considerably increased in patients with cholestasis. Ultraschall Med. 2014;35(4):364–7.
33. Eaton JE, Dzyubak B, Venkatesh SK, Smyrk TC, Gores GJ, Ehman RL, et al. Performance of magnetic resonance elastography in primary sclerosing cholangitis. J Gastroenterol Hepatol. 2016;31(6):1184–90.
34. Arena U, Vizzutti F, Corti G, Ambu S, Stasi C, Bresci S, et al. Acute viral hepatitis increases liver stiffness values measured by transient elastography. Hepatology. 2008;47(2):380–4.
35. Coco B, Oliveri F, Maina AM, Ciccorossi P, Sacco R, Colombatto P, et al. Transient elastography: a new surrogate marker of liver fibrosis influenced by major changes of transaminases. J Viral Hepat. 2007;14(5):360–9.
36. Sagir A, Erhardt A, Schmitt M, Häussinger D. Transient elastography is unreliable for detection of cirrhosis in patients with acute liver damage. Hepatology. 2008;47(2):592–5.
37. Millonig G, Friedrich S, Adolf S, Fonouni H, Golriz M, Mehrabi A, et al. Liver stiffness is directly influenced by central venous pressure. J Hepatol. 2010;52(2):206–10.
38. Bardou-Jacquet E, Legros L, Soro D, Latournerie M, Guillygomarc'h A, Le Lan C, et al. Effect of alcohol consumption on liver stiffness measured by transient elastography. World J Gastroenterol. 2013;19(4):516–22.
39. Mueller S, Millonig G, Sarovska L, Friedrich S, Reimann FM, Pritsch M, et al. Increased liver stiffness in alcoholic liver disease: differentiating fibrosis from steatohepatitis. World J Gastroenterol. 2010;16(8):966–72.
40. Trabut J-B, Thépot V, Nalpas B, Lavielle B, Cosconea S, Corouge M, et al. Rapid decline of liver stiffness following alcohol withdrawal in heavy drinkers. Alcohol Clin Exp Res. 2012;36(8):1407–11.
41. Wong GLH, Wong VWS, Choi PCL, Chan AWH, Chim AML, Yiu KKL, et al. Increased liver stiffness measurement by transient elastography in severe acute exacerbation of chronic hepatitis B. J Gastroenterol Hepatol. 2009;24(6):1002–7.
42. Boursier J, Ledinghen VD, Sturm N, Amrani L, Bacq Y, Sandrini J, et al. Precise evaluation of liver histology by computerized morphometry shows that steatosis influences liver stiffness measured by transient elastography in chronic hepatitis C. J Gastroenterol. 2014;49(3):527–37.
43. Gaia S, Carenzi S, Barilli AL, Bugianesi E, Smedile A, Brunello F, et al. Reliability of transient elastography for the detection of fibrosis in non-alcoholic fatty liver disease and chronic viral hepatitis. J Hepatol. 2011;54(1):64–71.
44. Arena U, Vizzutti F, Abraldes JG, Corti G, Stasi C, Moscarella S, et al. Reliability of transient elastography for the diagnosis of advanced fibrosis in chronic hepatitis C. Gut. 2008;57(9):1288–93.

45. Wong VW-S, Vergniol J, Wong GL-H, Foucher J, Chan HL-Y, Le Bail B, et al. Diagnosis of fibrosis and cirrhosis using liver stiffness measurement in nonalcoholic fatty liver disease. Hepatology. 2010;51(2):454–62.
46. Wong VW, Irles M, Wong GL, Shili S, Chan AW, Merrouche W, et al. Unified interpretation of liver stiffness measurement by M and XL probes in non-alcoholic fatty liver disease. Gut. 2019;68(11):2057–64.
47. Chen J, Yin M, Talwalkar JA, Oudry J, Glaser KJ, Smyrk TC, et al. Diagnostic performance of MR elastography and vibration-controlled transient elastography in the detection of hepatic fibrosis in patients with severe to morbid obesity. Radiology. 2016;283:418.
48. Wagner M, Corcuera-Solano I, Lo G, Esses S, Liao J, Besa C, et al. Technical failure of MR elastography examinations of the liver: experience from a large single-center study. Radiology. 2017;284:401.
49. de Franchis R, Baveno VIF. Expanding consensus in portal hypertension: report of the Baveno VI Consensus Workshop: stratifying risk and individualizing care for portal hypertension. J Hepatol. 2015;63(3):743–52.
50. Li Y, Huang YS, Wang ZZ, Yang ZR, Sun F, Zhan SY, et al. Systematic review with meta-analysis: the diagnostic accuracy of transient elastography for the staging of liver fibrosis in patients with chronic hepatitis B. Aliment Pharmacol Ther. 2016;43(4):458–69.
51. Friedrich-Rust M, Ong MF, Martens S, Sarrazin C, Bojunga J, Zeuzem S, et al. Performance of transient elastography for the staging of liver fibrosis: a meta-analysis. Gastroenterology. 2008;134(4):960–74.
52. Xiao G, Zhu S, Xiao X, Yan L, Yang J, Wu G. Comparison of laboratory tests, ultrasound, or magnetic resonance elastography to detect fibrosis in patients with nonalcoholic fatty liver disease: a meta-analysis. Hepatology. 2017;66(5):1486–501.
53. Nguyen-Khac E, Thiele M, Voican C, Nahon P, Moreno C, Boursier J, et al. Non-invasive diagnosis of liver fibrosis in patients with alcohol-related liver disease by transient elastography: an individual patient data meta-analysis. Lancet Gastroenterol Hepatol. 2018;3(9):614–25.
54. Poynard T, Halfon P, Castera L, Munteanu M, Imbert-Bismut F, Ratziu V, et al. Standardization of ROC curve areas for diagnostic evaluation of liver fibrosis markers based on prevalences of fibrosis stages. Clin Chem. 2007;53(9):1615–22.
55. Ransohoff DF, Feinstein AR. Problems of spectrum and bias in evaluating the efficacy of diagnostic tests. N Engl J Med. 1978;299(17):926–30.
56. Boursier J, Vergniol J, Guillet A, Hiriart JB, Lannes A, Le Bail B, et al. Diagnostic accuracy and prognostic significance of blood fibrosis tests and liver stiffness measurement by FibroScan in non-alcoholic fatty liver disease. J Hepatol. 2016;65(3):570–8.
57. Degos F, Perez P, Roche B, Mahmoudi A, Asselineau J, Voitot H, et al. Diagnostic accuracy of FibroScan and comparison to liver fibrosis biomarkers in chronic viral hepatitis: a multicenter prospective study (the FIBROSTIC study). J Hepatol. 2010;53(6):1013–21.
58. Hu X, Qiu L, Liu D, Qian L. Acoustic Radiation Force Impulse (ARFI) Elastography for noninvasive evaluation of hepatic fibrosis in chronic hepatitis B and C patients: a systematic review and meta-analysis. Med Ultrason. 2017;19(1):23–31.
59. Herrmann E, de Lédinghen V, Cassinotto C, Chu WCW, Leung VYF, Ferraioli G, et al. Assessment of biopsy-proven liver fibrosis by two-dimensional shear wave elastography: an individual patient data-based meta-analysis. Hepatology. 2018;67(1):260–72.
60. Xiao H, Shi M, Xie Y, Chi X. Comparison of diagnostic accuracy of magnetic resonance elastography and Fibroscan for detecting liver fibrosis in chronic hepatitis B patients: a systematic review and meta-analysis. PLoS One. 2017;12(11):e0186660.
61. Singh S, Venkatesh SK, Wang Z, Miller FH, Motosugi U, Low RN, et al. Diagnostic performance of magnetic resonance elastography in staging liver fibrosis: a systematic review and meta-analysis of individual participant data. Clin Gastroenterol Hepatol. 2015;13(3):440–51.e6.
62. Bota S, Herkner H, Sporea I, Salzl P, Sirli R, Neghina AM, et al. Meta-analysis: ARFI elastography versus transient elastography for the evaluation of liver fibrosis. Liver Int. 2013;33(8):1138–47.

63. Sporea I, Sirli R, Bota S, Popescu A, Sendroiu M, Jurchis A. Comparative study concerning the value of Acoustic Radiation Force Impulse Elastography (ARFI) in comparison with Transient Elastography (TE) for the assessment of liver fibrosis in patients with chronic hepatitis B and C. Ultrasound Med Biol. 2012;38(8):1310–6.

64. Ferraioli G, Tinelli C, Dal Bello B, Zicchetti M, Filice G, Filice C, et al. Accuracy of real-time shear wave elastography for assessing liver fibrosis in chronic hepatitis C: a pilot study. Hepatology. 2012;56(6):2125–33.

65. Leung VY-F, Shen J, Wong VW-S, Abrigo J, Wong GL-H, Chim AM-L, et al. Quantitative elastography of liver fibrosis and spleen stiffness in chronic hepatitis B carriers: comparison of shear-wave elastography and transient elastography with liver biopsy correlation. Radiology. 2013;269(3):910–8.

66. Cassinotto C, Boursier J, de Lédinghen V, Lebigot J, Lapuyade B, Cales P, et al. Liver stiffness in nonalcoholic fatty liver disease: a comparison of supersonic shear imaging, FibroScan, and ARFI with liver biopsy. Hepatology. 2016;63(6):1817–27.

67. Gerber L, Kasper D, Fitting D, Knop V, Vermehren A, Sprinzl K, et al. Assessment of liver fibrosis with 2-D shear wave elastography in comparison to transient elastography and acoustic radiation force impulse imaging in patients with chronic liver disease. Ultrasound Med Biol. 2015;41(9):2350–9.

68. Sporea I, Bota S, Jurchis A, Sirli R, Grădinaru-Tascău O, Popescu A, et al. Acoustic radiation force impulse and supersonic shear imaging versus transient elastography for liver fibrosis assessment. Ultrasound Med Biol. 2013;39(11):1933–41.

69. Dyvorne HA, Jajamovich GH, Bane O, Fiel MI, Chou H, Schiano TD, et al. Prospective comparison of magnetic resonance imaging to transient elastography and serum markers for liver fibrosis detection. Liver Int. 2016;36(5):659–66.

70. Huwart L, Sempoux C, Vicaut E, Salameh N, Annet L, Danse E, et al. Magnetic resonance elastography for the noninvasive staging of liver fibrosis. Gastroenterology. 2008;135(1):32–40.

71. Ichikawa S, Motosugi U, Morisaka H, Sano K, Ichikawa T, Tatsumi A, et al. Comparison of the diagnostic accuracies of magnetic resonance elastography and transient elastography for hepatic fibrosis. Magn Reson Imaging. 2015;33(1):26–30.

72. Imajo K, Kessoku T, Honda Y, Tomeno W, Ogawa Y, Mawatari H, et al. Magnetic resonance imaging more accurately classifies steatosis and fibrosis in patients with nonalcoholic fatty liver disease than transient elastography. Gastroenterology. 2016;150(3):626–37.e7.

73. Park CC, Nguyen P, Hernandez C, Bettencourt R, Ramirez K, Fortney L, et al. Magnetic resonance elastography vs transient elastography in detection of fibrosis and noninvasive measurement of steatosis in patients with biopsy-proven nonalcoholic fatty liver disease. Gastroenterology. 2017;152(3):598–607.e2.

74. Bohte AE, Niet A, Jansen L, Bipat S, Nederveen AJ, Verheij J, et al. Non-invasive evaluation of liver fibrosis: a comparison of ultrasound-based transient elastography and MR elastography in patients with viral hepatitis B and C. Eur Radiol. 2014;24(3):638–48.

75. Guo Y, Parthasarathy S, Goyal P, McCarthy RJ, Larson AC, Miller FH. Magnetic resonance elastography and acoustic radiation force impulse for staging hepatic fibrosis: a meta-analysis. Abdom Imaging. 2015;40(4):818–34.

76. Yoon JH, Lee JM, Joo I, Lee ES, Sohn JY, Jang SK, et al. Hepatic fibrosis: prospective comparison of MR elastography and US shear-wave elastography for evaluation. Radiology. 2014;273(3):772–82.

77. Cui J, Ang B, Haufe W, Hernandez C, Verna EC, Sirlin CB, et al. Comparative diagnostic accuracy of magnetic resonance elastography vs. eight clinical prediction rules for non-invasive diagnosis of advanced fibrosis in biopsy-proven non-alcoholic fatty liver disease: a prospective study. Aliment Pharmacol Ther. 2015;41(12):1271–80.

78. Ichikawa S, Motosugi U, Ichikawa T, Sano K, Morisaka H, Enomoto N, et al. Magnetic resonance elastography for staging liver fibrosis in chronic hepatitis C. Magn Reson Med Sci. 2012;11(4):291–7.

79. Kim D, Kim WR, Talwalkar JA, Kim HJ, Ehman RL. Advanced fibrosis in nonalcoholic fatty liver disease: noninvasive assessment with MR elastography. Radiology. 2013;268(2):411–9.

80. Venkatesh SK, Wang G, Lim SG, Wee A. Magnetic resonance elastography for the detection and staging of liver fibrosis in chronic hepatitis B. Eur Radiol. 2013;24(1):70–8.

81. Wu W-P, Chou C-T, Chen R-C, Lee C-W, Lee K-W, Wu H-K. Non-invasive evaluation of hepatic fibrosis: the diagnostic performance of magnetic resonance elastography in patients with viral hepatitis B or C. PLoS One. 2015;10(10):e0140068.

82. Rustogi R, Horowitz J, Harmath C, Wang Y, Chalian H, Ganger DR, et al. Accuracy of MR elastography and anatomic MR imaging features in the diagnosis of severe hepatic fibrosis and cirrhosis. J Magn Reson Imaging. 2012;35(6):1356–64.

83. Wang Y, Ganger DR, Levitsky J, Sternick LA, McCarthy RJ, Chen ZE, et al. Assessment of chronic hepatitis and fibrosis: comparison of MR elastography and diffusion-weighted imaging. Am J Roentgenol. 2011;196(3):553–61.

84. Hennedige TP, Hallinan JTPD, Leung FP, Teo LLS, Iyer S, Wang G, et al. Comparison of magnetic resonance elastography and diffusion-weighted imaging for differentiating benign and malignant liver lesions. Eur Radiol. 2016;26(2):398–406.

85. Ichikawa S, Motosugi U, Morisaka H, Sano K, Ichikawa T, Enomoto N, et al. MRI-based staging of hepatic fibrosis: comparison of intravoxel incoherent motion diffusion-weighted imaging with magnetic resonance elastography. J Magn Reson Imaging. 2015;42(1):204–10.

86. Park HS, Kim YJ, Yu MH, Choe WH, Jung SI, Jeon HJ. Three-Tesla magnetic resonance elastography for hepatic fibrosis: comparison with diffusion-weighted imaging and gadoxetic acid-enhanced magnetic resonance imaging. World J Gastroenterol. 2014;20(46):17558–67.

87. Wang Q-B, Zhu H, Liu H-L, Zhang B. Performance of magnetic resonance elastography and diffusion-weighted imaging for the staging of hepatic fibrosis: a meta-analysis. Hepatology. 2012;56(1):239–47.

88. Sasso M, Beaugrand M, de Ledinghen V, Douvin C, Marcellin P, Poupon R, et al. Controlled Attenuation Parameter (CAP): a novel VCTE™ guided ultrasonic attenuation measurement for the evaluation of hepatic steatosis: preliminary study and validation in a cohort of patients with chronic liver disease from various causes. Ultrasound Med Biol. 2010;36(11):1825–35.

89. Karlas T, Petroff D, Sasso M, Fan JG, Mi YQ, de Ledinghen V, et al. Individual patient data meta-analysis of controlled attenuation parameter (CAP) technology for assessing steatosis. J Hepatol. 2017;66(5):1022–30.

90. Eddowes PJ, Sasso M, Allison M, Tsochatzis E, Anstee QM, Sheridan D, et al. Accuracy of FibroScan controlled attenuation parameter and liver stiffness measurement in assessing steatosis and fibrosis in patients with nonalcoholic fatty liver disease. Gastroenterology. 2019;156(6):1717–30.

91. Siddiqui MS, Vuppalanchi R, Van Natta ML, Hallinan E, Kowdley KV, Abdelmalek M, et al. Vibration-controlled transient elastography to assess fibrosis and steatosis in patients with nonalcoholic fatty liver disease. Clin Gastroenterol Hepatol. 2019;17(1):156–63.e2.

92. Runge JH, Smits LP, Verheij J, Depla A, Kuiken SD, Baak BC, et al. MR spectroscopy-derived proton density fat fraction is superior to controlled attenuation parameter for detecting and grading hepatic steatosis. Radiology. 2018;286:547.

93. Weaver JB, Van Houten EEW, Miga MI, Kennedy FE, Paulsen KD. Magnetic resonance elastography using 3D gradient echo measurements of steady-state motion. Med Phys. 2001;28(8):1620–8.

94. Hirsch S, Guo J, Reiter R, Schott E, Büning C, Somasundaram R, et al. Towards compression-sensitive magnetic resonance elastography of the liver: sensitivity of harmonic volumetric strain to portal hypertension. J Magn Reson Imaging. 2014;39(2):298–306.

95. Glaser KJ, Manduca A, Ehman RL. Review of MR elastography applications and recent developments. J Magn Reson Imaging. 2012;36(4):757–74.

96. Loomba R, Cui J, Wolfson T, Haufe W, Hooker J, Szeverenyi N, et al. Novel 3D magnetic resonance elastography for the noninvasive diagnosis of advanced fibrosis in NAFLD: a prospective study. Am J Gastroenterol. 2016;111(7):986–94.

97. Shin SU, Lee J-M, Yu MH, Yoon JH, Han JK, Choi B-I, et al. Prediction of esophageal varices in patients with cirrhosis: usefulness of three-dimensional MR elastography with echo-planar imaging technique. Radiology. 2014;272(1):143–53.

98. Asbach P, Klatt D, Hamhaber U, Braun J, Somasundaram R, Hamm B, et al. Assessment of liver viscoelasticity using multifrequency MR elastography. Magn Reson Med. 2008;60(2):373–9.
99. Asbach P, Klatt D, Schlosser B, Biermer M, Muche M, Rieger A, et al. Viscoelasticity-based staging of hepatic fibrosis with multifrequency MR elastography. Radiology. 2010;257(1):80–6.
100. Klatt D, Hamhaber U, Asbach P, Braun J, Sack I. Noninvasive assessment of the rheological behavior of human organs using multifrequency MR elastography: a study of brain and liver viscoelasticity. Phys Med Biol. 2007;52(24):7281.
101. Etchell E, Jugé L, Hatt A, Sinkus R, Bilston LE. Liver stiffness values are lower in pediatric subjects than in adults and increase with age: a multifrequency MR elastography study. Radiology. 2016;283:222.

The Assessment of Portal Hypertension 11

Avik Majumdar, Giovanni Marasco, Amanda Vestito, Massimo Pinzani, and Davide Festi

11.1 General Concepts on the Pathophysiology of Portal Hypertension in Advanced Chronic Liver Disease

Portal hypertension (PH) and the relative clinical manifestations represent major complications of advanced chronic liver disease (ACLD) irrespective of the aetiology. Fundamentally, PH is caused by a progressive increase in the resistance to portal blood flow into the liver due to substantial angio-architectural changes associated with liver tissue fibrosis, neo-angiogenesis and increased vascular tone within the hepatic microcirculation. Intrahepatic vasoconstriction, due to an unbalanced predominance of vasoconstrictors, accounts for at least 25–30% of increased intrahepatic vascular resistance [1]. Phenotypic changes in hepatic cells, such as hepatic stellate cells (HSCs) and liver sinusoidal endothelial cells (LSECs), are known to play pivotal roles in causing an increased intrahepatic vascular resistance and have been extensively studied [2, 3]. HSCs are perisinusoidal pericyte-like cells located in the space of Disse. In response to liver injury, HSCs become activated and undergo a phenotypical transition into myofibroblast-like cells, with an exponential increase in the expression of pro-fibrogenic and pro-inflammatory genes [4]. In

Avik Majumdar, Giovanni Marasco, and Amanda Vestito contributed equally to this work.

A. Majumdar
AW Morrow Gastroenterology and Liver Centre, Royal Prince Alfred Hospital, Sydney, NSW, Australia

Central Clinical School, The University of Sydney, Sydney, NSW, Australia

G. Marasco · A. Vestito · D. Festi
Department of Medical and Surgical Sciences, University of Bologna, Bologna, Italy

M. Pinzani (✉)
UCL Institute for Liver and Digestive Health and Sheila Sherlock Liver Centre, Royal Free Hospital, London, UK
e-mail: m.pinzani@ucl.ac.uk

M. Fraquelli (ed.), *Elastography of the Liver and Beyond*,
https://doi.org/10.1007/978-3-030-74132-7_11

addition, activated HSCs become highly contractile, and their concentration around existing sinusoids, as well as their recruitment around newly formed venous vessels, contributes to the progressive increase in intrahepatic vascular resistance typical of cirrhosis [5]. LSECs represent the first line of defence protecting the liver from injury and play key homeostatic functions including the regulation of sinusoidal vascular tone. Chronic liver tissue injury is associated with the loss of the key specialised functions of LSECs leading to "endothelial dysfunction", which is primarily characterised by the inability of regulating sinusoidal blood flow (defective synthesis of nitric oxide and increased release of vasoconstrictors) but also by the promotion of inflammation and fibrogenesis [6]. LSECs as well as other liver endothelial cells are the main target of pro-angiogenetic growth factors with the development of an increased number of vessels in the fibrotic septa and the surrounding regenerative nodules [7]. As an ideal crossroad between fibrogenesis and angiogenesis, activated HSCs promote angiogenesis by releasing pro-angiogenic factors, such as angiopoietin and vascular endothelial growth factor (VEGF) [8].

It is important to stress that the relationship between the cirrhotic transformation of the liver and PH is extremely close and chronologically linear until extra-hepatic factors become determinant in the progression of PH. Indeed, the development of PH is progressively associated with an expansion of the splanchnic microcirculation due also to neo-angiogenesis, with a marked increase in the total portal blood flow reaching the liver [1, 3]. This leads to a further increase of PH, which, in turn, causes the opening of collateral vascular circuits with portal blood escaping into the systemic circulation. In a further phase of progression, the presence of arterial vasodilation in the splanchnic and systemic circulations leads to the so-called hyperdynamic circulation with an increase of cardiac output and consequent further increase in portal blood inflow and PH [1]. These pathophysiological considerations are of key relevance when evaluating the accuracy of non-invasive methods for the assessment of PH such as liver and spleen stiffness as will be expanded in this chapter.

11.1.1 The Standard Assessment of Portal Hypertension

The gold standard method for evaluating the severity of portal hypertension is the hepatic venous pressure gradient (HVPG), calculated through accessing the hepatic vein and subtracting the free hepatic vein pressure (FHVP) from the wedged hepatic vein pressure (WHVP) [9]. The normal HVPG is <5 mmHg, and although an HVPG 5–10 mmHg reflects an abnormal increase in portal pressure, complications only tend to occur for HVPG >10–12 mmHg [1]. In clinical practice, an HVPG >10 mmHg defines "clinically significant PH" (CSPH), while an HVPG >12 mmHg outlines "clinically severe PH". Patients with CSPH are at an increased risk of developing gastroesophageal varices, overt clinical decompensation (ascites, variceal haemorrhage and hepatic encephalopathy), postsurgical decompensation and hepatocellular carcinoma [1]. Although the technique of acquiring the HVPG values is relatively straightforward, specialist training is still required to achieve accurate measurements.

11.2 Liver Elastography (Transient, US-Based) as a Diagnostic and Prognostic Tool in PH

Liver elastography has evolved beyond its original purpose of staging liver fibrosis to provide important diagnostic and prognostic information in the setting of PH. Measurement of liver stiffness using vibration-controlled transient elastography (VCTE) remains the most studied elastography modality in the assessment of PH, with the role of point shear wave elastography (pSWE) and 2D-shear wave elastography (2D-SWE) still being established [10].

11.2.1 Clinically Significant Portal Hypertension and Liver Elastography

Liver elastography provides an indirect representation of the intrahepatic resistance component of PH in established ACLD. There is a strong linear correlation between VCTE and HVPG values of up to 10–12 mmHg [11, 12]. This correlation is less robust once HVPG exceeds this threshold, supporting the concept that alterations in portosystemic blood flow become the dominant pathophysiologic mechanism as portal pressure increases [12]. These alterations are influenced by factors including the hyperdynamic circulation, splanchnic vasodilatation and portosystemic shunting seen in clinically severe PH, which are not directly or indirectly quantified by liver elastography [10]. Therefore, liver elastography in isolation can determine the presence or absence of CSPH but cannot provide a direct approximation of HVPG values.

VCTE has very good diagnostic accuracy in detecting if CSPH is dichotomously present or absent. A meta-analysis of 11 studies with HVPG measurements found the summary area under the receiver operating characteristic curve (AUC) for VCTE to detect CSPH was 0.90. Lower cut-offs of VCTE (13.6–18 kPa) resulted in greater sensitivity (92%) for CSPH, with higher cut-offs (21–25 kPa) yielding higher specificity (91%) [13]. Furthermore, similar cut-off values for VCTE have been shown to stratify patients with potentially resectable hepatocellular carcinoma by the presence or absence of CSPH [14]. From these data, current consensus guidelines support a VCTE cut-off of >20–25 kPa for diagnosing CSPH [15–17].

Similar to fibrosis assessment using VCTE, the study populations in which CSPH has been investigated have had compensated ACLD (cACLD) predominantly due to chronic viral hepatitis, suggesting that more data in other aetiologies of liver disease is necessary. Other non-technical limitations of VCTE in assessing CSPH are that it cannot be used to assess the haemodynamic response to beta-blockers [18], nor can it predict resolution or reduction of PH after sustained virological response (SVR) in chronic hepatitis C virus (HCV) infection [19]. A recent follow-up study of 226 patients at 96-week post-SVR found that 30% still had CSPH on HVPG measurement despite VCTE values reducing to <13.6 kPa [20]. The diagnostic accuracy of VCTE in detecting CSPH can be improved in algorithms that involve various combinations of sonographic spleen size, spleen stiffness, laboratory values or clinical data.

In comparison to VCTE, there are limited studies investigating the relationship of either pSWE or 2D-SWE with HVPG. This is compounded by the fact that pSWE and 2D-SWE modalities both have several manufacturers with proprietary technology, making large validation studies difficult. A meta-analysis of CSPH measured by HVPG and liver elastography using either pSWE or 2D-SWE included nine studies (three studies using pSWE, six studies using 2D-SWE). The summary AUC for the detection of CSPH was 0.88 for both modalities of liver elastography [21]. In the four studies that included head-to-head comparisons of VCTE and SWE for detecting CSPH, there was no statistical difference in sensitivity or specificity; however, the values for VCTE (summary sensitivity 74% and specificity 81%) were lower than other published meta-analysis findings for VCTE alone [13]. The authors of the SWE meta-analysis acknowledged the limitation of combining different SWE modalities by several manufacturers, particularly in terms of defining a consistent cut-off value to predict CSPH. A recent individual patient meta-analysis of 328 patients that investigated 2D-SWE using Supersonic Imagine Aixplorer® found that a liver stiffness cut-off of <14 kPa can rule out CSPH with an AUC 0.88 [22]. However, the cohort was under-represented in terms of compensated cirrhosis. Unlike VCTE, there is currently insufficient data to support cut-offs for either pSWE or 2D-SWE that can rule in or rule out CSPH [17]. Both pSWE and 2D-SWE are incorporated to standard B-mode ultrasound (US) machines and hence offer technical advantages over VCTE by allowing the operator to visualise and position the region of interest in real time. This overcomes some of the applicability issues experienced in obese patients undergoing VCTE and allows liver elastography to be performed at the same time as routine US screening for hepatocellular carcinoma. Therefore, although pSWE and 2D-SWE are both promising tools in the assessment of PH, both require further study.

11.2.2 Gastroesophageal Varices and Liver Elastography

Unlike the detection of CSPH, liver elastography alone has limited use in the detection or risk stratification of gastroesophageal varices. The role of VCTE has been explored extensively in this setting by focussing on the detection or exclusion of high-risk or large varices, which are also termed varices needing treatment (VNT). A meta-analysis of 15 studies examining VCTE alone found that the summary sensitivity and specificity was 84% and 62% for detecting any varices and 78% and 76% for large varices, respectively [23]. This low diagnostic accuracy was attributed to variations in VCTE cut-offs in the included studies across various aetiologies of chronic liver disease.

In 2015, the Baveno VI consensus meeting proposed that liver stiffness measurement (LSM) of <20 kPa using VCTE combined with a platelet count >150 × 10^9 cells/L could safely exclude VNT and, therefore, patients meeting these criteria could avoid regular surveillance endoscopy due to a low perceived risk of bleeding [23]. Since then, the Baveno VI criteria have been widely studied and also have been modified in attempts to improve clinical utility [24–26]. A meta-analysis of 8469 participants from 30 studies found that the summary sensitivity and specificity for Baveno VI criteria for VNTs was 97% and 32%, respectively. By comparison, the "expanded" Baveno VI criteria (VCTE <25 kPa and platelet count <110 × 10^9 cells/L) had a summary sensitivity and specificity of 90% and 51%, respectively. In a hypothetical cohort of 1000 patients with a VNT prevalence of 20%, the use of the Baveno VI criteria would result in 262 spared endoscopies, but six patients with VNT would be missed, compared to the expanded Baveno VI criteria which would result in 428 spared endoscopies but at the cost of 20 patients with VNT being missed [27]. A subsequent decision curve analysis of these data favoured the latter strategy [28]. Validating pSWE and 2D-SWE for the detection or exclusion of VNT results in the same challenges as diagnosing CSPH using these modalities. There is a paucity of data regarding liver elastography alone using either pSWE or 2D-SWE for the detection of varices; however, progress has been made in terms of using these modalities for measurement of spleen stiffness [29].

Liver elastography using VCTE can detect or exclude CSPH and, when used in combination with platelet count, can safely avoid variceal surveillance endoscopies. These simple applications of VCTE have revolutionised hepatology clinical practice. Although pSWE and 2D-SWE are promising modalities, larger validation studies are required before defined cut-off values can be applied in the clinical setting for CSPH or gastroesophageal varices. Both pSWE and 2D-SWE liver stiffness measurement (LSM) can readily be combined with spleen stiffness to provide better diagnostic accuracy and will be discussed in the next section.

11.3 The Spleen in Advanced Chronic Liver Disease

In the last decade, several authors have focused their attention on the study of spleen-related parameters [30]. Indeed, chronic PH causes spleen congestion, hyperplasia, angiogenesis, fibrogenesis, enlargement and hyperactivation of the lymphoid tissue [31, 32]. Taken together, these factors may better mirror the PH-related hyperdynamic circulation. According to this pathophysiological hypothesis, spleen stiffness measurement (SSM) has been proposed [33, 34] as a non-invasive tool (NIT) to assess the presence and degree of PH and oesophageal varices (EV).

11.3.1 Spleen Stiffness Measurement Techniques

The evaluation of SSM has often been reported concomitantly with the evaluation of LSM [35]. US elastography and magnetic resonance elastography are the methods most commonly used. Thereafter, the US device analyzes the feedback generated by the tissue and depending on its stiffness to the shear wave [36, 37]. To date, no validated algorithm exists for the specific evaluation of SSM as all studies evaluating SSM use the standardised criteria that were already present for assessing LSM. Moreover, several factors may influence SSM feasibility: first, the spleen anatomical location is deeper than that of the liver, and this may reduce the acoustic window; second, feasibility is dependent on the spleen diameter and the fat thickness between the US probe and the spleen [33]. For these reasons, most of the studies carried out with VCTE, which is the most common technique for evaluating SSM, used US guidance for better targeting the spleen parenchyma [38, 39] and pre-existing LSM feasibility and validity recommendations (M probe, patient lying supine or prone, fasting period of at least 6 h, success rate >60%, IQR >30% and at least ten valid measurements) [38]. Another possible limitation of SSM by VCTE is the ceiling effect of the upper limit value of stiffness set at 75 kPa, likely due to the fact that the VCTE probe was initially designed for the liver. Indeed, the spleen is stiffer than the liver, and this could limit further stratification of PH for values above 75 kPa. To overcome this limit, a prospective multicentre study [39] using a novel spleen-dedicated FibroScan® (SSM@100 Hz) concluded that SSM@100 Hz accuracy for ruling out large EV (AUC 0.782) was higher than that reached with the standard LSM probe (SSM@50 Hz, AUC 0.720, $p = 0.027$). However, SSM by VCTE still remains the most used technique mainly due to high inter- and intra-observer agreement (0.89 and 0.94, respectively) [40, 41] and an acceptable failure rate (around 15–20%) [40]. Similar to LSM, several other US modalities beyond VCTE have been used for SSM leading to difficult comparisons of the different thresholds obtained in each study [42]. For example, pSWE allows direct assessment of spleen stiffness in a region of interest chosen by the operator, thus avoiding the influence of ascites, obesity or narrow intercostal spaces [43, 44] and leading to an overall feasibility of 85–100%. However, low inter-and intra-observer agreement has been reported [45, 46]. On the other hand, the newer elastography techniques of 2D-SWE and real-time two-dimensional shear wave elastography (RT-2D-SWE) have a similar feasibility range to pSWE but with higher intra- and inter-operator reproducibility [47].

11.3.2 Spleen Stiffness and Fibrosis Degree Evaluation

During the natural history of chronic liver disease, structural changes driven by PH occur in the spleen, which enlarges not merely due to congestion. The degree of liver cirrhosis degree influences the degree of PH, which in turn influences the spleen structural changes and its stiffness.

Since the prognosis of patients with ACLD is largely dependent on the stage of liver fibrosis and the presence of cirrhosis, several authors have postulated that SSM might be useful in determining liver fibrosis as surrogate of LSM or liver biopsy, when these methods are unfeasible or with unreliable results. Recently, it was reported that spleen stiffness was increased already in early chronic liver disease when compared to healthy subjects [48]. Another study by Chen et al. [49] using SSM to classify patients according to METAVIR fibrosis (METAVIR F) scores reported AUC 0.839 (95% CI: 0.780–0.898) for METAVIR F1 vs. F2–4, AUC 0.936

(95% CI: 0.898–0.975) for F1–2 vs. F3–4 and AUC 0.932 (95% CI: 0.893–0.971) for F1–3 vs. F4. In parallel, Leung et al. [50] defined specific SSM cut-off points for discriminating the different liver fibrosis stages: F1 19.4 kPa, F2 19.8 kPa, F3 20.6 kPa and F4 22 kPa. Several other studies [40, 50–52] have confirmed similar results. However, SSM thresholds for defining the presence of liver cirrhosis are still not yet validated and suffer from wide variability (ranging from 22 to 46 kPa or from 2.51 to 3.32 m/s) [35].

11.4 Spleen Elastography as a Diagnostic and Prognostic Tool in Portal Hypertension

Several attempts have been made to replace HVPG as the gold standard for assessing PH in cirrhotic patients [53]. The morphological remodelling of the spleen in patients with PH has justified the use of SSM as another surrogate parameter of PH in cirrhosis [31, 33]. SSM is able to more accurately reflect the dynamic changes concerning the splanchnic circulation occurring in advanced stages of cirrhosis than LSM [54]. In 2002, Colecchia et al. [33] demonstrated a strong correlation between SSM and HVPG values in a series of 113 consecutive HCV-related cirrhotic patients, suggesting that the increase in SS is closely related to PH progression.

The first meta-analysis to support the possibility of using SSM for the diagnosis of CSPH [55] found good accuracy with a summary sensitivity and specificity of 0.88 (95% CI 0.7–0.96) and 0.84 (95% CI 0.72–0.92), respectively. Other authors have tried to assess SSM with other US elastography methods beyond VCTE. Attia et al. [56] assessed the use of SSM by pSWE in 78 patients with compensated ACLD (cACLD) documenting that SSM could identify an HVPG $\geq$10 mmHg (cut-off 2.32 m/s) and an HVPG $\geq$12 mmHg (cut-off 2.53 m/s) with high accuracy (AUC 0.97 and 0.95, respectively). In a large prospective multicentre study using 2D-SWE, Jansen and colleagues [57] proposed an algorithm to rule out and rule in CSPH, with cut-offs of 21.7 kPa for LSM and 35.6 kPa for SSM.

11.4.1 Spleen Stiffness and Gastroesophageal Varices

Recently, the possibility of detecting the presence and the degree of EV using SSM in cirrhotic patients was explored. Indeed, several studies have shown that SSM was more accurate when compared to other non-invasive parameters in identifying patients with EV and different degrees of PH [33, 34, 58]. For example, Colecchia et al. [33] demonstrated that SSM was more accurate than LSM in predicting the presence of EV. Similarly, Stefanescu et al. [34] confirmed these results on the usefulness of SSM. Notably in the latter study, a comparison between SSM performance in detecting EV with other validated non-invasive parameters was also carried out, confirming the superiority of SSM [34]. A cut-off value of 46.4 kPa was proposed for identifying EV. Ma et al. [59], in a recent meta-analysis of 16 studies performed with different ultrasound-elastography methods, confirmed that SSM was more accurate than LSM in predicting the presence of EV. Recently, Colecchia et al. [60] reported that a combined algorithm using Baveno VI criteria and SSM (cut-off 46 kPa) was able to safely spare a greater number of unneeded endoscopies in patients with cACLD. Indeed, when the proposed algorithm combining Baveno VI criteria and SSM was applied, the proportion of spared endoscopies doubled and the rate of missed VNT safely remained less than 5%. A recent retrospective study reporting a sequential combination of the Baveno VI criteria and SSM measured by supersonic shear imaging (SSI) reported similar results [61].

Interestingly, SSM may be useful even when dynamically assessed, similarly to HVPG. Two recent studies reported SSM to predict the response to non-selective beta-blockers for EV bleeding prophylaxis [62, 63]. In the latter study [63], a SSM reduction $\geq 10\%$ was able to assess haemodynamic response, in parallel with HVPG.

11.4.2 Spleen Stiffness and Hepatic Decompensation

The presence, degree and time progression of CSPH are the main predictors of hepatic decompensation in patients with cirrhosis [64]. SSM is an accurate surrogate marker of PH and, therefore, was recently proposed as a tool for predicting hepatic decompensation and mortality in patients with cirrhosis [65]. Early recognition of patients with compensated cirrhosis at high risk for developing decompensation is necessary to allow the initiation of preventative strategies that are able to prolong patient survival [66]. Although patients with compensated cirrhosis have a median survival of 12 years, patients with decompensated cirrhosis have a median survival of 2 years [67]. In a previous report, HVPG showed a greater discriminative ability compared with serum albumin, model for end-stage liver disease (MELD) and Child-Pugh score for decompensation. Patients with an HVPG less than 10 mmHg had a 90% probability of not developing hepatic decompensation over a median follow-up period of 4 years [68]. In a study by Colecchia et al. [61], SSM by TE and MELD were independently associated with the risk of hepatic decompensation; patients with a SSM >54 kPa showed higher risk of developing liver-related complications within 2 years of enrolment. In line with these results, Takuma et al. [69] found that in a series of 393 ACLD patients, those with SSM <3.25 m/s had a 98.8% probability of not developing hepatic decompensation. Conversely, SSM >3.43 m/s was able to predict mortality over a median follow-up period of 44.6 months [69]. Recently, the ability of SSM in predicting hepatic decompensation was also tested [70] in a cohort of HCV patients undergoing treatment with direct-acting antiviral agents (DAAs). In this cohort, SSM ≥ 54 kPa was independently associated with decompensation, despite achievement of SVR or history of decompensation. Interestingly, dynamic assessment of SSM identified that a SSM reduction <10% after antiviral therapy was directly linked to the risk of decompensation after SVR.

11.4.3 Spleen Stiffness in Monitoring Outcome After Interventional Procedure for PH

The prognostic value of SSM has been also proposed for the evaluation of transjugular intrahepatic portosystemic shunt (TIPS) function in decompensated cirrhotic patients [71]. TIPS is an established intervention in the treatment of complications of PH such as bleeding from gastroesophageal varices, ascites or hepatorenal syndrome by reducing portal pressure. Although determination of the portosystemic pressure gradient is considered the reference standard for diagnosing and monitoring portal hypertension, its use in monitoring TIPS is restricted to tertiary centres and limited by invasiveness [72]. Among non-invasive ultrasound imaging techniques, colour Doppler sonography is widely used for surveillance of TIPS patency by measurement of intra-stent flow velocity [73]. However, anatomic conditions sometimes make sonographic flow measurements inside the TIPS difficult. A decrease in SSM values after TIPS implantation is a useful additional parameter in monitoring proper TIPS function. Gao et al. [74] showed a statistically significant difference in SSM values before and after TIPS implantation ($p < 0.001$) using SWE. Notably, SSM significantly decreased after TIPS implantation on post-interventional Day 1 and 28 in patients with patent stents, while LSM decreased simultaneously without statistical significance. In line with these results, Buechter et al. [75] showed that SSM variations after TIPS were similar to those of HVPG. Indeed, a high degree of PH according to HVPG before TIPS implantation was associated with a median SSM value of 67.1 kPa (standard deviation [SD] 17.3 kPa), whereas after TIPS, HVPG decreased together with SSM (44.7 kPa [SD 18.5 kPa], $p < 0.05$). This prompt decrease in both HVPG and SSM values is not surprising as haemodynamic changes in the portal venous circulation occur immediately after TIPS placement. These data demonstrated that SSM reflects portal pressure excellently, even when rapid changes occur.

In conclusion, SSM evaluation is a promising tool to be used alone or in association with other non-invasive markers, for monitoring patients with ACLD during follow-up and for stratifying the risk of developing PH-related complications.

References

1. Turco L, Garcia-Tsao G. Portal hypertension: pathogenesis and diagnosis. Clin Liv Dis. 2019;23:573–87.
2. Pinzani M, Gentilini P. Biology of hepatic stellate cells and their possible relevance in the pathogenesis of portal hypertension in cirrhosis. Semin Liver Dis. 1999;19:397–410.
3. Brusilovskaya K, Königshofer P, Schwabl P, Reiberger T. Vascular targets for the treatment of portal hypertension. Semin Liver Dis. 2019;39:483–501.
4. Parola M, Pinzani M. Liver fibrosis: pathophysiology, pathogenetic targets and clinical issues. Mol Asp Med. 2019;65:37–55.
5. Pinzani M, Failli P, Ruocco C, Casini A, Milani S, Baldi E, Giotti A, Gentilini P. Fat-storing cells as liver-specific pericytes. Spatial dynamics of agonist-stimulated intracellular calcium transients. J Clin Invest. 1992;90:642–6.

6. Gracia-Sancho J, Marrone G, Fernández-Iglesias A. Hepatic microcirculation and mechanisms of portal hypertension. Nat Rev Gastroenterol Hepatol. 2019;16:221–34.

7. Fernández M, Semela D, Bruix J, Colle I, Pinzani M, Bosch J. Angiogenesis in liver disease. J Hepatol. 2009;50:604–20.

8. Novo E, Cannito S, Zamara E, et al. Proangiogenic cytokines as hypoxia-dependent factors stimulating migration of human hepatic stellate cells. Am J Pathol. 2007;170:1942–53.

9. Maurice J, Pinzani M. The stratification of cirrhosis. Hepatol Res. 2020;50:535–41.

10. Berzigotti A. Non-invasive evaluation of portal hypertension using ultrasound elastography. J Hepatol. 2017;67:399. https://doi.org/10.1016/j.jhep.2017.02.003.

11. Carrión JA, Navasa M, Bosch J, Bruguera M, Gilabert R, Forns X. Transient elastography for diagnosis of advanced fibrosis and portal hypertension in patients with hepatitis C recurrence after liver transplantation. Liver Transpl. 2006;12:1791–8.

12. Vizzutti F, Arena U, Romanelli RG, et al. Liver stiffness measurement predicts severe portal hypertension in patients with HCV-related cirrhosis. Hepatology. 2007;45:1290–7.

13. You MW, Kim KW, Pyo J, Huh J, Kim HJ, Lee SJ, Park SH. A meta-analysis for the diagnostic performance of transient elastography for clinically significant portal hypertension. Ultrasound Med Biol. 2017;43:59–68.

14. Llop E, Berzigotti A, Reig M, Erice E, Reverter E, Seijo S, Abraldes JG, Bruix J, Bosch J, García-Pagan JC. Assessment of portal hypertension by transient elastography in patients with compensated cirrhosis and potentially resectable liver tumors. J Hepatol. 2012;56:103–8.

15. de Franchis R. Expanding consensus in portal hypertension: report of the Baveno VI Consensus Workshop: stratifying risk and individualizing care for portal hypertension. J Hepatol. 2015;63:743–52.

16. Castera L, et al. EASL-ALEH Clinical Practice Guidelines: non-invasive tests for evaluation of liver disease severity and prognosis. J Hepatol. 2015;63(1):237–64.

17. Ferraioli G, Wong VW-S, Castera L, Berzigotti A, Sporea I, Dietrich CF, Choi BI, Wilson SR, Kudo M, Barr RG. Liver ultrasound elastography: an update to the world federation for ultrasound in medicine and biology guidelines and recommendations. Ultrasound Med Biol. 2018;44:2419–40.

18. Reiberger T, Ferlitsch A, Payer BA, Pinter M, Homoncik M, Peck-Radosavljevic M. Non-selective β-blockers improve the correlation of liver stiffness and portal pressure in advanced cirrhosis. J Gastroenterol. 2012;47:561–8.

19. Lens S, Alvarado-Tapias E, Mariño Z, et al. Effects of all-oral anti-viral therapy on HVPG and systemic hemodynamics in patients with hepatitis C virus-associated cirrhosis. Gastroenterology. 2017;153:1273–1283.e1.

20. Lens S, Baiges A, Alvarado E, et al. Clinical outcome and hemodynamic changes following HCV eradication with oral antiviral therapy in patients with clinically significant portal hypertension. J Hepatol. 2020;73:1415. https://doi.org/10.1016/j.jhep.2020.05.050.

21. Suh CH, Kim KW, Park SH, Lee SS, Kim HS, Tirumani SH, Lee JG, Pyo J. Shear wave elastography as a quantitative biomarker of clinically significant portal hypertension: a systematic review and meta-analysis. Am J Roentgenol. 2018;210:W185–95.

22. Thiele M, Hugger MB, Kim Y, et al. 2D shear wave liver elastography by Aixplorer to detect portal hypertension in cirrhosis: an individual patient data meta-analysis. Liver Int. 2020;40:1435–46.

23. Pu K, Shi JH, Wang X, Tang Q, Wang XJ, Tang KL, Long ZQ, Hu XS. Diagnostic accuracy of transient elastography (FibroScan) in detection of esophageal varices in patients with cirrhosis: a meta-analysis. World J Gastroenterol. 2017;23:345–56.

24. Augustin S, Pons M, Maurice JB, et al. Expanding the Baveno VI criteria for the screening of varices in patients with compensated advanced chronic liver disease. Hepatology. 2017;66:1980–8.

25. Tosetti G, Primignani M, La Mura V, et al. Evaluation of three "beyond Baveno VI" criteria to safely spare endoscopies in compensated advanced chronic liver disease. Dig Liver Dis. 2019;51:1135–40.

26. Abraldes JG, Bureau C, Stefanescu H, et al. Noninvasive tools and risk of clinically significant portal hypertension and varices in compensated cirrhosis: the "anticipate" study. Hepatology. 2016;64:2173–84.
27. Stafylidou M, Paschos P, Katsoula A, Malandris K, Ioakim K, Bekiari E, Haidich AB, Akriviadis E, Tsapas A. Performance of Baveno VI and expanded Baveno VI criteria for excluding high-risk varices in patients with chronic liver diseases: a systematic review and meta-analysis. Clin Gastroenterol Hepatol. 2019;17:1744–1755.e11.
28. Majumdar A, Tsochatzis EA. Curve your enthusiasm: the decision to use expanded or original Baveno VI criteria to exclude high-risk varices. Clin Gastroenterol Hepatol. 2020;18:1243–4.
29. Paternostro R, Reiberger T, Bucsics T. Elastography-based screening for esophageal varices in patients with advanced chronic liver disease. World J Gastroenterol. 2019;25:308.
30. Colecchia A, Marasco G, Taddia M, Montrone L, Eusebi LH, Mandolesi D, Schiumerini R, Di Biase AR, Festi D. Liver and spleen stiffness and other noninvasive methods to assess portal hypertension in cirrhotic patients: a review of the literature. Eur J Gastroenterol Hepatol. 2015;27:992–1001.
31. Mejias M, Garcia-Pras E, Gallego J, Mendez R, Bosch J, Fernandez M. Relevance of the mTOR signaling pathway in the pathophysiology of splenomegaly in rats with chronic portal hypertension. J Hepatol. 2010;52:529–39.
32. Bolognesi M, Merkel C, Sacerdoti D, Nava V, Gatta A. Role of spleen enlargement in cirrhosis with portal hypertension. Dig Liver Dis. 2002;34:144–50.
33. Colecchia A, Montrone L, Scaioli E, et al. Measurement of spleen stiffness to evaluate portal hypertension and the presence of esophageal varices in patients with HCV-related cirrhosis. Gastroenterology. 2012;143:646–54.
34. Stefanescu H, Grigorescu M, Lupsor M, et al. Spleen stiffness measurement using Fibroscan for the noninvasive assessment of esophageal varices in liver cirrhosis patients. J Gastroenterol Hepatol. 2011;26:164–70.
35. Colecchia A, Ravaioli F, Marasco G, Festi D. Spleen stiffness by ultrasound elastography. In: Diagnostic methods for cirrhosis and portal hypertension. New York, NY: Springer; 2018. https://doi.org/10.1007/978-3-319-72628-1_8.
36. Bamber J, Cosgrove D, Dietrich CF, et al. EFSUMB guidelines and recommendations on the clinical use of ultrasound elastography. Part 1: Basic principles and technology. Ultraschall Med. 2013;34:169–84.
37. Krankenhaus C, Mergentheim B, Royal T, et al. EFSUMB Guidelines and Recommendations on the Clinical use of liver ultrasound elastography, Update 2017 (long version). Ultraschall Med. 2017;38(4):e16–47.
38. Bonino F, Arena U, Brunetto MR, et al. Liver stiffness, a non-invasive marker of liver disease: a core study group report. Antivir Ther. 2010;15(Suppl 3):69–78.
39. Stefanescu H, Marasco G, Calès P, et al. A novel spleen-dedicated stiffness measurement by FibroScan® improves the screening of high-risk esophageal varices. Liver Int. 2020;40:175.
40. Fraquelli M, Giunta M, Pozzi R, et al. Feasibility and reproducibility of spleen transient elastography and its role in combination with liver transient elastography for predicting the severity of chronic viral hepatitis. J Viral Hepat. 2014;21:90–8.
41. Goldschmidt I, Brauch C, Poynard T, Baumann U. Spleen stiffness measurement by transient elastography to diagnose portal hypertension in children. J Pediatr Gastroenterol Nutr. 2014;59:197–203.
42. Piscaglia F, Salvatore V, Mulazzani L, et al. Differences in liver stiffness values obtained with new ultrasound elastography machines and fibroscan: a comparative study. Dig Liver Dis. 2017;49:802. https://doi.org/10.1016/j.dld.2017.03.001.
43. Bota S, Herkner H, Sporea I, Salzl P, Sirli R, Neghina AM, Peck-Radosavljevic M. Meta-analysis: ARFI elastography versus transient elastography for the evaluation of liver fibrosis. Liver Int. 2013;33:1138–47.
44. Hudson JM, Milot L, Parry C, Williams R, Burns PN. Inter- and intra-operator reliability and repeatability of shear wave elastography in the liver: a study in healthy volunteers. Ultrasound Med Biol. 2013;39:950–5.

45. Cabassa P, Ravanelli M, Rossini A, Contessi G, Almajdalawi R, Maroldi R. Acoustic radiation force impulse quantification of spleen elasticity for assessing liver fibrosis. Abdom Imaging. 2015;40:738–44.

46. Ferraioli G, Tinelli C, Lissandrin R, Zicchetti M, Bernuzzi S, Salvaneschi L, Filice C, Elastography Study Group. Ultrasound point shear wave elastography assessment of liver and spleen stiffness: effect of training on repeatability of measurements. Eur Radiol. 2014;24:1283–9.

47. Cassinotto C, Charrie A, Mouries A, et al. Liver and spleen elastography using supersonic shear imaging for the non-invasive diagnosis of cirrhosis severity and oesophageal varices. Dig Liver Dis. 2015;47:695–701.

48. Grgurevic I, Cikara I, Horvat J, Lukic IK, Heinzl R, Banic M, Kujundzic M, Brkljacic B. Noninvasive assessment of liver fibrosis with acoustic radiation force impulse imaging: increased liver and splenic stiffness in patients with liver fibrosis and cirrhosis. Ultraschall Med. 2011;32:160–6.

49. Chen SH, Li YF, Lai HC, Kao JT, Peng CY, Chuang PH, Su WP, Chiang IP. Noninvasive assessment of liver fibrosis via spleen stiffness measurement using acoustic radiation force impulse sonoelastography in patients with chronic hepatitis B or C. J Viral Hepat. 2012;19:654–63.

50. Leung VY, Shen J, Wong VW, et al. Quantitative elastography of liver fibrosis and spleen stiffness in chronic hepatitis B carriers: comparison of shear-wave elastography and transient elastography with liver biopsy correlation. Radiology. 2013;269:910–8.

51. Bota S, Sporea I, Sirli R, Popescu A, Dănilă M, Sendroiu M, Focşa M. Spleen assessment by Acoustic Radiation Force Impulse Elastography (ARFI) for prediction of liver cirrhosis and portal hypertension. Med Ultrason. 2010;12:213–7.

52. Ye X-P, Ran H-T, Cheng J, Zhu Y-F, Zhang D-Z, Zhang P, Zheng Y-Y. Liver and spleen stiffness measured by acoustic radiation force impulse elastography for noninvasive assessment of liver fibrosis and esophageal varices in patients with chronic hepatitis B. J Ultrasound Med. 2012;31:1245–53.

53. Garcia-Tsao G, Abraldes JG, Berzigotti A, Bosch J. Portal hypertensive bleeding in cirrhosis: risk stratification, diagnosis, and management: 2016 practice guidance by the American Association for the study of liver diseases. Hepatology. 2017;65:310–35.

54. Singh S, Muir AJ, Dieterich DT, Falck-Ytter YT. American gastroenterological association institute technical review on the role of elastography in chronic liver diseases. Gastroenterology. 2017;152:1544–77.

55. Song J, Huang J, Huang H, Liu S, Luo Y. Performance of spleen stiffness measurement in prediction of clinical significant portal hypertension: a meta-analysis. Clin Res Hepatol Gastroenterol. 2018;42:216–26.

56. Attia D, Schoenemeier B, Rodt T, Negm AA, Lenzen H, Lankisch TO, Manns M, Gebel M, Potthoff A. Evaluation of liver and spleen stiffness with acoustic radiation force impulse quantification elastography for diagnosing clinically significant portal hypertension. Ultraschall Med. 2015;36:603–10.

57. Jansen C, Bogs C, Verlinden W, et al. Algorithm to rule out clinically significant portal hypertension combining shear-wave elastography of liver and spleen: a prospective multicentre study. Gut. 2016;65:1057–8.

58. Sharma P, Kirnake V, Tyagi P, Bansal N, Singla V, Kumar A, Arora A. Spleen stiffness in patients with cirrhosis in predicting esophageal varices. Am J Gastroenterol. 2013;108:1101–7.

59. Ma X, Wang L, Wu H, Feng Y, Han X, Bu H, Zhu Q. Spleen stiffness is superior to liver stiffness for predicting esophageal varices in chronic liver disease: a meta-analysis. PLoS One. 2016;11:e0165786.

60. Colecchia A, Ravaioli F, Marasco G, Colli A, Dajti E, Di Biase AR, Bacchi Reggiani ML, Berzigotti A, Pinzani M, Festi D. A combined model based on spleen stiffness measurement and Baveno VI criteria to rule out high-risk varices in advanced chronic liver disease. J Hepatol. 2018;69:308. https://doi.org/10.1016/j.jhep.2018.04.023.

61. Cho YS, Kim Y, Sohn JH. Application of supersonic shear imaging to the Baveno VI criteria and a combination model with spleen stiffness measurement to rule out high-risk varices

in compensated advanced chronic liver disease. Ultraschall der Medizin. 2020; https://doi.org/10.1055/a-1168-6271.

62. Kim HY, So YH, Kim W, Ahn DW, Jung YJ, Woo H, Kim D, Kim MY, Baik SK. Non-invasive response prediction in prophylactic carvedilol therapy for cirrhotic patients with esophageal varices. J Hepatol. 2019;70:412–22.

63. Marasco G, Dajti E, Ravaioli F, et al. Spleen stiffness measurement for assessing the response to β-blockers therapy for high-risk esophageal varices patients. Hepatol Int. 2020;14:850. https://doi.org/10.1007/s12072-020-10062-w.

64. Ripoll C, Groszmann R, Garcia-Tsao G, et al. Hepatic venous pressure gradient predicts clinical decompensation in patients with compensated cirrhosis. Gastroenterology. 2007;133:481–8.

65. Ravaioli F, Montagnani M, Lisotti A, Festi D, Mazzella G, Azzaroli F. Noninvasive assessment of portal hypertension in advanced chronic liver disease: an update. Gastroenterol Res Pract. 2018;2018:1–11.

66. Muir AJ. Understanding the complexities of cirrhosis. Clin Ther. 2015;37:1822–36.

67. D'amico G, Morabito A, Pagliaro L, Marubini E. Survival and prognostic indicators in compensated and decompensated cirrhosis. Dig Dis Sci. 1986;31:468–75.

68. Ripoll C, Zipprich A, Garcia-Tsao G. Prognostic factors in compensated and decompensated cirrhosis. Curr Hepat Rep. 2014;13:171–9.

69. Takuma Y, Morimoto Y, Takabatake H, Toshikuni N, Tomokuni J, Sahara A, Matsueda K, Yamamoto H. Measurement of spleen stiffness with acoustic radiation force impulse imaging predicts mortality and hepatic decompensation in patients with liver cirrhosis. Clin Gastroenterol Hepatol. 2017;15:1782–1790.e4.

70. Dajti E, Ravaioli F, Colecchia A, et al. Spleen stiffness measurements predict the risk of hepatic decompensation after direct-acting antivirals in HCV cirrhotic patients. Ultraschall der Medizin. 2020; https://doi.org/10.1055/a-1205-0367.

71. Ran H-T, Ye X-P, Zheng Y-Y, Zhang D-Z, Wang Z-G, Chen J, Madoff D, Gao J. Spleen stiffness and splenoportal venous flow: assessment before and after transjugular intrahepatic portosystemic shunt placement. J Ultrasound Med. 2013;32:221–8.

72. Siramolpiwat S. Transjugular intrahepatic portosystemic shunts and portal hypertension-related complications. World J Gastroenterol. 2014;20:16996–7010.

73. Ricci P, Cantisani V, Lombardi V, Alfano G, D'Ambrosio U, Menichini G, Marotta E, Drudi FM. Is color-Doppler US a reliable method in the follow-up of transjugular intrahepatic portosystemic shunt (TIPS)? J Ultrasound. 2007;10:22–7.

74. Gao J, Zheng X, Zheng YY, Zuo GQ, Ran HT, Auh YH, Waldron L, Chan T, Wang ZG. Shear wave elastography of the spleen for monitoring transjugular intrahepatic portosystemic shunt function: a pilot study. J Ultrasound Med. 2016;35:951–8.

75. Buechter M, Manka P, Theysohn JM, Reinboldt M, Canbay A, Kahraman A. Spleen stiffness is positively correlated with HVPG and decreases significantly after TIPS implantation. Dig Liver Dis. 2018;50:54–60.

Assessing Disease Severity and Prognosis

12

Élise Vuille-Lessard, Ahmed Y. Elmahdy, and Annalisa Berzigotti

12.1 Introduction

The natural history of advanced chronic liver disease (ACLD) can be divided in two very different stages. The first is devoid of the typical complications of cirrhosis and portal hypertension, usually completely asymptomatic and termed "compensated." Survival in this stage of the disease is good (5-year survival 90–98.5%) [1], and mortality is usually unrelated to liver disease (except for that related to hepatocellular carcinoma). This phase is followed by a "decompensated" stage characterized by the onset of ascites, and/or variceal bleeding and/or hepatic encephalopathy, which often recur and pose patients at high risk of further complications and death (5-year survival depending on the type and number of decompensation and liver function ranges 40–80% once entered in this stage) [1]. The onset of the first clinical decompensation is driven by the presence of portal hypertension (see previous chapter) and by additional factors such as reduction in liver function (low albumin, increased bilirubin, and INR) and presence of obesity [2]. Several other factors can play a role in aggravating the prognosis and accelerating the course of the disease (e.g., alcohol consumption; genetic factors). In the era of effective antiviral therapies, it has become clear as well that the removal of the main etiological agent of liver damage can positively modify the natural history of ACLD, preventing clinical decompensation and even reverting from a decompensated to a (re-) compensated stage. The complexity of this changing scenario underlines how prognostic stratification has to take into account several factors. However, it is known since years that the severity of liver fibrosis (even beyond the presence of cirrhosis) and portal hypertension are major factors to be considered to identify those patients at the

É. Vuille-Lessard · A. Y. Elmahdy · A. Berzigotti (✉)
Hepatology, University Clinic for Visceral Surgery and Medicine (UVCM), Inselspital, University Hospital of Bern, University of Bern, Berne, Switzerland

Department of Biomedical Research (DBMR), University of Bern, Berne, Switzerland
e-mail: annalisa.berzigotti@insel.ch

© Springer Nature Switzerland AG 2021
M. Fraquelli (ed.), *Elastography of the Liver and Beyond*,
https://doi.org/10.1007/978-3-030-74132-7_12

highest risk of clinical decompensation and death. Liver stiffness measurement (LSM) has been robustly validated not only as a diagnostic test for assessing liver fibrosis but also as a prognostic test. Spleen stiffness measurement (SSM) has been more recently added to the diagnostic armamentarium of hepatologists. This chapter summarizes the current evidence regarding the prognostic significance of both tests in patients with advanced chronic liver disease.

12.2 Prediction of First Clinical Decompensation

12.2.1 Liver Stiffness

The previous chapter described how LSM correlates with HVPG and how it can well discriminate between patients with and without CSPH. This observation justifies why LSM also holds prognostic value for the development of first clinical decompensation. Table 12.1 summarizes the most important studies reporting on the prediction of first clinical decompensation and LSM measured by different ultrasound elastography techniques.

Initial studies such as that of Grgurevic et al. [22] showed that patients with decompensated cirrhosis had a higher LSM by 2D-SWE SSI than compensated patients (35.3 kPa vs. 18.3 kPa, adjusted difference 65%, 95% CI 43–90%; $p < 0.001$) [23]. A prospective, cross-sectional study showed that LSM by vibration-controlled transient elastography (VCTE also commonly known as transient elastography, TE) and by 2D-SWE SSI were significantly different in patients with compensated, previously decompensated, and currently decompensated cirrhosis (for TE, 15.9 kPa, 29.9 kPa, and 39.3 kPa, respectively; for 2D-SWE SSI, 15.2 kPa, 25.2 kPa, and 35.9 kPa, respectively), suggesting that LSM is a dynamic parameter and can improve between episodes of decompensation.

Moreover, multiple long-term follow-up studies have shown that a higher baseline LSM is associated with a higher risk of decompensation over time in patients with compensated cirrhosis and performs similarly as the HVPG and better than histology. This was confirmed by a recent systematic review and meta-analysis of 62 cohort studies including 43,817 patients with compensated cirrhosis [24] that concluded to a pooled RR of 7.33 (95% CI 3.84–14.00) for decompensation in patients with a higher baseline LSM by TE. This was in a dose-dependent fashion: for each kPa increase in baseline LSM by TE, there was an 8% and 7% increase in the risk of hepatic decompensation and liver-related events (LREs, a composite outcome of HCC, hepatic decompensation, all-cause, and/or liver-related mortality), respectively. The risk increased the most at lower ranges of baseline LSM and then showed a slight decrease above 25 kPa, corresponding to a lesser magnitude of effect when very high LSM values were reached. Two other meta-analyses yielded similar results [25, 26]. In one of them [25], a 5-kPa increase in LSM was associated with a 53% increase in the risk of developing LREs (RR 1.53; 95% CI 1.41–1.65), with stabilization of the risk at approximately 34.5 kPa. The progression of LSM over time in HIV/HCV-coinfected patients [27] and its lack of improvement after

Table 12.1 Accuracy of LSM and SSM using elastography techniques to predict complications and mortality in CLD

Study (year)	Method used	N included (% cirrhosis)	Etiology	Median follow-up (months)	Complications[a] rate	Complications[a] AUROC (selected cut-off[b])	Overall/liver-related mortality[c] rate	Overall/liver-related mortality AUROC (selected cut-off)
LSM								
Robic et al. [3] (2011)	TE	100 (65%)	Mixed	16	41%	0.84 (21.1 kPa)	N/A	N/A
Vergniol et al. [4] (2011)	TE	1457 (18%)	HCV	47	N/A	N/A	5.3%/2.7%	0.82/N/A (N/A)
Chon et al. [5] (2012)	TE	1126 (18%)	HBV	31	6%	0.82 (N/A)	N/A	N/A
Kim et al. [6] (2012)	TE	217 (100%)	HBV	42	12%	0.77 (18 kPa)	N/A	N/A
Kim et al. [7] (2012)	TE	128 (86%)	HBV	28	14.8%	0.72 (19 kPa)	N/A	N/A
Merchante et al. [8] (2012)	TE	239 (93%)	HIV-HCV	20	13%	0.72 (40 kPa)	6%/4.2%	0.602/0.728 (N/A)
De Ledinghen et al. [9] (2013)	TE	600 (23%)	HBV	50	N/A	N/A	4.8%/2.8%	0.80/N/A (20 kPa)
Corpechot et al. [10] (2014)	TE	168 (14%)	PSC	47	14%	N/A	3.6%/3.0%	N/A (18.5 kPa)
Pang et al. [11] (2014)	TE	2052 (15%)	Mixed	16	3.4%	N/A (20 kPa)	0.8%/N/A	0.67/N/A (N/A)
Pérez-Latorre et al. [12] (2014)	TE	60 (53%)	HCV/HIV, HCV	42	25%	0.85 (25 kPa; 40 kPa)	10%/N/A	N/A
Wang et al. [13] (2014)	TE	220 (100%)	Mixed	37	22.3%	0.929 (21 kPa)	N/A	N/A
Kitson et al. [14] (2015)	TE	95 (93%)	Mixed	15	30%	0.73 (34.5 kPa)	14%/10%	N/A

(continued)

Table 12.1 (continued)

Study (year)	Method used	N included (% cirrhosis)	Etiology	Median follow-up (months)	Complications[a] rate	Complications[a] AUROC (selected cut-off[b])	Overall/ liver-related mortality[c] rate	Overall/liver-related mortality AUROC (selected cut-off)
Park et al. [15] (2015)	TE	151 (40%)	HBV	60	11.9%	N/A	2%/2%	0.70/N/A (N/A)
Wong et al. [16] (2015)	TE	1555 (32%)	HBV	69	7.6%	N/A	3.6%/1.7%	N/A
Dillon et al. [17] (2018)	TE	259 (100%)	Mixed	36	8.1%	N/A (21 kPa; 35 kPa)	N/A	N/A
Wu et al. [18] (2020)	SSI	430 (14%)	HBV	48	6.7%	0.86 (N/A)	N/A	N/A
Shili-Masmoudi et al. [19] (2020)	TE	2251 (13% with LSM >12 kPa)	NAFLD	27	0.9%	N/A	2.4%/N/A	0.797/N/A (12 kPa)
SSM								
Colecchia et al. [20] (2014)	TE	92 (100%)	HCV	24	32.6%	0.85 (54 kPa)	N/A	N/A
Takuma et al. [21] (2017)	pSWE	393 (100%; 71% compensated)	Mixed	45	12.5% (in compensated patients)	0.843 (in compensated patients) (3.25 m/s)	17%/N/A	0.824 (3.41 m/s in compensated patients; 3.53 m/s in decompensated patients)

AUROC area under the receiver operating characteristic curve, *HBV* hepatitis B virus, *HCV* hepatitis C virus, *HIV* human immunodeficiency virus, *LSM* liver stiffness measurement, *N/A* not applicable, *NAFLD* non-alcoholic fatty liver disease, *NPV* negative predictive value, *PSC* primary sclerosing cholangitis, *SSM* spleen stiffness measurement, *SSI* supersonic imagine, *pSWE* point shear wave elastography, *TE* transient elastography

[a]Includes decompensation events +/− HCC, OLT, and death depending on the study

[b]Selection criteria vary (combination of best sensitivity and specificity, or PPV/NPV, or based on prior studies, or dual cut-off with prediction of no events vs. events or "low risk" vs. "high risk" of events)

[c]Included OLT in some studies

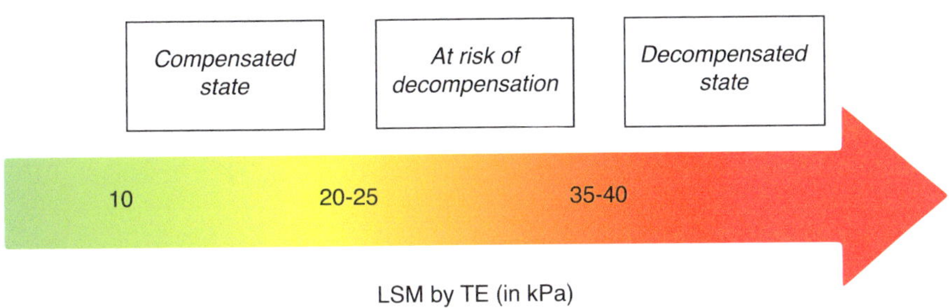

Fig. 12.1 Cut-off values of LSM by TE (in kPa) corresponding to compensated, at risk of decompensation, and decompensated stages of ACLD

direct-acting antiviral (DAA) therapy in patients with compensated HCV cirrhosis [28] were also found to have a prognostic value for decompensation, which supports the longitudinal use of LSM.

The LSM by TE cut-off value that identifies current decompensation (including a "pre-decompensated" stage, i.e., ascites only detectable by US) seems to be around 35–40 kPa (Fig. 12.1) [12, 22, 23]. As for the cut-off value that predicts the occurrence of decompensation, it seems to be similar to the one that predicts CSPH, i.e., approximately 20–25 kPa [3, 7, 11–13, 17, 28], with overall AUC in the 0.86–0.88 range [18, 29]. LSM by 2D-SWE seems to perform as well as LSM by TE in predicting hepatic decompensation [18], and similar cut-off values have been proposed [23]. Data is lacking for LSM by pSWE.

Some studies have tried to identify specific cut-off values for each decompensation event, specifically variceal bleeding and ascites [22, 29–31], but no agreement has been reached so far, probably reflecting the poor correlation of LSM with the portal pressure in more severe PH. This issue might be partly resolved by the use of SSM, as discussed below.

Most of the studies assessing the prognostic ability of LSM were done in patients with viral etiologies of cirrhosis such as HCV [12, 32], HCV/HIV coinfection [8, 12, 33], and HBV [5, 6], but the association has also been found in NAFLD [19] and PSC [10], and other study cohorts had mixed etiologies. Patients with cirrhosis and HCV/HIV coinfection seem to have a particularly steep rise in the risk of decompensation with increasing LSM [24].

LSM by MRE has also been associated with hepatic decompensation as a single measurement [34–36] and with progression over time [37].

Since post-hepatectomy liver failure (PHLF)/clinical decompensation is the leading cause of death after HCC resection, the prognostic ability of preoperative LSM in this context has been a topic of interest [38]. For instance, Wu et al. observed a significantly different LSM (by TE) in patients who did and did not develop postoperative liver decompensation (19.1 kPa vs. 11.9 kPa; $p = 0.03$) [39], while Cescon et al. proposed a cut-off value of 15.7 kPa (by TE) to identify high-risk patients [40] and Shen et al. 11.75 kPa (by 2D-SWE) [41]. Another study, using LSM by pSWE, reached the same conclusion, with the most performant model combining LSM with the remnant liver volume rate [42]. On the other hand, Procopet et al. found that LSM had a similar performance as HVPG in predicting decompensation at 3 months but could not predict adequately post-hepatectomy liver failure [43]. A nomogram based on LSM by TE (as well as age, MELD score, and albumin), the CCI (Comprehensive Complication Index), was recently developed by Serenari et al. to help predicting postoperative liver failure following HCC resection (AUC 0.751) [44].

As for TE-based CAP, data is inconclusive. Our group recently showed that a CAP >220 dB/m with M probe was associated with an increased risk of clinical decompensation and bacterial infections independently of LSM in patients with cACLD [45]. Two other studies however could not confirm this association [46, 47], and a bicentric study focusing on obese patients studied with XL probe suggested that CAP below 220 dB/m (possibly indicating a more advanced disease in NASH by absence of steatosis) would be an additional risk factor for decompensation in this population [48].

12.2.2 Spleen Stiffness

A high spleen stiffness has been associated with a higher risk of hepatic decompensation. For instance, in a study by Meister et al., all patients who developed hepatic decompensation ($n = 12$) had a baseline SSM by TE ≥ 39 kPa [49], while Colecchia et al. suggested a cut-off value of 54 kPa [20]. A SSM by SSI ≥ 31.7 kPa has been associated with a 2.70-fold higher risk of event occurrence in patients with compensated cirrhosis over a follow-up period of 18–48 months, with borderline significance ($p = 0.056$) after adjustment for age and MELD [23]. The evolution of SSM over time can also identify patients at risk of complications [50], supporting the longitudinal use of SSM, as it is for LSM.

As discussed in the previous chapter, SSM potentially has multiple advantages over LSM in the assessment of PH, which reflects in its prognostic accuracy. Indeed, SSM outperformed LSM in predicting clinical decompensation in a few studies. Takuma et al. observed that SSM by pSWE performed better than LSM (as well as Child-Pugh and MELD scores) in predicting hepatic decompensation in patients with compensated cirrhosis (HR 14.5; 95% CI 5.8–36.2), with a 14.5-fold risk increase for each SS unit increase and with an optimal cut-off value of 3.25 m/s (NPV of 98.8% and accuracy of 68.9%) [21]. The same group showed that SSM but not LSM (by pSWE) was independently associated with an increased risk of variceal bleeding, with a AUC of 0.857 (maximal NPV at a cut-off value of 3.48 m/s) [51]. Wang et al. showed that a SSM by TE cut-off value of 55.2 kPa had a sensitivity of 90% in predicting variceal bleeding [29], while Buechter et al. found that a SSM cut-off value of 42.6 kPa had a 97% NPV for this complication [31]. In another study, SSM but not LSM (by pSWE) correlated with the presence of ascites (AUC 0.80; 95% CI 0.63–0.98) [52].

As for the ability of SSM to predict PHLF, data is inconclusive [39, 53]. However, interestingly, SSM predicted the development of hepatic decompensation after radiofrequency ablation in patients with HCC in a recent study [54]. However, a study showed that survival after liver resection was lower in patients with LSM $\geq$16.2 kPa, while SSM was not significantly different between those who survived and those who did not [39].

12.2.3 Combination Tests

A few studies have observed that liver and spleen elastography have a prognostic ability to predict decompensation when combined together or with other scores or biomarkers. In a retrospective study of 143 patients, the combination of LSM (cut-off value, 20.8 kPa) and SSM (cut-off value, 42.6 kPa) by TE (LSSM) had a 100% NPV (sensitivity, 100%; specificity, 55%) in identifying those who had prior esophageal variceal bleeding, better than when taken separately [31].

In a large cohort of patients with HBV- or HCV-associated cirrhosis followed for a median of 61.2 months, achieving a "favorable Baveno VI status" (i.e., LSM <20 kPa and PLT >150 $\times$ 10^9/L) after SVR was associated with the absence of PH progression (defined as the onset of VNT- or PH-related bleeding) as well as survival [55]. A study in patients with compensated HBV cirrhosis showed that patients with LSPS 1.1–2.5 and $\geq$2.5 had a higher risk of hepatic decompensation (HR 5.8; $p = 0.004$ and HR 13.6; $p < 0.001$, respectively) compared to those with LSPS <1.1 [6], and Chon et al. found that LSPS had an AUC of 0.848 in predicting decompensation in patients with chronic hepatitis C [5]. A recent study showed that combining LSM and hyaluronic acid (specifically $\geq$200 ng/mL at baseline) provided could better predict complications in patients with chronic hepatitis C than LSM alone [56].

Our group has recently shown that in patients with cACLD and overweight or obesity, LSM, LSPS, and PH risk score have an excellent diagnostic accuracy (using XL probe) to predict the first clinical decompensation (AUC 0.848, 0.881, and 0.890, respectively) [48].

As for liver failure after HCC resection, it could also be predicted by the platelet to spleen stiffness ratio (PSR) [57] and the liver stiffness-spleen size-to-platelet ratio score (LSPS) [53].

12.3   Prediction of Further Clinical Decompensation

LSM and SSM correlate well with outcomes in compensated cirrhosis, but data for decompensated cirrhosis are scarce. A study in patients with alcoholic cirrhosis and refractory ascites did not show any association between baseline LSM (by TE and pSWE) or SSM (by pSWE) and incidence of events or transplant-free survival, regardless if patients were treated with TIPS insertion or with conservative therapy [58]. This could be explained by the limited correlation of stiffness and PH in very advanced liver disease, for both liver and spleen.

The utility of elastography in patients with decompensated cirrhosis also lies in the assessment of the response to treatment. For instance, a change in SSM was shown to have a good performance in predicting response to NSBB in patients with

HRV [59], and patients treated with propranolol who had a decrease in LSM had a lower risk of undergoing liver transplantation or death irrespective of HVPG [60].

Elastography has also been proven useful to monitor patients post TIPS. Jansen et al. showed that an increase in LSM post TIPS reflects inflammation and predicts organ failure and mortality [61]. Multiple studies observed a significant decrease in SSM following TIPS, by both TE [62–64] and pSWE [65, 66], proposing it as a tool to identify TIPS dysfunction. An exception is when there is concurrent embolization or thrombosis of competitive shunts, where SSM may increase post TIPS [67]. An increase in SSM by VTQ after BRTO could also predict the exacerbation of EV in a recent study [68].

LSM and SSM could also be used as prognostic markers in non-cirrhotic PH in various contexts. For instance, LSM was shown to be able predict the development of sinusoidal obstruction syndrome (SOS) in patients undergoing hematopoietic stem cell transplantation (HSCT) before the occurrence of clinical signs [69]. A study showed that patients with extrahepatic portal vein obstruction (EHPVO) who had a history of variceal bleeding had a higher SSM by TE than those who did not (60.4 kPa vs. 30.3 kPa, respectively) [70].

Interestingly, a case series of seven patients with BCS suggested that extremely high (75 kPa) LSM and SSM values at diagnosis could be associated with the development of recurrent decompensation events and need for TIPS or OLT [71]. The authors also suggest that a lack of improvement in LSM could help differentiating those patients who have BCS-related cirrhosis and remain at risk of decompensation from those who recovered.

12.4 Prediction of Development of Hepatocellular Carcinoma

Hepatocellular carcinoma (HCC) is one of the most common malignant tumors in the world, and its incidence is increasing worldwide [72]. HCC is diagnosed mostly at a late stage, where treatment options are still limited, which explains the overall low 5-year survival (12%). Early diagnosis allows a curative treatment with much higher 5-year survival rates [73], and ultrasound screening is therefore suggested in patients at high risk of developing HCC.

Irrespective of the etiology of liver disease, the highest incidence of HCC is observed in patients with cirrhosis. It has been reported that up to one in three patients with cirrhosis develops HCC in a lifetime. In addition, the vast majority of patients with HCC but no cirrhosis show significant or severe fibrosis on histology. In compensated patients, the identification of subjects at risk of HCC is therefore strictly related to a correct staging of liver fibrosis and in particular to the diagnosis of advanced chronic liver disease [73].

Ultrasound elastography proved to be accurate in assessing the degree of liver fibrosis and diagnosing cACLD and liver cirrhosis. In addition, it is noninvasive and reproducible and can be repeated easily in the follow-up, providing dynamic data potentially improving the prediction of risk. Based on these assumptions, liver stiffness measurement by different ultrasound elastography techniques (mostly transient elastography) has been used in studies addressing HCC development risk in patients with chronic liver disease of different etiologies, mostly in studies from Asia [74, 75]. Not unexpectedly, liver stiffness correlated with the risk of developing HCC in patients with HCV and HBV chronic liver disease. In the first report about this topic, Masuzaki et al. reported this association first in 2008 in patients with HCV [76]. In a second study [77], the same group followed up 866 patients with chronic hepatitis C for 3 years and divided them into five groups according to LSM values <10, 10.1–15, 15.1–20, 20.1–25, and >25 kPa. Cumulative incidence rates at 1, 2, and 3 years differed significantly among the five groups and increased with increasing LS values. Similar results have been obtained in studies looking at patients with chronic hepatitis B. In the largest published so far, Jung et al. prospectively followed 1130 chronic hepatitis B patients for a median of 30.7 months [78]. Of them, 57 patients developed HCC. On multivariate analysis, basal LS by TE value >8 kPa was an independent predictor of HCC development with HRs of 3.07, 4.68, 5.55, and 6.60 and LS values of 8–13 kPa, 13–18 kPa, 18–23 kPa, and >23 kPa, respectively. In addition, the authors dynamically evaluated the association between changes in LS values and changes in the risk of HCC development by serial LS measuring during follow-up. Patients with basal LS and serial LS values <13 kPa were significantly at lower risk than patients with basal and serial LS >13 kPa ($p < 0.001$). Several additional papers confirmed these results; the most relevant of the last 5 years are summarized in Table 12.2.

Less data is available regarding patients with viral hepatitis C who have been treated successfully and viral hepatitis B under successful viral suppression. Hamada et al. retrospectively evaluated 196 patients who achieved SVR using LS by 2D shear wave elastography (SWE). Among them, eight patients developed HCC after SVR (median time 28 months, range 6–46 months). Univariate and multivariate analysis showed that LS at SVR24 was independently associated with the development of HCC. ROC analysis identified LS ≥11 kPa as a cut-off value for predicting the development of HCC, with a negative predictive value of 0.989 [72].

Rinaldi et al. prospectively followed 258 patients with HCV cirrhosis who received DAAs aiming at studying the association between pre-treatment LSM by TE and development of HCC after SVR. Baseline LSM was significantly higher in patients who developed HCC than patients who did not (37.2 kPa vs. 23.9 kPa; $p < 0.0001$). On multivariate analysis, pre-therapy LSM was an independent predictor of HCC development. The best cut-off was 27.8 kPa (sensitivity 72% and specificity 65%) [79].

Since LSM decreases rapidly during and after treatment with DAAs, which has been attributed to changes in intrahepatic inflammation, Ravaioli et al. retrospectively evaluated 139 patients with HCV cirrhosis treated with DAAs to assess whether the difference in LSM at the end of DAA treatment (EOT) vs. pre-therapy (ΔLSM) could provide additional information on the risk of developing HCC. During a median follow-up of 15 months (IQR 12–19), 20 patients developed HCC. The ΔLSM was significantly lower in patients who developed HCC than patients who did not. On multivariate analysis, ΔLSM lower than −30% (HR 5.360; 95% CI 1.561–18.405; $p = 0.008$) was an independent predictor of HCC development after

Table 12.2 Main studies of the last 5 years using ultrasound elastography techniques to predict HCC in CLD

Study (year)	Region	N included patients	Etiology	Median follow-up (months)	N who developed HCC	AUROC LSM	Selected cut-off (kPa)
Kim et al. (2015)	Asia	2876	HBV	48.9	52	0.532	13.0
Wang et al. (2016)	Asia	278	HCV	91.2	18	0.781	12.0
Adler et al. (2016)	Europe	432	Mixed	31.3	41	N/A	20.0
Bihari et al. (2016)	Asia	964	HBV	N/A	14	0.767	N/A
Seo et al. (2016)	Asia	381	HBV	48.1	34	0.745	N/A
Jeon et al. (2017)	Asia	540	HBV	54.1	81	0.598	13.0
Li et al. (2017)	Asia	1200	HBV	48	156	N/A	N/A
D'Ambrosio et al. (2018)	Europe	404	HCV	36	24	N/A	N/A
Hamada et al. (2018)	Asia	196	HCV (pre-post DAAs)	26	8	N/A	11
Ravaioli al. (2018)	Europe	139	HCV (pre-post DAAs)	15	20	N/A	<−30%[a]
Rinaldi et al. (2019)	Europe	258	HCV (pre-post DAAs)	12	35	0.691	27.8
Wang et al. (2019)	Asia	371	HBV	67.2	27	0.636	21.5
Degasperi et al. (2019)	Europe	546	HCV (SVR)	25	28	N/A	30.0
Izumi et al. (2019)	Asia	419	HCV	30	32	0.806	8.0
Izumi et al. (2019)	Asia	377	HBV	27	23	0.795	6.2
Izumi et al. (2019)	Asia	258	NAFLD	30	33	0.698	5.4
Pons et al. (2019)	Europe	572	HCV (SVR)	33	25	N/A	N/A
Nakagomi et al. (2019)	Asia	1146	HCV	78	190	N/A	N/A
Papatheodoridis et al. (2020)	Europe	1427	HBV (on entecavir or tenofovir)	8.4 years	33	N/A	12.0

AUROC area under the receiver operating characteristic curve, *DAA* direct-acting antiviral, *HBV* hepatitis B virus, *HCC* hepatocellular carcinoma, *HCV* hepatitis C virus, *LSM* liver stiffness measurement, *N/A* not applicable, *NAFLD* non-alcoholic fatty liver disease, *SVR* sustained virologic response
[a]Change in LSM less than −30% was an independent predictor of HCC development after DAA treatment

DAA treatment. It was suggested that monitoring HCV patients with LSM at EOT and subsequently calculating the ΔLS may therefore improve the ultrasound-based screening for HCC identification after DAA treatment [80].

A study from Beijing followed up 438 chronic hepatitis B patients with compensated cirrhosis. Patients were on entecavir-based antiviral therapy, and LSM was measured every 26 weeks for 2 years. The researchers aimed at defining the relationship between the percentage of change in LSM and liver-related events (LRE). Sixteen patients had episodes of decompensation and 18 developed a HCC. Patients who did not develop LRE had a median LSM of 17.8 kPa, 12.3 kPa, 10.6 kPa, and 10.2 kPa at Week 0, 26, 52, and 78, respectively, with a decrease in the first 26 weeks of 30.9%. Patients who developed LRE had a median LSM of 20.9 kPa, 18.6 kPa, 20.4 kPa, and 20.3 kPa at Week 0, 26, 52, and 78 with a decrease in the first 26 weeks of 11%. The percentage of change in LSM from Week 26 vs. baseline was statistically different between the two groups ($p = 0.004$), suggesting that not only baseline value but improvement or worsening of liver stiffness possibly due to the existence of comorbidities impacts the risk of HCC and might be used for risk stratification [81].

These observations led to the creation of models integrating liver stiffness together with other variables independently predicting HCC risk. In a study from Japan conducted in 1808 patients with CLD, LS by pSWE (ARFI virtual touch quantification) >1.33 m/s, FPG >110 mg/dL, sex (male), age >55 years, and alpha-fetoprotein (AFP) >5 ng/mL were independently associated with HCC development. Using these five parameters, the VFMAP score could be calculated (0 if below or 1 if above the cut-off; range 0–5). Findings were a low score with 0–1 points ($n = 478$), intermediate score with 2–3 points ($n = 673$), and high score with 4–5 points ($n = 172$). The 3 and 5 years cumulative incidence rates of HCC were 0% and 0.3% in the low-score group, 3.0% and 3.5% in the intermediate-score group, and 11.7% and 14.8% in the high-score group ($p < 0.001$ among groups). The hazard ratios for the incidence of HCC in the intermediate- and high-score groups were 17.37 (95% CI 2.35–128.40; $p = 0.005$) and 66.82 (95% CI 9.01–495.80; $p < 0.001$), respectively, compared to the low-score group. The AUC of VFMAP scores was 0.82 (95% CI 0.76–0.87). When using a VFMAP score cut-off level of 3, the NPV for excluding HCC development in 5 years was 98.2% [82].

In South Korea, scientists assessed the efficiency of four models in predicting HCC in treated chronic hepatitis B patients at two different time points with a 6-month interval. CU-HCC model included age, serum albumin level, total bilirubin level, HBV DNA level, and cirrhosis. REACH-B model included gender, age, alanine aminotransferase (ALT) level, hepatitis B e antigen (HBeAg) status, and HBV DNA level. LSM-HCC model included LSM assessed by TE, together with age, serum albumin level, and HBV DNA level. Modified REACH-B (mREACH-B) model included the LSM value instead of HBV DNA. All four models significantly predicted the HCC development at the two different time points; however, the change in their values between the two time points did not [83].

However, it remains unclear how to translate these findings into clinical practice, and until new data become available, according to the current guidelines, all patients with cirrhosis prior to treatment should be kept on ultrasound surveillance for HCC every 6 months lifelong [84]. Whether ultrasound screening intervals could be safely modified according to risk stratification remains open to future studies.

12.4.1 Prediction of HCC Recurrence After Treatment

Lee et al. retrospectively evaluated the association between preoperative LSM values and de novo HCC recurrence in 111 HCC patients who had a resection surgery. In this study, 47 patients had de novo HCC recurrence. On multivariate analysis, preoperative LSM was an independent predictor of HCC recurrence, and patients with LSM >13.0 kPa had a significantly higher risk than patients with LSM <13.0 kPa ($p < 0.05$) [74].

Another prospective study evaluated 133 HCC patients with available preoperative LSM who had a curative resection. During a median follow-up of 25 months (range 3–54.6), 62 had HCC recurrence. On multivariate analysis, preoperative LSM was one of the independent predictors of recurrence (HR 1.034; 95% CI 1.007–1.061; $p < 0.05$). A cut-off value of 13.4 kPa was the best to discriminate the risk of recurrence at 1, 2, and 3 years ($p = 0.009$) [74]. A study from Kyungpook National University followed prospectively 138 patients with HCC who underwent radiofrequency ablation (RFA) for a median of 21.9 months (range 3–60). LS was assessed by pSWE (Virtual Touch ARFI) and TE before the intervention. On multivariate analysis, LSM by both techniques were independent predictors of HCC recurrence. The optimal cut-off value for pSWE was 1.6 m/s, while it was 14 kPa for TE [85].

12.5 Survival

LSM has been repeatedly shown to be a very good predictor of survival in viral CLD such as in HBV [9], HCV [4], and HCV/HIV [33] cirrhosis, and a rise in LSM over time has been associated with a poorer survival compared to a decrease in LSM in patients with chronic hepatitis C [86]. Additionally, a recent cohort study showed that baseline LSM was an independent predictor of overall survival in NAFLD patients [19].

A recent systematic review and meta-analysis showed that for each kPa increase in baseline LSM, there was an 8% increase in all-cause mortality and a 11% increase in liver-related mortality [24]. Another recent meta-analysis found similar results (RR 1.06; 95% CI 1.06–1.07 for LREs and RR 1.06; 95% CI 1.04–1.07 for all-cause mortality) [25], while the RR was slightly higher in an earlier meta-analysis (RR 1.22; 95% CI 1.05–1.43) [26]. The meta-analysis by Shen et al. also showed that, compared with the reference of 5 kPa, the pooled RR (95% CI) was 1.34 (0.86–2.07) for 8.5 kPa, 3.25 (1.90–5.56) for 13.5 kPa, 7.72 (4.51–13.22) for 19.8 kPa, and 14.25 (8.22–24.73) for 37.5 kPa, respectively [24]. The plot showed a steep increase in the risk of all-cause mortality for baseline LSM below 24.1 kPa and then turned into a relatively stable increase. Takuma et al. showed that SSM by pSWE was also an excellent predictor of mortality in patients with both compensated and decompensated cirrhosis, with optimal cut-off values of 3.41 m/s and 3.53 m/s, respectively [21]. LSM by MRE has also been associated with survival [34].

12.6 Conclusion

Liver stiffness, and to lesser extent spleen stiffness, can be considered validated predictors of clinical decompensation and survival in patients with compensated advanced chronic liver disease of different etiologies. Even if cut-off values vary among the different studies, it seems evident that models including liver stiffness and possibly spleen stiffness together with other noninvasive variables and clinical characteristics might be already calculated to improve risk stratification in this population. In addition to "static" baseline measurements, "dynamic," repeated measurements over time could be used, allowing to better understand the evolution or regression of the underlying liver disease, which relates to prognosis. The creation of such predictive models and the subsequent calibration in the different etiologies and settings remain an unmet need that could potentially move the field forward allowing individualization of care.

Liver stiffness measurement has emerged as well as predictor of hepatocellular carcinoma, likely since this parameter integrates fibrosis severity, inflammation, and indirectly portal hypertension, which play a role in the pathogenesis of HCC. In this field, predictive models taking into account this parameter have already been calculated and validated, but pragmatic trials comparing different surveillance strategies according to different LSM risk categories have not been performed and would be highly needed to assess whether imaging could be restricted to the middle-high-risk cases.

Acknowledgement *Financial Support*: Élise Vuille-Lessard is supported by a Clinical Hepatology Fellowship of the Canadian Association for the Study of the Liver (CASL-CLF 2020–2021). Ahmed Y. Elmahdy is supported by a Swiss Government Excellence Scholarship (ESKAS 2019.0832).

References

1. D'Amico G, Morabito A, D'Amico M, Pasta L, Malizia G, Rebora P, et al. Clinical states of cirrhosis and competing risks. J Hepatol. 2018;68(3):563–76.
2. Berzigotti A, Garcia-Tsao G, Bosch J, Grace ND, Burroughs AK, Morillas R, et al. Obesity is an independent risk factor for clinical decompensation in patients with cirrhosis. Hepatology. 2011;54(2):555–61.
3. Robic MA, Procopet B, Metivier S, Peron JM, Selves J, Vinel JP, et al. Liver stiffness accurately predicts portal hypertension related complications in patients with chronic liver disease: a prospective study. J Hepatol. 2011;55(5):1017–24.

4. Vergniol J, Foucher J, Terrebonne E, Bernard PH, le Bail B, Merrouche W, et al. Noninvasive tests for fibrosis and liver stiffness predict 5-year outcomes of patients with chronic hepatitis C. Gastroenterology. 2011;140(7):1970–9, 9.e1–3.

5. Chon YE, Jung ES, Park JY, Kim DY, Ahn SH, Han KH, et al. The accuracy of noninvasive methods in predicting the development of hepatocellular carcinoma and hepatic decompensation in patients with chronic hepatitis B. J Clin Gastroenterol. 2012;46(6):518–25.

6. Kim BK, Park YN, Kim DY, Park JY, Chon CY, Han KH, et al. Risk assessment of development of hepatic decompensation in histologically proven hepatitis B viral cirrhosis using liver stiffness measurement. Digestion. 2012;85(3):219–27.

7. Kim SU, Lee JH, Kim DY, Ahn SH, Jung KS, Choi EH, et al. Prediction of liver-related events using fibroscan in chronic hepatitis B patients showing advanced liver fibrosis. PLoS One. 2012;7(5):e36676.

8. Merchante N, Rivero-Juárez A, Téllez F, Merino D, José Ríos-Villegas M, Márquez-Solero M, et al. Liver stiffness predicts clinical outcome in human immunodeficiency virus/hepatitis C virus-coinfected patients with compensated liver cirrhosis. Hepatology. 2012;56(1):228–38.

9. de Ledinghen V, Vergniol J, Barthe C, Foucher J, Chermak F, Le Bail B, et al. Non-invasive tests for fibrosis and liver stiffness predict 5-year survival of patients chronically infected with hepatitis B virus. Aliment Pharmacol Ther. 2013;37(10):979–88.

10. Corpechot C, Gaouar F, El Naggar A, Kemgang A, Wendum D, Poupon R, et al. Baseline values and changes in liver stiffness measured by transient elastography are associated with severity of fibrosis and outcomes of patients with primary sclerosing cholangitis. Gastroenterology. 2014;146(4):970–9; quiz e15–6.

11. Pang JX, Zimmer S, Niu S, Crotty P, Tracey J, Pradhan F, et al. Liver stiffness by transient elastography predicts liver-related complications and mortality in patients with chronic liver disease. PLoS One. 2014;9(4):e95776.

12. Perez-Latorre L, Sanchez-Conde M, Rincon D, Miralles P, Aldamiz-Echevarria T, Carrero A, et al. Prediction of liver complications in patients with hepatitis C virus-related cirrhosis with and without HIV coinfection: comparison of hepatic venous pressure gradient and transient elastography. Clin Infect Dis. 2014;58(5):713–8.

13. Wang JH, Chuah SK, Lu SN, Hung CH, Kuo CM, Tai WC, et al. Baseline and serial liver stiffness measurement in prediction of portal hypertension progression for patients with compensated cirrhosis. Liver Int. 2014;34(9):1340–8.

14. Kitson MT, Roberts SK, Colman JC, Paul E, Button P, Kemp W. Liver stiffness and the prediction of clinically significant portal hypertension and portal hypertensive complications. Scand J Gastroenterol. 2015;50(4):462–9.

15. Park MS, Kim SU, Kim BK, Park JY, Kim DY, Ahn SH, et al. Prognostic value of the combined use of transient elastography and fibrotest in patients with chronic hepatitis B. Liver Int. 2015;35(2):455–62.

16. Wong GL, Chan HL, Yu Z, Wong CK, Leung C, Ho PP, et al. Noninvasive assessments of liver fibrosis with transient elastography and Hui index predict survival in patients with chronic hepatitis B. J Gastroenterol Hepatol. 2015;30(3):582–90.

17. Dillon A, Galvin Z, Sultan AA, Harman D, Guha IN, Stewart S. Transient elastography can stratify patients with Child-Pugh A cirrhosis according to risk of early decompensation. Eur J Gastroenterol Hepatol. 2018;30(12):1434–40.

18. Wu M, Wu L, Jin J, Wang J, Li S, Zeng J, et al. Liver stiffness measured with two-dimensional shear-wave elastography is predictive of liver-related events in patients with chronic liver disease due to hepatis B viral infection. Radiology. 2020;295:353.

19. Shili-Masmoudi S, Wong GL, Hiriart JB, Liu K, Chermak F, Shu SS, et al. Liver stiffness measurement predicts long-term survival and complications in non-alcoholic fatty liver disease. Liver Int. 2020;40(3):581–9.

20. Colecchia A, Colli A, Casazza G, Mandolesi D, Schiumerini R, Reggiani LB, et al. Spleen stiffness measurement can predict clinical complications in compensated HCV-related cirrhosis: a prospective study. J Hepatol. 2014;60(6):1158–64.

21. Takuma Y, Morimoto Y, Takabatake H, Toshikuni N, Tomokuni J, Sahara A, et al. Measurement of spleen stiffness with acoustic radiation force impulse imaging predicts mortality and hepatic decompensation in patients with liver cirrhosis. Clin Gastroenterol Hepatol. 2017;15(11):1782–90.e4.
22. Cassinotto C, Charrie A, Mouries A, Lapuyade B, Hiriart JB, Vergniol J, et al. Liver and spleen elastography using supersonic shear imaging for the non-invasive diagnosis of cirrhosis severity and oesophageal varices. Dig Liver Dis. 2015;47(8):695–701.
23. Grgurević I, Bokun T, Mustapić S, Trkulja V, Heinzl R, Banić M, et al. Real-time two-dimensional shear wave ultrasound elastography of the liver is a reliable predictor of clinical outcomes and the presence of esophageal varices in patients with compensated liver cirrhosis. Croat Med J. 2015;56(5):470–81.
24. Shen Y, Wu SD, Wu L, Wang SQ, Chen Y, Liu LL, et al. The prognostic role of liver stiffness in patients with chronic liver disease: a systematic review and dose-response meta-analysis. Hepatol Int. 2019;13(5):560–72.
25. Wang J, Li J, Zhou Q, Zhang D, Bi Q, Wu Y, et al. Liver stiffness measurement predicted liver-related events and all-cause mortality: a systematic review and nonlinear dose-response meta-analysis. Hepatol Commun. 2018;2(4):467–76.
26. Singh S, Fujii LL, Murad MH, Wang Z, Asrani SK, Ehman RL, et al. Liver stiffness is associated with risk of decompensation, liver cancer, and death in patients with chronic liver diseases: a systematic review and meta-analysis. Clin Gastroenterol Hepatol. 2013;11(12):1573–84. e1-2; quiz e88–9.
27. Merchante N, Téllez F, Rivero-Juárez A, Ríos-Villegas MJ, Merino D, Márquez-Solero M, et al. Progression of liver stiffness predicts clinical events in HIV/HCV-coinfected patients with compensated cirrhosis. BMC Infect Dis. 2015;15:557.
28. Pons M, Rodriguez-Tajes S, Esteban JI, Marino Z, Vargas V, Lens S, et al. Non-invasive prediction of liver-related events in patients with HCV-associated compensated advanced chronic liver disease after oral antivirals. J Hepatol. 2020;72(3):472–80.
29. Wang XK, Wang P, Zhang Y, Qi SL, Chi K, Wang GC. A study on spleen transient elastography in predicting the degree of esophageal varices and bleeding. Medicine (Baltimore). 2019;98(9):e14615.
30. Merchante N, Rivero-Juárez A, Téllez F, Merino D, Ríos-Villegas MJ, Ojeda-Burgos G, et al. Liver stiffness predicts variceal bleeding in HIV/HCV-coinfected patients with compensated cirrhosis. AIDS. 2017;31(4):493–500.
31. Buechter M, Kahraman A, Manka P, Gerken G, Jochum C, Canbay A, et al. Spleen and liver stiffness is positively correlated with the risk of esophageal variceal bleeding. Digestion. 2016;94(3):138–44.
32. Bloom S, Kemp W, Nicoll A, Roberts SK, Gow P, Dev A, et al. Liver stiffness measurement in the primary care setting detects high rates of advanced fibrosis and predicts liver-related events in hepatitis C. J Hepatol. 2018;69(3):575–83.
33. Macías J, Mancebo M, Márquez M, Merino D, Téllez F, Rivero A, et al. Low risk of liver decompensation among human immunodeficiency virus/hepatitis C virus-coinfected patients with mild fibrosis in the short term. Hepatology. 2015;61(5):1503–11.
34. Lee DH, Lee JM, Chang W, Yoon JH, Kim YJ, Lee JH, et al. Prognostic role of liver stiffness measurements using magnetic resonance elastography in patients with compensated chronic liver disease. Eur Radiol. 2018;28(8):3513–21.
35. Asrani SK, Talwalkar JA, Kamath PS, Shah VH, Saracino G, Jennings L, et al. Role of magnetic resonance elastography in compensated and decompensated liver disease. J Hepatol. 2014;60(5):934–9.
36. Idilman IS, Low HM, Bakhshi Z, Eaton J, Venkatesh SK. Comparison of liver stiffness measurement with MRE and liver and spleen volumetry for prediction of disease severity and hepatic decompensation in patients with primary sclerosing cholangitis. Abdom Radiol (NY). 2020;45:701.

37. Eaton JE, Sen A, Hoodeshenas S, Schleck CD, Harmsen WS, Gores GJ, et al. Changes in liver stiffness, measured by magnetic resonance elastography, associated with hepatic decompensation in patients with primary sclerosing cholangitis. Clin Gastroenterol Hepatol. 2019;18:1576.
38. Berzigotti A, Reig M, Abraldes JG, Bosch J, Bruix J. Portal hypertension and the outcome of surgery for hepatocellular carcinoma in compensated cirrhosis: a systematic review and meta-analysis. Hepatology. 2015;61(2):526–36.
39. Wu D, Chen E, Liang T, Wang M, Chen B, Lang B, et al. Predicting the risk of postoperative liver failure and overall survival using liver and spleen stiffness measurements in patients with hepatocellular carcinoma. Medicine (Baltimore). 2017;96(34):e7864.
40. Cescon M, Colecchia A, Cucchetti A, Peri E, Montrone L, Ercolani G, et al. Value of transient elastography measured with FibroScan in predicting the outcome of hepatic resection for hepatocellular carcinoma. Ann Surg. 2012;256(5):706–12; discussion 12–3.
41. Shen Y, Zhou C, Zhu G, Shi G, Zhu X, Huang C, et al. Liver stiffness assessed by shear wave elastography predicts postoperative liver failure in patients with hepatocellular carcinoma. J Gastrointest Surg. 2017;21(9):1471–9.
42. Nishio T, Taura K, Koyama Y, Tanabe K, Yamamoto G, Okuda Y, et al. Prediction of posthepatectomy liver failure based on liver stiffness measurement in patients with hepatocellular carcinoma. Surgery. 2016;159(2):399–408.
43. Procopet B, Fischer P, Horhat A, Mois E, Stefanescu H, Comsa M, et al. Good performance of liver stiffness measurement in the prediction of postoperative hepatic decompensation in patients with cirrhosis complicated with hepatocellular carcinoma. Med Ultrason. 2018;20(3):272–7.
44. Serenari M, Han KH, Ravaioli F, Kim SU, Cucchetti A, Han DH, et al. A nomogram based on liver stiffness predicts postoperative complications in patients with hepatocellular carcinoma. J Hepatol. 2020;73:855.
45. Margini C, Murgia G, Stirnimann G, De Gottardi A, Semmo N, Casu S, et al. Prognostic significance of controlled attenuation parameter in patients with compensated advanced chronic liver disease. Hepatol Commun. 2018;2(8):929–40.
46. Scheiner B, Steininger L, Semmler G, Unger LW, Schwabl P, Bucsics T, et al. Controlled attenuation parameter does not predict hepatic decompensation in patients with advanced chronic liver disease. Liver Int. 2019;39(1):127–35.
47. Liu K, Wong VW, Lau K, Liu SD, Tse YK, Yip TC, et al. Prognostic value of controlled attenuation parameter by transient elastography. Am J Gastroenterol. 2017;112(12):1812–23.
48. Mendoza Y, Cocciolillo S, Murgia G, Chen T, Margini C, Sebastiani G, et al. Noninvasive markers of portal hypertension detect decompensation in overweight or obese patients with compensated advanced chronic liver disease. Clin Gastroenterol Hepatol. 2020;18:3017.
49. Meister P, Dechêne A, Büchter M, Kälsch J, Gerken G, Canbay A, et al. Spleen stiffness differentiates between acute and chronic liver damage and predicts hepatic decompensation. J Clin Gastroenterol. 2018;53:457.
50. Zhang Y, Mao DF, Zhang MW, Fan XX. Clinical value of liver and spleen shear wave velocity in predicting the prognosis of patients with portal hypertension. World J Gastroenterol. 2017;23(45):8044–52.
51. Takuma Y, Nouso K, Morimoto Y, Tomokuni J, Sahara A, Takabatake H, et al. Prediction of oesophageal variceal bleeding by measuring spleen stiffness in patients with liver cirrhosis. Gut. 2016;65(2):354–5.
52. Mori K, Arai H, Abe T, Takayama H, Toyoda M, Ueno T, et al. Spleen stiffness correlates with the presence of ascites but not esophageal varices in chronic hepatitis C patients. Biomed Res Int. 2013;2013:857862.
53. Marasco G, Colecchia A, Dajti E, Ravaioli F, Cucchetti A, Cescon M, et al. Prediction of posthepatectomy liver failure: role of SSM and LSPS. J Surg Oncol. 2019;119(3):400–1.
54. Lee PC, Chiou YY, Chiu NC, Chen PH, Liu CA, Kao WY, et al. Liver stiffness measured by acoustic radiation force impulse elastography predicted prognoses of hepatocellular carcinoma after radiofrequency ablation. Sci Rep. 2020;10(1):2006.

55. Thabut D, Bureau C, Layese R, Bourcier V, Hammouche M, Cagnot C, et al. Validation of Baveno VI criteria for screening and surveillance of esophageal varices in patients with compensated cirrhosis and a sustained response to antiviral therapy. Gastroenterology. 2019;156(4):997–1009.e5.
56. Hansen JF, Christiansen KM, Staugaard B, Moessner BK, Lillevang S, Krag A, et al. Combining liver stiffness with hyaluronic acid provides superior prognostic performance in chronic hepatitis C. PLoS One. 2019;14(2):e0212036.
57. Peng W, Li JW, Zhang XY, Li C, Wen TF, Yan LN, et al. A novel model for predicting posthepatectomy liver failure in patients with hepatocellular carcinoma. PLoS One. 2019;14(7):e0219219.
58. Lindner F, Mühlberg R, Wiegand J, Tröltzsch M, Hoffmeister A, Keim V, et al. Predictive value of liver and spleen stiffness in advanced alcoholic cirrhosis with refractory ascites. Z Gastroenterol. 2018;56(6):561–8.
59. Kim HY, So YH, Kim W, Ahn DW, Jung YJ, Woo H, et al. Non-invasive response prediction in prophylactic carvedilol therapy for cirrhotic patients with esophageal varices. J Hepatol. 2019;70(3):412–22.
60. Piecha F, Mandorfer M, Peccerella T, Ozga AK, Poth T, Vonbank A, et al. Pharmacological decrease of liver stiffness is pressure-related and predicts long-term clinical outcome. Am J Physiol Gastrointest Liver Physiol. 2018;315(4):G484–G94.
61. Jansen C, Moller P, Meyer C, Kolbe CC, Bogs C, Pohlmann A, et al. Increase in liver stiffness after transjugular intrahepatic portosystemic shunt is associated with inflammation and predicts mortality. Hepatology. 2018;67(4):1472–84.
62. Ran HT, Ye XP, Zheng YY, Zhang DZ, Wang ZG, Chen J, et al. Spleen stiffness and splenoportal venous flow: assessment before and after transjugular intrahepatic portosystemic shunt placement. J Ultrasound Med. 2013;32(2):221–8.
63. Gao J, Zheng X, Zheng YY, Zuo GQ, Ran HT, Auh YH, et al. Shear wave elastography of the spleen for monitoring transjugular intrahepatic portosystemic shunt function: a pilot study. J Ultrasound Med. 2016;35(5):951–8.
64. Buechter M, Manka P, Theysohn JM, Reinboldt M, Canbay A, Kahraman A. Spleen stiffness is positively correlated with HVPG and decreases significantly after TIPS implantation. Dig Liver Dis. 2018;50(1):54–60.
65. Attia D, Rodt T, Marquardt S, Hinrichs J, Meyer BC, Gebel M, et al. Shear wave elastography prior to transjugular intrahepatic portosystemic shunt may predict the decrease in hepatic vein pressure gradient. Abdom Radiol (NY). 2019;44(3):1127–34.
66. De Santis A, Nardelli S, Bassanelli C, Lupo M, Iegri C, Di Ciesco CA, et al. Modification of splenic stiffness on acoustic radiation force impulse parallels the variation of portal pressure induced by transjugular intrahepatic portosystemic shunt. J Gastroenterol Hepatol. 2018;33(3):704–9.
67. Novelli PM, Cho K, Rubin JM. Sonographic assessment of spleen stiffness before and after transjugular intrahepatic portosystemic shunt placement with or without concurrent embolization of portal systemic collateral veins in patients with cirrhosis and portal hypertension: a feasibility study. J Ultrasound Med. 2015;34(3):443–9.
68. Takuma Y, Morimoto Y, Takabatake H, Tomokuni J, Sahara A, Matsueda K, et al. Changes in liver and spleen stiffness by virtual touch quantification technique after balloon-occluded retrograde transvenous obliteration of gastric varices and exacerbation of esophageal varices: a preliminary study. Ultraschall Med. 2020;41(2):157–66.
69. Colecchia A, Ravaioli F, Sessa M, Alemanni VL, Dajti E, Marasco G, et al. Liver stiffness measurement allows early diagnosis of veno-occlusive disease/sinusoidal obstruction syndrome in adult patients who undergo hematopoietic stem cell transplantation: results from a monocentric prospective study. Biol Blood Marrow Transplant. 2019;25:995.
70. Sharma P, Mishra SR, Kumar M, Sharma BC, Sarin SK. Liver and spleen stiffness in patients with extrahepatic portal vein obstruction. Radiology. 2012;263(3):893–9.

71. Dajti E, Ravaioli F, Colecchia A, Marasco G, Vestito A, Festi D. Liver and spleen stiffness measurements for assessment of portal hypertension severity in patients with Budd Chiari syndrome. Can J Gastroenterol Hepatol. 2019;2019:1673197.

72. Hamada K, Saitoh S, Nishino N, Fukushima D, Horikawa Y, Nishida S, et al. Shear wave elastography predicts hepatocellular carcinoma risk in hepatitis C patients after sustained virological response. PLoS One. 2018;13(4):e0195173.

73. Bruix J, Reig M, Sherman M. Evidence-based diagnosis, staging, and treatment of patients with hepatocellular carcinoma. Gastroenterology. 2016;150(4):835–53.

74. Park MS, Han KH, Kim SU. Non-invasive prediction of development of hepatocellular carcinoma using transient elastography in patients with chronic liver disease. Expert Rev Gastroenterol Hepatol. 2014;8(5):501–11.

75. Marasco G, Colecchia A, Silva G, Rossini B, Eusebi LH, Ravaioli F, et al. Non-invasive tests for the prediction of primary hepatocellular carcinoma. World J Gastroenterol. 2020;26(24):3326–43.

76. Masuzaki R, Tateishi R, Yoshida H, Yoshida H, Sato S, Kato N, et al. Risk assessment of hepatocellular carcinoma in chronic hepatitis C patients by transient elastography. J Clin Gastroenterol. 2008;42(7):839–43.

77. Masuzaki R, Tateishi R, Yoshida H, Goto E, Sato T, Ohki T, et al. Prospective risk assessment for hepatocellular carcinoma development in patients with chronic hepatitis C by transient elastography. Hepatology. 2009;49(6):1954–61.

78. Jung KS, Kim SU, Ahn SH, Park YN, Kim DY, Park JY, et al. Risk assessment of hepatitis B virus-related hepatocellular carcinoma development using liver stiffness measurement (FibroScan). Hepatology. 2011;53(3):885–94.

79. Rinaldi L, Guarino M, Perrella A, Pafundi PC, Valente G, Fontanella L, et al. Role of liver stiffness measurement in predicting hcc occurrence in direct-acting antivirals setting: a real-life experience. Dig Dis Sci. 2019;64(10):3013–9.

80. Ravaioli F, Conti F, Brillanti S, Andreone P, Mazzella G, Buonfiglioli F, et al. Hepatocellular carcinoma risk assessment by the measurement of liver stiffness variations in HCV cirrhotics treated with direct acting antivirals. Dig Liver Dis. 2018;50(6):573–9.

81. Wu S, Kong Y, Piao H, Jiang W, Xie W, Chen Y, et al. On-treatment changes of liver stiffness at week 26 could predict 2-year clinical outcomes in HBV-related compensated cirrhosis. Liver Int. 2018;38(6):1045–54.

82. Aoki T, Iijima H, Tada T, Kumada T, Nishimura T, Nakano C, et al. Prediction of development of hepatocellular carcinoma using a new scoring system involving virtual touch quantification in patients with chronic liver diseases. J Gastroenterol. 2017;52(1):104–12.

83. Jeon MY, Lee HW, Kim SU, Kim BK, Park JY, Kim DY, et al. Feasibility of dynamic risk prediction for hepatocellular carcinoma development in patients with chronic hepatitis B. Liver Int. 2018;38(4):676–86.

84. European Association for the Study of the Liver. EASL Clinical Practice Guidelines: management of hepatocellular carcinoma. J Hepatol. 2018;69(1):182–236.

85. Yoon JS, Lee YR, Kweon YO, Tak WY, Jang SY, Park SY, et al. Comparison of acoustic radiation force impulse elastography and transient elastography for prediction of hepatocellular carcinoma recurrence after radiofrequency ablation. Eur J Gastroenterol Hepatol. 2018;30(10):1230–6.

86. Vergniol J, Boursier J, Coutzac C, Bertrais S, Foucher J, Angel C, et al. Evolution of non-invasive tests of liver fibrosis is associated with prognosis in patients with chronic hepatitis C. Hepatology. 2014;60(1):65–76.

Part III

Extrahepatic Diseases: Pancreas

Pancreas: Transabdominal Ultrasound-Based Elastography

13

Clara Benedetta Conti and Roberta Pozzi

13.1 Introduction

Nowadays, elastography is widely used in the evaluation of many tissues, from the liver (where the liver stiffness assessment of fibrosis has even updated the routine use of liver biopsy in patients with chronic liver diseases) to the assessment of lymph nodes, prostate, thyroid, breasts, and spleen.

These achievements in the noninvasive evaluation of tissue stiffness have raised the physicians' interest about investigating the potential feasibility and clinical applicability of pancreatic stiffness (PS). Basically, by using ultrasound-based methods, PS can be measured through transabdominal elastography or echoendoscopic elastography. This chapter aims to provide a comprehensive overview of the application of transabdominal elastography to the pancreas.

Transient elastography (FibroScan, EchoSense), largely used for the assessment of liver stiffness, cannot be applied to the pancreas as this organ is located deep in the abdomen and difficult to explore without proper visualization to correctly place the probe. Therefore, the application of transabdominal elastography to the pancreas needs an elastographic software module incorporated in the ultrasound (US) machine, in order to properly apply elastography to the tissue under the US B-mode guidance. This way a physician can perfectly target the pancreas during the parenchymal stiffness measurement. However, this is not the only reason to perform a complete pancreatic US examination before performing PS assessment. Indeed, the pancreas dimensions (head, corpus), the echo pattern, and the pancreatic duct diameter should also be evaluated as they provide very useful additional information. For example, US scan can help to find signs of chronic pancreatitis, such as calcifications, duct irregularities, pseudocysts, or lesions (solid, cysts). The presence of large

C. B. Conti (✉)
Gastroenterology and Digestive Endoscopy, ASST Cremona, Cremona, Italy

R. Pozzi
Internal Medicine Unit, ASST Lecco, Lecco, Italy

© Springer Nature Switzerland AG 2021
M. Fraquelli (ed.), *Elastography of the Liver and Beyond*,
https://doi.org/10.1007/978-3-030-74132-7_13

cysts or ductal pancreatic irregularities may interfere with measurement acquisition. Moreover, elastographic measurements require an excellent US window, not always easy to obtain, especially in obese patients or in the presence of large-volume ascites. This difficulty can be avoided just by setting the region of interest (ROI) in a space free of liquid. Conversely, obesity may interfere with PS measurement as a consequence of the deep location of the organ. In this case, a physician may find it impossible to correctly position the ROI and, thus, to acquire the measurement. Apart from these possible technical problems, measuring PS is usually a quick and easy task to perform. The measurements should be performed with the patient in supine position, fasting conditions (for at least 6 h). The number of measurements to be performed is ideally five to ten, and it usually takes around 10 min [1–8]. The patient should stop breathing in an indifferent breathing phase while each measurement is made, in order not to affect the measurement value as it occurs in the inspiration phase of breathing.

PS assessment has been proposed to characterize both pancreatic tumors and benign pancreatic diseases [1]. Regarding the different techniques, in the available studies, the methods that are commonly applied are both ultrasound strain elastography and ultrasound shear wave elastography (SWE). The strain method is only qualitative and depends on color maps to display the magnitude of strain in a tissue. Thus, it is a highly operator-dependent method. In the case of strain elastography, in fact, quantitative analysis can be achieved by the use of the strain ratio, defined as the ratio of the strain of a reference tissue divided by the strain of the target tissue. However, there is no consensus yet on where to set the reference area in the pancreas. During pancreatic cancer assessment, some investigators have set the reference area on a non-tumorous area inside the pancreatic parenchyma, whereas others have set it on a red area around the pancreas which was estimated as fat; but this latter consideration is not supported by any evidence. Conversely, SWE consists in a quantitative method, which is considered as the most informative method to assess PS. In the available literature, the PS value of the normal parenchyma at shear wave speed is about 1.4 m/s [2] and seems to increase with age [3, 4]. However, a precise stiffness cut-off value to define the normal pancreatic parenchyma is still missing or needs standardization.

13.2 Pancreatic Stiffness Measurement in Benign Pancreatic Diseases

13.2.1 Chronic Pancreatitis and Alcohol-Related Disease

In the setting of chronic pancreatitis (CP), the values of PS resulted significantly higher compared to healthy volunteers in the study by Yashima et al. [5]. The authors assessed the pancreatic stiffness by using Acoustic Radiation Force Impulse (ARFI) transabdominal elastography in 46 patients (76% with alcohol-related CP, 70% with calcifications or signs of advanced disease) and in a control group including 52 healthy volunteers (HV). The authors found stiffness values significantly higher in patients with CP than in HV in every part of the pancreas (head, corpus, and tail), although the measurements were demanding in the tail of the organ. Actually, the feasibility of the technique resulted good in the body, fair in the head, and low in the tail: 75%, 69%, and 42%, respectively. They determined a SWE cut-off value of 1.40 m/s for diagnosing chronic pancreatitis and reported sensitivity, specificity, PPV, and NPV of 75%, 72%, 69%, and 78%, respectively, for diagnosing chronic pancreatitis. Alcoholic etiology ($r^2 = 0.142$) and a decreased BMI ($r^2 = 0.107$) were found to be significantly associated to high stiffness values.

Similarly, in a study by our group, 52 CP patients and 42 healthy subjects underwent PS measurement by using point-SWE [6]. In this study, feasibility was excellent (98%). PS was significantly higher in CP patients than HV ($p = 0.001$). Significantly higher values in the CP group were also observed in patients with longer disease duration (>10 years vs. ≤10 years) ($p = 0.01$), on chronic analgesic drugs ($p < 0.05$), and with lower body weight ($p < 0.05$, $r = -0.38$). At multivariate analysis, all the three variables resulted independently associated with the PS value. The intraclass correlation coefficient (ICC) for PS was 0.77. These results, even if limited and derived from small samples, showed an excellent level of feasibility of the technique and good reproducibility. Strong correlation between clinical outcome and PS in the CP setting is lacking, but elastography may have a future potential role in the stratification of CP patients by severity.

In this direction, in another study by using point-SWE, Kawada et al. [7] prospectively investigated a cohort of 85 patients with alcoholic abuse, to identify a possible high-risk group for pancreatic cancer. Of the 85 patients, five patients, including obese patients, were excluded because the pancreas was not clearly visualized at US, and other six patients with an already known diagnosis of pancreatic cancer were excluded because of a markedly dilated main pancreatic duct accompanied with severe atrophic pancreas. Fourteen patients were excluded because the shear wave velocity IQR/median was higher than 40%. Thus, the analysis was limited to 60 patients: among them, 18 patients (21%) with pancreatic cancer were identified. A 100% success rate was achieved at the head, body, and tail of the pancreas in 80%, 83%, and 68% of the patients, respectively. The comparison between patients with and without cancer did not reach statistical significance, but stiffness values were associated with a severe (>60 g ethanol/day) amount of alcohol intake ($p = 0.005$). In another study by our group, PS was measured in 87 patients with alcohol-related liver and/or pancreatic disease resulting significantly higher than HV ($p < 0.001$). The feasibility of the technique was excellent, and the only variable that significantly correlated with the PS value at multivariate analysis was the presence of liver cirrhosis ($p = 0.005$). Reproducibility was fair, but patients were mostly obese or with decompensated cirrhosis [8]. The amount of alcohol intake did not correlate with the PS value. However, differently from the population in the Kawada study [6], all the patients told of homogeneous severe alcohol abuse. These results, even if limited, open up to the interesting possibility to use elastography to detect and monitor alcohol-related pancreatic damage earlier.

Figure 13.1 summarizes the main available studies focusing on the role of PS in chronic pancreatitis and alcohol-related diseases. The values of PS in healthy volunteers and patients are illustrated by the histograms.

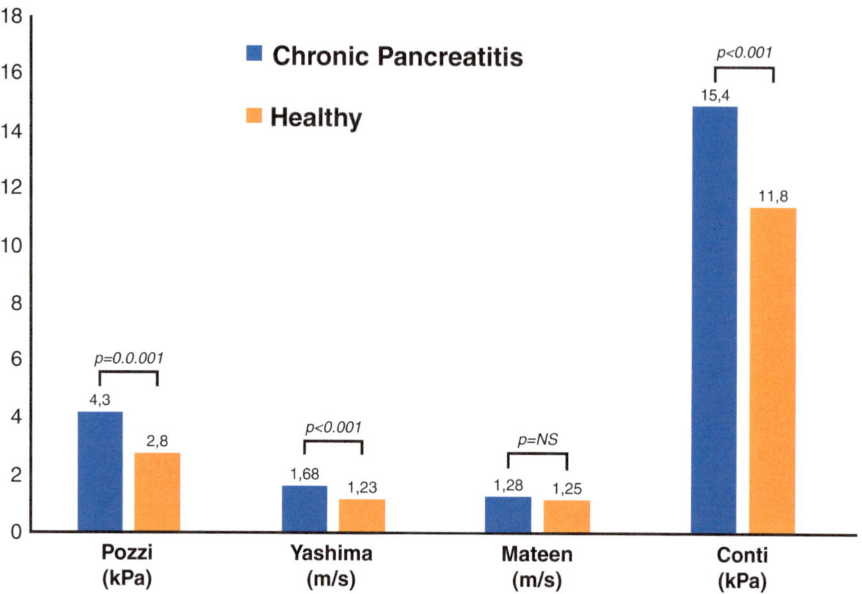

Fig. 13.1 Main studies focusing on the role of PS in chronic pancreatitis and alcohol-related diseases. The values of PS in healthy volunteers and patients are illustrated by the histograms

13.2.2 Acute Pancreatitis

The application of PS in acute pancreatitis is an interesting topic. However, the few available studies offered little and conflicting data. In detail, a study that investigated PS values in 44 acute pancreatitis and 210 HV did not find any statistically significant difference between the two groups [9]. Conversely, a study that evaluated 166 patients divided into normal, chronic, and acute pancreatitis group found different mean PS values: 1.28 m/s, 1.25 m/s, and 3.28 m/s for the normal pancreas, chronic, and acute pancreatitis, respectively. The authors concluded that PS may have a role in the diagnosis of acute pancreatitis, to assess the extent of inflammation or to identify necrosis and to monitor a patient's response to treatment [10]. Another study [11] compared PS by using ARFI with CT scan in 41 patients. The results appeared promising, as PS measurement showed very high accuracy (97.1% sensitivity, 92.9% specificity) for the diagnosis of acute pancreatitis. Again, a significant difference in PS values between patients with acute pancreatitis and HV was found (1.27 ± 0.50 m/s vs. 1.00 ± 0.17 m/s, $p = 0.001$, respectively) by Sanjeevi et al. [12]. The authors of this latter study found a positive correlation between PS and the number of pain episodes ($p = 0.026$) reported by the patients and a negative correlation with BMI ($p = 0.002$). Nevertheless, these observations need validation in larger samples, and further studies are thus necessary.

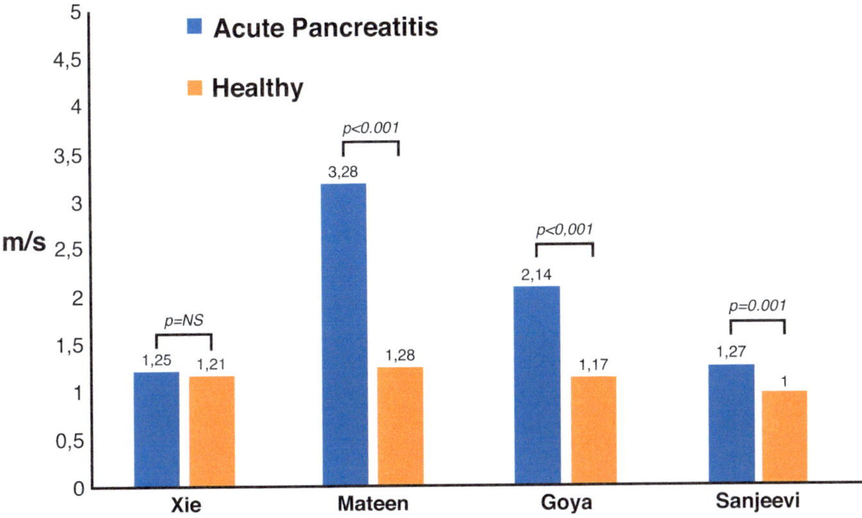

Fig. 13.2 Main studies focusing on the role of PS in acute pancreatitis. The values of PS in healthy volunteers and patients are illustrated by the histograms

Figure 13.2 summarizes the main available studies focusing on the role of PS in acute pancreatitis. The values of PS in healthy volunteers and patients are illustrated by the histograms.

13.2.3 Application in Surgery

A further interesting application of PS is its preoperative measurement to predict the incidence of postoperative pancreatic juice fistula (PF) and the risk of surgical complications [13]. Indeed, in the study by Harada et al. [14], PS turned out to be a good index for estimating pancreatic fibrosis and predicting postoperative PF in 17 patients. Similarly, the shear wave velocity (SWV) of the pancreas was preoperatively measured by ARFI in 62 patients undergoing pancreatic resection. SWV directly correlated with the degree of pancreatic fibrosis ($p < 0.001$) and inversely with postoperative amylase concentrations and the daily output of pancreatic juice. Multivariate analysis showed that low stiffness values were independent predictors of postoperative PF (odds ratio 38.3; 95% CI 5.82–445; $p = 0.001$) [15]. Another study found clinically relevant fistulae in eight patients, in a group of 25 patients who had undergone pancreaticoduodenectomy or distal pancreatectomy. No statistically significant difference was found between the fistula and non-fistula groups. Only in the sub-analysis of the group of patients who had undergone pancreaticoduodenectomy, ARFI values were significantly lower in the patients with fistulas than in those without [16].

13.2.4 Cystic Fibrosis and Diabetes

Regarding the application of PS in the cystic fibrosis setting, a German study [17] investigated liver and pancreatic stiffness in 106 patients. The patients with pancreatic insufficiency had significantly lower pancreas ARFI values as compared to those without. Similar results were found in a cohort of 27 CF patients who underwent PS measurement by pSWE: significantly lower SW velocities were found in CF patients than in HV [18]. Conversely, another study that investigated 22 CF patients found that the mean SWV of the pancreas was significantly higher than that of the HV [19].

Regarding the potential application of PS measurement to the diabetic population, the studies focusing on type 2 diabetes investigated the chance of predicting the presence of microangiopathy through PS measurement. In detail, a study measured PS in 213 type 2 diabetic patients with or without known microangiopathy. The pancreatic SWV increased significantly in patients with microangiopathy ($p < 0.01$) and resulted correlated with the number of microvascular complications. Therefore, the authors suggested that the SWV in the pancreatic body may be considered as a potential marker for diabetic microangiopathy [20]. Similar results were found by Öztürk et al. [21], who confirmed that an increased SWV in the pancreatic body was significantly related to the presence of microangiopathy [21].

The evaluation of type 1 diabetes, conversely, has focused on the possible PS use as a marker of severity of the disease. However, in a pilot study, no significant PS difference was found between patients and HV. In fact, the patients showed higher values than HV only in the tail segment [22]. Similar results were found in a larger study that assessed kidney and pancreatic stiffness in children with type 1 diabetes [23]. Conversely, another study on 60 children with type 1 diabetes made use of strain elastography. ROC analysis yielded a pathological pancreas cut-off value of 2.24 (AUC = 0.999, $p < 0.001$; sensitivity, 0.983; specificity, 1.00) for the strain ratio. The strain ratio in patients was significantly higher than in HV and significantly correlated with age and disease duration ($p < 0.001$) [24].

Therefore, for the purpose of evaluating such diseases as CF or type 1 diabetes in the pediatric population, PS appears promising and useful, it being a noninvasive, repeatable, and largely available technique. However, the results of the studies are still scanty and conflicting to support the routine use of this method as a surrogate marker of pancreatic damage in these settings: further studies are needed.

13.3 Pancreatic Stiffness Measurement in Focal Pancreatic Lesions

The application of PS in the evaluation of pancreatic lesions aims to help in the differential diagnosis between benign and neoplastic lesions and among different types of pancreatic cancer (PC). Few studies in literature have focused on the transabdominal evaluation of pancreatic masses in this setting. However, some promising evidence is available to support the noninvasive assessment of pancreatic lesions' stiffness and corroborate the histological diagnosis.

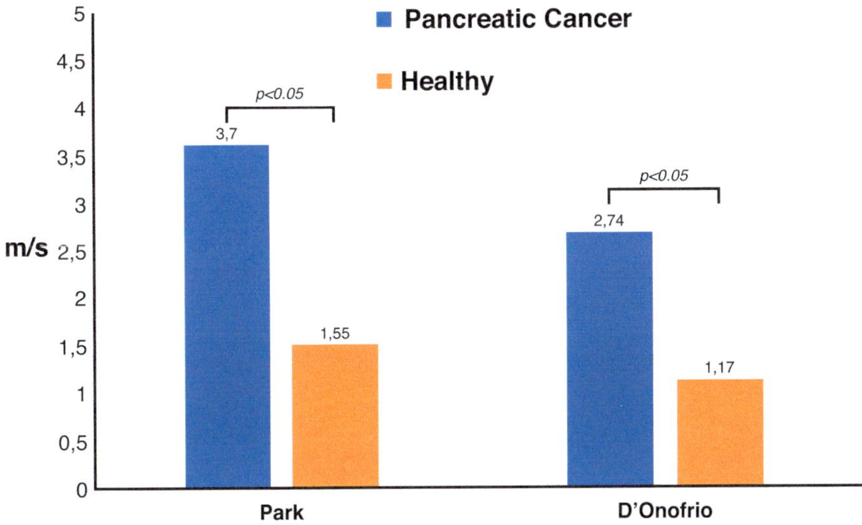

Fig. 13.3 Main studies focusing on the role of PS in predicting pancreatic cancer. The values of PS in healthy volunteers and patients are illustrated in the histograms

Figure 13.3 summarizes the main available studies focusing on the role of PS in predicting pancreatic cancer. The values of PS in healthy volunteers and patients are illustrated in the histograms.

13.3.1 Evaluation of Solid Lesions

D'Onofrio et al. [25] prospectively evaluated 123 pancreatic lesions. The median SWV for adenocarcinoma (ADK) was 2.74 m/s. In the HV group, the median SWV value was 1.17 m/s. The difference between the PS of ADK and the normal pancreas was statistically significant ($p < 0.05$). Moreover, good sensitivity (73.3%) and specificity (83.3%) were obtained for the characterization of mucinous cystic lesions. Another study performed ARFI elastography in 26 patients, with 27 focal solid pancreatic lesions: eight benign (focal pancreatitis and autoimmune pancreatitis) and 19 malignant (16 ADK, two metastases, one neuroendocrine tumor). No statistical difference was found in the mean SWV between benign and malignant lesions. However, the mean SWV difference values between the lesions and background parenchyma of the malignant lesions (1.5 ± 0.8 m/s) were higher than those of the benign lesions (0.4 ± 0.3 m/s; $p = 0.011$) [26]. Furthermore, a preliminary Phase I and a prospective Phase II studies were conducted. In the Phase I study, five patients with PC, two with endocrine tumor, five with chronic pancreatitis, and 14 with intraductal papillary mucinous neoplasm were investigated. In the Phase II study, 53 consecutive patients were enrolled. In the Phase I study, the colorimetric scale evaluated the normal parenchyma, which resulted homogeneously colored and

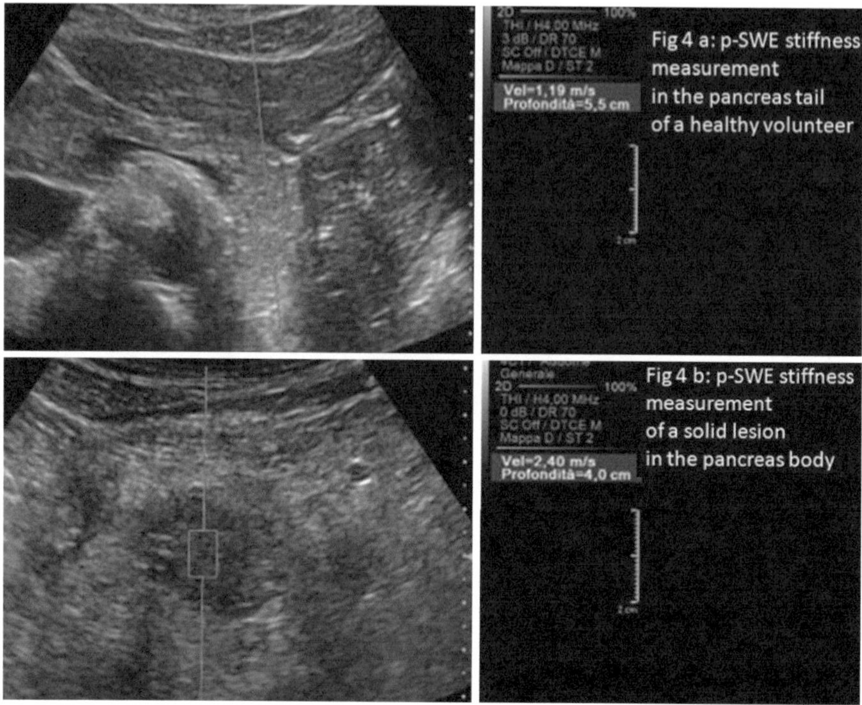

Fig. 13.4 Pancreatic stiffness measurement by point SWE in a healthy volunteer (**a**) and in a focal pancreatic solid lesion (**b**)

PC, which resulted as a markedly hard area with soft spots inside. Conversely, neuroendocrine tumors appeared as uniform and soft. Chronic pancreatitis did not show a peculiar pattern. In the Phase II study, the authors identified 77.4% of the lesions and observed 60.0% of the cancers, 100% of the endocrine tumors, and 92.0% of the cases of chronic pancreatitis [27].

Figure 13.4 illustrates the PS measurement by point SWE in a healthy volunteer (a) and in a focal pancreatic solid lesion (b).

13.3.2 Evaluation of Cystic Lesions

Regarding the stiffness evaluation of cystic lesions, PS assessment seems to have a remarkable role in their histologic characterization. Indeed, a study investigated 38 patients with pancreatic cystic focal lesions (diameter >3 cm and located at a 5.5 cm depth). The sensitivity, specificity, positive predictive value, negative predictive value, and accuracy for the differential diagnosis between mucinous and non-mucinous cystic lesions were 68.8%, 77.3%, 68.8%, 77.3%, and 73.7%, respectively; by the second method, the values were 37.5%, 100%, 100%, 68.8%, and 73.3% [28]. Similarly, other studies with small samples have shown encouraging results as regards the application of PS measurement in distinguishing mucinous from non-mucinous lesions [29–31].

In conclusion, the method seems to be good at distinguishing between solid benign and malignant masses. Similarly, the stiffness assessment of pancreatic cystic lesions seems to be promising in helping physicians to distinguish between mucinous and non-mucinous lesions. However, further studies are required to largely corroborate the use of the technique in these settings.

13.4 Limitations of Transabdominal PS Assessment

There are many limitations in transabdominal PS determination and its widespread use in clinical practice. The most important are anatomical limitations related to the deep location to the organ, as already described, in the presence of obesity or large-volume ascites or ductal abnormalities. Regarding the clinical application of the PS measurement to benign pathological conditions, the method remains a promising tool, but strong, univocal, and agreed results are still lacking. Even if pancreatic biopsy in absence of a target lesion is not routinely performed, the lack of it as the reference standard to assess chronic, acute pancreatitis, or alcoholic pancreatic damage still remains the main methodological limitation of the studies.

The use of PS measurement in the differential diagnosis of pancreatic lesions, even if promising, still requires further evidence.

References

1. Dietrich CF, Hocke M. Elastography of the pancreas, current view. Clin Endosc. 2019;52(6):533–40. https://doi.org/10.5946/ce.2018.156.
2. Gallotti A, D'Onofrio M, Pozzi MR. Acoustic radiation force impulse (ARFI) technique in ultrasound with virtual touch tissue quantification of the upper abdomen. Radiol Med. 2010;115:889–97. https://doi.org/10.1007/s11547-010-0504-5.
3. Kawada N, Tanaka S. Elastography for the pancreas: current status and future perspective. World J Gastroenterol. 2016;22(14):3712–24. https://doi.org/10.3748/wjg.v22.i14.3712.
4. Janssen J, Papavassiliou I. Effect of aging and diffuse chronic pancreatitis on pancreas elasticity evaluated using semiquantitative EUS elastography. Ultraschall Med. 2014;35:253–8. https://doi.org/10.1055/s-0033-1355767.
5. Yashima Y, Sasahira N, Isayama H, Kogure H, Ikeda H, Hirano K, et al. Acoustic radiation force impulse elastography for noninvasive assessment of chronic pancreatitis. J Gastroenterol. 2012;47:427–32. https://doi.org/10.1007/s00535-011-0491-x.
6. Pozzi R, Parzanese I, Baccarin A, Giunta M, Conti CB, Cantù P, et al. Point shear-wave elastography in chronic pancreatitis: a promising tool for staging disease severity. Pancreatology. 2017;17(6):905–10. https://doi.org/10.1016/j.pan.2017.10.003.
7. Kawada N, Tanaka S, Uehara H, Ohkawa K, Yamai T, Takada R, et al. Potential use of point shear wave elastography for the pancreas: a single center prospective study. Eur J Radiol. 2014;83:620–4. https://doi.org/10.1016/j.ejrad.2013.11.029.
8. Conti CB, Weiler N, Casazza G, Schrecker C, Schneider M, Mücke MM, et al. Feasibility and reproducibility of liver and pancreatic stiffness in patients with alcohol-related liver disease. Dig Liver Dis. 2019;51(7):1023–9. https://doi.org/10.1016/j.dld.2018.12.017.

9. Xie J, Zou L, Yao M, Xu G, Zhao L, Xu H, et al. A preliminary investigation of normal pancreas and acute pancreatitis elasticity using virtual touch tissue quantification (VTQ) imaging. Med Sci Monit. 2015;21:1693–9. https://doi.org/10.12659/MSM.892239.

10. Mateen MA, Muheet KA, Mohan RJ, Rao P, Majaz H, Rao GV, et al. Evaluation of ultrasound based acoustic radiation force impulse (ARFI) and eSie touch sonoelastography for diagnosis of inflammatory pancreatic diseases. JOP. 2012;13:36–44. PMID: 22233945.

11. Göya C, Hamidi C, Hattapoğlu S, Cetinçakmak MG, Teke M, Degirmenci MS, et al. Use of acoustic radiation force impulse elastography to diagnose acute pancreatitis at hospital admission: comparison with sonography and computed tomography. J Ultrasound Med. 2014;33:1453–60. https://doi.org/10.7863/ultra.33.8.1453.

12. Sanjeevi R, John RA, Kurien RT, Dutta AK, Simon EG, David D, et al. Acoustic radiation force impulse imaging of pancreas in patients with early onset idiopathic recurrent acute pancreatitis. Eur J Gastroenterol Hepatol. 2020;32:950. https://doi.org/10.1097/MEG.0000000000001732.

13. Săftoiu A, Gilja OH, Sidhu PS, Dietrich CF, Cantisani V, Amy D, et al. The EFSUMB guidelines and recommendations for the clinical practice of elastography in non-hepatic applications: update 2018. Ultraschall Med. 2019;40(4):425–53. https://doi.org/10.1055/a-0838-9937.

14. Harada N, Yoshizumi T, Maeda T, Kayashima H, Ikegami T, Harimoto N, et al. Preoperative pancreatic stiffness by real-time tissue elastography to predict pancreatic fistula after pancreaticoduodenectomy. Anticancer Res. 2017;37(4):1909–15. https://doi.org/10.21873/anticanres.11529.

15. Hatano M, Watanabe J, Kushihata F, Tohyama T, Kuroda T, Koizumi M, et al. Quantification of pancreatic stiffness on intraoperative ultrasound elastography and evaluation of its relationship with postoperative pancreatic fistula. Int Surg. 2015;100(3):497–502. https://doi.org/10.9738/INTSURG-D-14-00040.1.

16. Lee TK, Kang CM, Park MS, Choi SH, Chung YE, Choi JY, et al. Prediction of postoperative pancreatic fistulas after pancreatectomy: assessment with acoustic radiation force impulse elastography. J Ultrasound Med. 2014;33(5):781–6. https://doi.org/10.7863/ultra.33.5.781.

17. Friedrich-Rust M, Schlueter N, Smaczny C, Eickmeier O, Rosewich M, Feifel K, et al. Non-invasive measurement of liver and pancreas fibrosis in patients with cystic fibrosis. Cyst Fibros. 2013;12(5):431–9. https://doi.org/10.1016/j.jcf.2012.12.013.

18. Pfahler MHC, Kratzer W, Leichsenring M, Graeter T, Schmidt SA, Wendlik I, et al. Point shear wave elastography of the pancreas in patients with cystic fibrosis: a comparison with healthy controls. Abdom Radiol (NY). 2018;43(9):2384–90. https://doi.org/10.1007/s00261-018-1479-2.

19. Sağlam D, Demirbaş F, Bilgici MC, Yücel S, Çaltepe G, Eren E. Can point shear wave elastography be used as an early indicator of involvement?: evaluation of the pancreas and liver in children with cystic fibrosis. J Ultrasound Med. 2020;39:1769. https://doi.org/10.1002/jum.15281.

20. He Y, Jin Y, Li X, Wu L, Jin C. Quantification of pancreatic elasticity in type 2 diabetes: a new potential imaging marker for evaluation of microangiopathy. Eur J Radiol. 2020;124:108827. https://doi.org/10.1016/j.ejrad.2020.108827.

21. He Y, Wang H, Li XP, Zheng JJ, Jin CX. Pancreatic elastography from acoustic radiation force impulse imaging for evaluation of diabetic microangiopathy. Am J Roentgenol. 2017;209(4):775–80. https://doi.org/10.2214/AJR.16.17626.

22. Püttmann S, Koch J, Steinacker JP, Schmidt SA, Seufferlein T, Kratzer W, et al. Ultrasound point shear wave elastography of the pancreas: comparison of patients with type 1 diabetes and healthy volunteers - results from a pilot study. BMC Med Imaging. 2018;18(1):52. https://doi.org/10.1186/s12880-018-0295-z.

23. Sağlam D, Bilgici MC, Kara C, Yılmaz GC, Çamlıdağ İ. Acoustic radiation force impulse elastography in determining the effects of type 1 diabetes on pancreas and kidney elasticity in children. Am J Roentgenol. 2017;209(5):1143–9. https://doi.org/10.2214/AJR.17.18170.

24. Öztürk M, Yildirim R. Evaluation of pancreas with strain elastography in children with type 1 diabetes mellitus. Pol J Radiol. 2017;82:767–72. https://doi.org/10.12659/PJR.904118.

25. D'Onofrio M, De Robertis R, Crosara S, Poli C, Canestrini S, Demozzi E, et al. Acoustic radiation force impulse with shear wave speed quantification of pancreatic masses: a prospective study. Pancreatology. 2016;16(1):106–9. https://doi.org/10.1016/j.pan.2015.12.003.
26. Park MK, Jo J, Kwon H, Cho JH, Oh JY, Noh MH, et al. Usefulness of acoustic radiation force impulse elastography in the differential diagnosis of benign and malignant solid pancreatic lesions. Ultrasonography. 2014;33(1):26–33. https://doi.org/10.14366/usg.13017.
27. Uchida H, Hirooka Y, Itoh A, Kawashima H, Hara K, Nonogaki K, et al. Feasibility of tissue elastography using transcutaneous ultrasonography for the diagnosis of pancreatic diseases. Pancreas. 2009,38(1):17–22. https://doi.org/10.1097/MPA.0b013e318184db78.
28. D'Onofrio M, Crosara S, Canestrini S, Demozzi E, De Robertis R, Salvia R, et al. Virtual analysis of pancreatic cystic lesion fluid content by ultrasound acoustic radiation force impulse quantification. J Ultrasound Med. 2013;32(4):647–51. https://doi.org/10.7863/jum.2013.32.4.647.
29. D'Onofrio M, Gallotti A, Martone E, Pozzi MR. Solid appearance of pancreatic serous cystadenoma diagnosed as cystic at ultrasound acoustic radiation force impulse imaging. JOP. 2009;10(5):543–6.
30. D'Onofrio M, Gallotti A, Mucelli RP. Pancreatic mucinous cystadenoma at ultrasound acoustic radiation force impulse (ARFI) imaging. Pancreas. 2010;39(5):684–5. https://doi.org/10.1097/MPA.0b013e3181c34d19.
31. D'Onofrio M, Gallotti A, Falconi M, Capelli P, Mucelli RP. Acoustic radiation force impulse ultrasound imaging of pancreatic cystic lesions: preliminary results. Pancreas. 2010;39(6):939–40. https://doi.org/10.1097/MPA.0b013e3181d36244.

Endoscopic Ultrasound Elastography in Pancreatic Diseases

EUS-EG in Pancreatic Diseases

Federica Cavalcoli, Roberta Elisa Rossi, and Sara Massironi

14.1 Introduction

Elastography is an imaging modality for the evaluation of tissue stiffness, by using ultrasound. Pathologic processes such as cancerization and fibrosis alter tissue elasticity and therefore induce changes in elastographic appearance [1]. Neoplastic lesions are known to be stiffer (or less elastic) than surrounding healthy tissue; therefore, they could be characterized in elasticity-based imaging. Ultrasound elastography has been used to differentiate malignant from benign neoplasms in several organs, such as breast, thyroid, cervix, and liver. More recently also the pancreas has been a field of application of this technique, due to the increasingly widespread use of endoscopic ultrasound (EUS), in several different pancreatic diseases, including neoplasms, and inflammatory processes, that can modify the tissue stiffness. Endoscopic ultrasound elastography (EUS-EG) has been proposed in the evaluation of both focal lesions and parenchymal diseases [2]. Concerning focal lesions, EUS-EG is a promising imaging technique with a high degree of accuracy for the differential diagnosis of solid pancreatic tumors, and the recent introduction of the second generation EUS-EG allows not only for qualitative analysis of tissue stiffness but also for the quantitative one [1, 3]. EUS-EG is classified into two categories, based on the different mechanical properties: EUS strain elastography (EUS-SE) and EUS shear wave measurement (EUS-SWM) [4, 5]. EUS-SE evaluates tissue stiffness by measuring the relative tissue distortion within a region of

F. Cavalcoli
Gastroenterology and Endoscopy Unit, Istituti Clinici Zucchi, Monza, Italy

R. E. Rossi
Gastrointestinal Surgery and Liver Transplantation Unit, Fondazione IRCCS Istituto Nazionale dei Tumori and Department of Pathophysiology and Organ Transplant, Università degli Studi di Milano, Milan, Italy

S. Massironi (✉)
Gastroenterology Unit, San Gerardo Hospital, University of Milano – Bicocca, Monza, Italy

© Springer Nature Switzerland AG 2021
M. Fraquelli (ed.), *Elastography of the Liver and Beyond*,
https://doi.org/10.1007/978-3-030-74132-7_14

interest (ROI) when applying pressure, giving therefore a visual pattern that lacks objectivity and reproducibility. Therefore, it is necessary to use strain ratio (SR) or strain histogram (SH) analysis to have quantitative parameters [5–7]. EUS-SWM is based on the properties of a shear wave and involves a technique to measure the velocity of the shear wave [4, 8]. Theoretically, greater tissue elasticity corresponds to faster shear wave propagation.

14.2 Focal Lesions

14.2.1 Pancreatic Ductal Adenocarcinoma

The diagnosis of solid pancreatic lesions is challenging. Up to 40% of such lesions are due to pancreatic ductal adenocarcinoma (PDAC), the remaining being represented by several entities including neuroendocrine neoplasms (NENs), metastases, focal pancreatitis, and small solid-appearing serous cystadenomas [9]. Pancreatic cancer is characterized by a dismal prognosis, mainly because of its aggressive behavior and the difficulty in early diagnosis [10]. Surgical resection represents the only potential cure, but small pancreatic cancers are often lately diagnosed so that only less than 15% of patients can undergo surgery with curative purpose. Therefore, an accurate differential diagnosis between benign and malignant pancreatic masses is crucial for making clinical decisions.

Available radiologic and endoscopic methods such as transabdominal ultrasound, computerized tomography (CT), magnetic resonance imaging (MRI), positron emission tomography (PET), or endoscopic retrograde cholangiopancreatography (ERCP) are all characterized by limited sensitivity for recognizing early pancreatic tumors as they often fail in accurately differentiating malignant from benign lesions. Endoscopic ultrasound-guided fine-needle aspiration (EUS-FNA) has been recognized to be the most accurate technique in this setting [11]. EUS-EG has been increasingly used for the evaluation of solid pancreatic lesions and has been largely reported as a useful supplemental method to EUS-guided FNA [12–17], particularly in those cases where the FNA results are inconclusive. Of note, EUS-EG has the relevant advantage of potentially causing no additional adverse risk [10]. On qualitative elastography, the normal pancreas appears elastographically soft (homogenously green) in most cases, being this finding highly reproducible [18–20]. Conversely, malignant pancreatic lesions are generally harder than adjacent pancreatic tissue, due to the presence of fibrosis and marked desmoplasia [18]. A five-score classification was firstly reported based on the color patterns of lesions (Fig. 14.1), according to Giovannini et al. [19, 21], with a sensitivity of 100% and a specificity of 67%. In detail, a green pattern is considered to be suggestive of soft homogeneous tissue, namely, normal pancreatic tissue, while blue lesions with heterogeneity might suggest hard tissue and, therefore, PDAC. In this scoring system, scores 3–5 were considered indicative of malignancy. A four-score classification has also been used, which varies from homogenous green to homogeneous and heterogeneous blue, suggestive of a pancreatic neuroendocrine tumor and

Elastic score	Elastography	Pattern	Condition
1	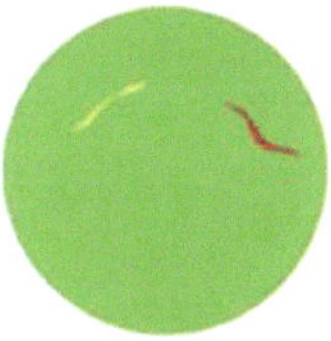	Distortion for entire low echo area	Normal pancreas
2	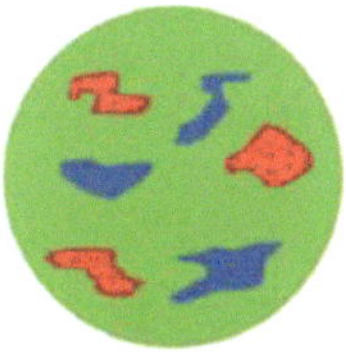	No distortion on low echo area even for a part	Fibrosis, chronic pancreatitis
3	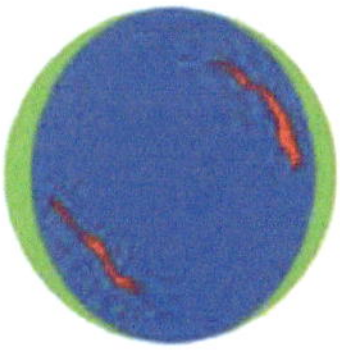	Distortion at the edge of low echo area, even for a part	Small adenocarcinoma
4	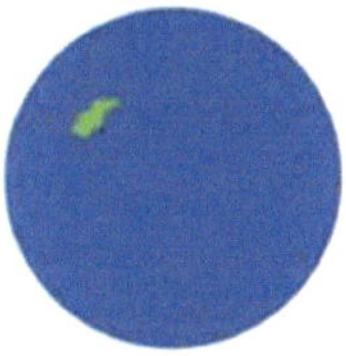	No distortion for entire low echo area	Endocrine tumor
5	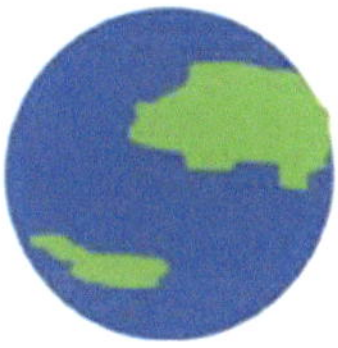	No distortion on low echo area and surrounding	Advanced adenocarcinoma

Fig. 14.1 Classification of elastography findings proposed by Giovannini et al. [19]. (Image adapted from [21]. License: http://creativecommons.org/licenses/by-nc/4.0/)

pancreatic adenocarcinoma, respectively [22]. Based on this score, the diagnostic sensitivity, specificity, and overall accuracy of EUS-EG for diagnosing malignancy were reported to be 100%, 85.5%, and 94%, respectively [22]. In a recent multi-center study [9], including 218 patients with solid pancreatic lesions $\leq$15 mm in size and a definite diagnosis, on elastography, 50% of lesions were stiffer than the surrounding pancreatic parenchyma (stiff lesions), and 50% were less stiff or of similar stiffness (soft lesions). The high stiffness values had a sensitivity of 84% and specificity of 67% for the diagnosis of malignancy. Furthermore, for the diagnosis of PDAC, the sensitivity and specificity were 96% and 64%, respectively, thus high-lighting that in patients with small solid pancreatic lesions, EUS-EG can rule out malignancy with a high level of certainty if the lesion appears soft, although a stiff lesion can be either benign or malignant.

On the other hand, some authors reported poor results for qualitative EUS-EG, observing a poor accuracy in distinguishing pancreatic malignancy from chronic pancreatitis [4, 23, 24]. Taken into account that qualitative elastography is largely based on the subjective interpretation of the elastographic pattern, the diagnostic accuracy is variable among different studies [4].

Quantitative EUS-EG can be based on both strain ratio (SR) and strain histogram (SH) without differences regarding the accuracy of the two techniques for the differentiation between benign and malignant pancreatic masses [1]. In a prospective study including 86 consecutive patients who underwent EUS for the evaluation of solid pancreatic masses, the SR was significantly higher among patients with pancreatic malignant tumors compared with those with inflammatory masses. The sensitivity and specificity of SR for detecting pancreatic malignancies were 100% and 92.9%, respectively [3]. In detail, A SR higher than 6.04 was reported to be 100% sensitive for classification of tumors as being malignant, being the specificity improved to 100% with an SR higher than 15.41. Of note, it was also possible to differentiate pancreatic cancers from neuroendocrine tumors with 100% sensitivity and 88% specificity, respectively [3]. Available studies proposed a cut-off of 175 for mean SH, with satisfactory results in terms of sensitivity (approximately 90–100%), specificity (66–100%), and accuracy (85–90%) [18, 25–27]. However, in the study by Schrader et al. [27], reporting excellent results in terms of both sensitivity and specificity for malignancy detection (100%), the control group was represented by normal control pancreatic parenchyma, instead of different consecutive pancreatic lesions or chronic pancreatitis, which must be considered as a bias of that study overestimating operative characteristics.

Although qualitative EUS elastography is considered to be more operator-dependent, according to a recent meta-analysis [10], both qualitative and quantitative EUS-EG have high accuracy in the detection of malignant pancreatic masses. However, specificity was not satisfactory (approximately 60%) with both methods. Previous studies [28–31] reported that the combination of contrast-enhanced ultrasound (CEUS) and EUS-EG might improve the specificity, although further studies are needed to confirm these preliminary observations. In details, in a prospective study [28], including 54 patients with chronic pancreatitis ($n = 21$) and pancreatic adenocarcinoma ($n = 33$), the sensitivity, specificity, and accuracy of the combined techniques for differentiation of hypovascular hard masses suggestive of pancreatic carcinoma were 75.8%, 95.2%, and 83.3%, respectively.

A prompt diagnosis of pancreatic adenocarcinoma is, indeed, needed given the poor prognosis of this type of cancer; however, it is challenging. When there is strong clinical suspicion of pancreatic cancer, but the biopsy is inconclusive or negative, a hard focal lesion on elastography should guide clinical management by indicating repeat EUS-FNA or direct referral to surgery. Qualitative EUS seems more operator-dependent, even if superimposable results have been reported for both techniques. However, accuracy is not fully satisfactory, and this is due to the difficult differential diagnosis between pancreatic cancer and other malignancy and/

or chronic pancreatitis. The combination of EUS elastography and CEUS might be a viable solution to improve specificity, but further studies are needed to draw more solid conclusions.

14.2.2 Pancreatic Neuroendocrine Neoplasms

The diagnosis of pancreatic neuroendocrine neoplasms (pNENs), especially non-functioning pNENs, represents a significant diagnostic challenge since these tumors have a nonspecific clinical presentation and more than half of them are detected incidentally, usually during diagnostic imaging studies or endoscopic procedures performed for other indications [32]. Among pancreatic solid lesions, after adeno-carcinomas and inflammatory masses, pNENs, even if rare in incidence, represent a relatively frequent finding during the EUS examination. Ultrasound imaging using elastography is an increasingly available technique allowing one to assess focal lesion's hardness [1].

At qualitative EUS-EG, NENs appear as well-defined "blue lesions" (Fig. 14.2), indicating stiff lesions. In a study by Iglesias-Garcia et al. [3], different kind of pancreatic solid lesions in 86 consecutive patients were analyzed (49 PDAC, 27 inflammatory masses, six pNENs, two metastatic cell lung cancers, one pancreatic lymphoma, and one pancreatic solid pseudopapillary tumor) and compared with 20 controls. Normal pancreatic tissue showed a mean strain ratio of 1.68 (95% CI: 1.59–1.78). Inflammatory masses exhibited a strain ratio (mean 3.28) that was significantly higher than that of the normal pancreas but lower than that of pancreatic adenocarcinoma (mean 18.12). The highest strain ratio was found among endocrine tumors (mean 52.34). On the other hand, in another more recent study by Ignee [9],

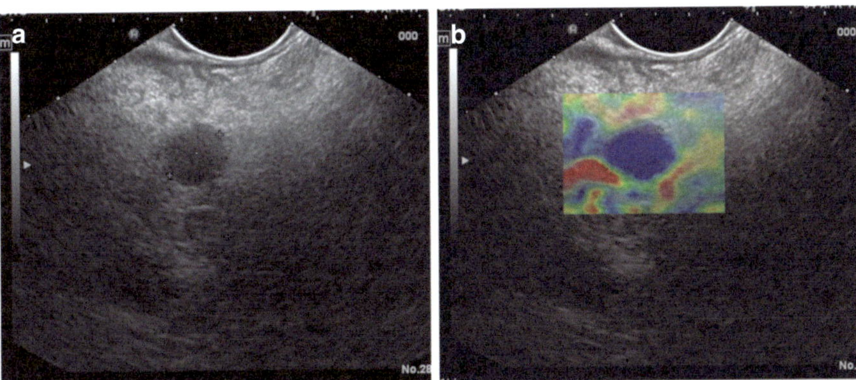

Fig. 14.2 Qualitative diagnosis in endoscopic ultrasound strain elastography (EUS-SE). B-mode image (left, **a**) of a small pancreatic lesion shows a 9 mm hypoechoic, rounded, well-defined pancreatic lesion. Endoscopic ultrasound strain elastography (EUS-SE) (right, **b**) demonstrated a "blue lesion"; that means that the lesion is stiffer compared to surrounding pancreatic tissue, suggesting a possible neuroendocrine neoplasm. Subsequent biopsy resulted in the diagnosis of a G1, well-differentiated pancreatic neuroendocrine tumor

NENs were diagnosed in 114/218 patients (52%). A stiff lesion was seen in 36% of patients with NETs, while 64% showed a soft lesion compared to the surrounding pancreatic parenchyma.

In summary, qualitative and quantitative EUS-EG is useful as a complementary tool used to differentiate between benign and malignant pancreatic lesions [3]. According to the recommendations of the European Federation of Societies for Ultrasound in Medicine and Biology (EFSUMB), EUS elastography may be helpful in making therapeutic decisions in cases where fine-needle biopsy performed during EUS has no diagnostic value [33]. However, elastography alone cannot replace the cytological assessment.

14.3 Parenchymal Diseases

The normal pancreas has been demonstrated with high reproducibility to be a homogeneous soft tissue at EUS-EG [19, 34], while parenchymal pancreatic diseases may result in diffuse alterations of pancreas or mass-forming lesions.

14.3.1 Chronic Pancreatitis

Chronic pancreatitis (CP) is characterized by chronic, progressive pancreatic inflammation and scarring and irreversible pancreatic damage leading to a permanent impairment of exocrine and endocrine functions. With an estimated annual prevalence and incidence of 52.4/100,000 and 14.0/100,000, CP is currently considered as an important healthcare problem [35]. Since the introduction of the Rosemont classification based on morphological criteria, EUS has assumed a key role in the diagnosis of CP [36] (Table 14.1). However, Rosemont morphological criteria present some pitfalls in the diagnosing of non-advanced disease [18]. EUS-EG can provide additional relevant information on tissue stiffness providing an objective evaluation of CP [37, 38].

In 2013 a prospective study on 191 patients [38] observed a significant direct linear correlation between the mean pancreatic SR and the number of EUS criteria for CP ($r = 0.813$). Overall, EUS-EG showed a diagnostic accuracy of 91.1% (cut-off SR of 2.25). In this study, the SR was measured in the head, body, and tail of the pancreas and compared with a soft reference area corresponding to the normal surrounding gut wall; the mean value was used for analysis. Similarly, Kuwahara et al. observed a significant correlation between the Rosemont criteria staging and mean pancreatic elastographic values ($p < 0.001$), as well a significant negative correlation between mean pancreatic elastographic values and the number of EUS features (rs $= -0.59, p < 0.001$) [7].

More recently, Yamashita et al. reported the mean EUS-SWM to be significantly correlated with the presence of Rosemont criteria and the number of EUS features [39]. The authors also observed EUS-SWM values to be suggestive for chronic pancreatitis, being significantly higher than normal control. Diagnostic operative

Table 14.1 Rosemont endoscopic ultrasound criteria (divided in major and minor) for the diagnosis of chronic pancreatitis

Criteria	Feature	Definition
Major A	Hyperechoic foci with shadowing	Echogenic structures ≥2 mm in length and width that shadow
Major B	Lobularity with honeycombing	Well-circumscribed, ≥5 mm structures with enhancing rim and relatively echo-poor center, contiguous ≥3 lobules
Minor	Lobularity without honeycombing	Well-circumscribed, ≥5 mm structures with enhancing rim and relatively echo-poor center, noncontiguous three lobules
Minor	Hyperechoic foci without shadowing	Echogenic structures foci ≥2 mm in both length and width with no shadowing
Minor	Cysts	Anechoic, rounded/elliptical structures with or without septations
Minor	Stranding	Hyperechoic lines of ≥3 mm in length in at least two different directions concerning the imaged plane
Major A	MPD calculi	Echogenic structure(s) within MPD with acoustic shadowing
Minor	Irregular MPD contour	Uneven or irregular outline and ectatic course
Minor	Dilated side branches	Three or more tubular anechoic structure each measuring ≥1 mm in width, budding from the MPD
Minor	MPD dilation	≥3.5 mm body or >1.5 mm tail
Minor	Hyperechoic MPD margin	Echogenic, distinct structure greater than 50% of entire MPD in the body and tail

characteristics for CP, with a cut-off value of 2.19, were very encouraging, with a sensitivity of 100%, a specificity of 94%, and the overall diagnostic accuracy of 97%.

Moreover, a direct relationship was found between SR values and the probability of both pancreatic exocrine failure [40] and endocrine insufficiency [39].

In conclusion, current data suggest EUS-EG is a promising diagnostic tool for CP, although the optimal diagnostic cut-off value for CP has not been identified yet. The significative correlation between SR and endocrine and exocrine insufficiency may be of value in tailoring the medical substitutive treatment.

14.3.2 Autoimmune Pancreatitis

Autoimmune pancreatitis (AIP) is a rare condition with a hypothesized autoimmune mechanism, accounting for up to 10% of chronic pancreatitis cases [41]. AIP is characterized by diffuse or focal enlargement of the pancreas and diffuse irregular narrowing of the main pancreatic duct. The main biochemical feature of AIP is an increase of serum gamma globulin, including IgG and particularly IgG4 [41]. However, some patients present with atypical imaging with a "mass-forming" picture that requires differentiation from pancreatic cancer. In such cases, a 2-week steroid trial may be helpful in confirming the diagnosis, because AIP shows a dramatic response to steroid therapy. On the other hand, it is not always easy to

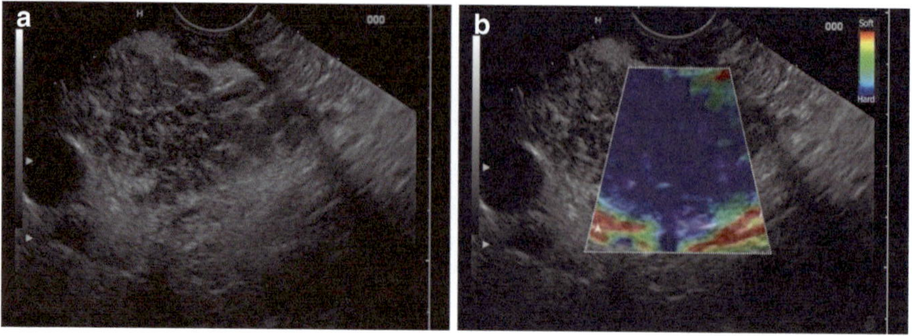

Fig. 14.3 Qualitative endoscopic ultrasound strain elastography in autoimmune pancreatitis: B-mode image (left, **a**) shows an enlarged, heterogeneous, course, and hypoechoic pancreas. Endoscopic ultrasound strain elastography (EUS-SE) (right, **b**) demonstrated the entire pancreas as a homogenously blue tissue stiffer than the normal pancreatic gland

evaluate the treatment response over a short period, and relapse may occur [42]. Therefore, mass-forming AIP represents a clinical challenge for the physician. Establishing a correct diagnosis of AIP can prevent the consequences of progressive disease and unnecessary surgery [43–47].

EUS-EG has been demonstrated to be helpful for the diagnosis of AIP [48]. Typically, at elastography, AIP presents with a diffuse, homogeneous, pattern of small spotted, mainly blue, color signals that are evenly spread over all the pancreatic parenchyma even in presence of mass-forming autoimmune pancreatitis [49] (Fig. 14.3). Thus, the unique finding of a homogenous stiffness of the whole organ has high diagnostic accuracy for AIP, as compared with PDAC in which the increase of stiffness is limited to the lesion. More recently, Ohno et al. suggested EUS-SWM as a method for assessment of AIP activity in patients undergoing steroid therapy [8]. The authors observed, in a series of six AIP patients on steroid therapy, a significant decrease of mean share wave elastography (3.32 m/s before steroid treatment vs. 2.46 m/s after steroid treatment, $p = 0.023$), suggesting EUS-SWM as an objective method for disease activity evaluation. Moreover, a recent study investigating the usefulness of EUS-EG combined with strain ratio (SR) in the estimation of the short-term treatment effect of AIP showed a high diagnostic capability of SR in identifying the steroid response at 2 weeks [48], even if the exact cut-off point varies between the reports.

14.4 Conclusion

EUS-EG allows the assessment of pancreatic tissue stiffness, and it has been demonstrated to be able to rule out malignancy with a high level of certainty in small pancreatic lesions when displayed as soft homogenous tissue. In the case of a small lesion with a very hard pattern, a pNEN should be hypothesized. In larger pancreatic lesions (>30 mm), the results are less convincing, mainly due to the heterogenicity of the lesions but also because of concomitant changes of the surrounding pancreatic parenchyma [9].

To date, elastography still presents some limitations in the differential diagnosis between focal pancreatitis and PDAC since chronic focal pancreatitis can also be stiffer than the otherwise healthy pancreatic parenchyma. Finally, strain elastography is also useful in the diagnosing of parenchymal diffuse such as chronic pancreatitis and autoimmune pancreatitis in which the entire organ shows stiffer tissue properties. The current role of EUS-SWM remains to be clarified.

In conclusion, EUS-EG represents a useful tool compared to EUS alone, providing relevant information on tissue stiffness for characterization of both focal lesion and parenchymal disease. In the study of focal lesions, EUS-EG may have a key role in cases in which EUS-FNA results inconclusive. Concerning parenchymal disease, EUS-EG provides a quantitative analysis of tissue stiffness allowing an objective evaluation of pancreatic disease at diagnosis and during follow-up.Conflict of Interest StatementNo conflicting interests (including but not limited to commercial, personal, political, intellectual, or religious interests) to declare.

References

1. Iglesias-Garcia J, et al. Endoscopic ultrasound elastography. Endosc Ultrasound. 2012;1(1):8–16.
2. Mondal U, et al. Endoscopic ultrasound elastography: current clinical use in pancreas. Pancreas. 2016;45(7):929–33.
3. Iglesias-Garcia J, et al. Quantitative endoscopic ultrasound elastography: an accurate method for the differentiation of solid pancreatic masses. Gastroenterology. 2010;139(4):1172–80.
4. Ohno E, et al. Diagnostic performance of endoscopic ultrasonography-guided elastography for solid pancreatic lesions: shear-wave measurements versus strain elastography with histogram analysis. Dig Endosc. 2020;33:629.
5. Hirooka Y, et al. JSUM ultrasound elastography practice guidelines: pancreas. J Med Ultrason (2001). 2015;42(2):151–74.
6. Itoh Y, et al. Quantitative analysis of diagnosing pancreatic fibrosis using EUS-elastography (comparison with surgical specimens). J Gastroenterol. 2014;49(7):1183–92.
7. Kuwahara T, et al. Quantitative diagnosis of chronic pancreatitis using EUS elastography. J Gastroenterol. 2017;52(7):868–74.
8. Ohno E, et al. Feasibility and usefulness of endoscopic ultrasonography-guided shear-wave measurement for assessment of autoimmune pancreatitis activity: a prospective exploratory study. J Med Ultrason (2001). 2019;46(4):425–33.
9. Ignee A, et al. Endoscopic ultrasound elastography of small solid pancreatic lesions: a multicenter study. Endoscopy. 2018;50(11):1071–9.
10. Zhang B, et al. Endoscopic ultrasound elastography in the diagnosis of pancreatic masses: a meta-analysis. Pancreatology. 2018;18(7):833–40.
11. Huang C, et al. Clinical features of patients infected with 2019 novel coronavirus in Wuhan, China. Lancet. 2020;395(10223):497–506.
12. Pei Q, et al. Diagnostic value of EUS elastography in differentiation of benign and malignant solid pancreatic masses: a meta-analysis. Pancreatology. 2012;12(5):402–8.
13. Li X, et al. Endoscopic ultrasound elastography for differentiating between pancreatic adenocarcinoma and inflammatory masses: a meta-analysis. World J Gastroenterol. 2013;19(37):6284–91.

14. Hu DM, Gong TT, Zhu Q. Endoscopic ultrasound elastography for differential diagnosis of pancreatic masses: a meta-analysis. Dig Dis Sci. 2013;58(4):1125–31.
15. Mei M, et al. EUS elastography for diagnosis of solid pancreatic masses: a meta-analysis. Gastrointest Endosc. 2013;77(4):578–89.
16. Xu W, et al. Endoscopic ultrasound elastography for differentiation of benign and malignant pancreatic masses: a systemic review and meta-analysis. Eur J Gastroenterol Hepatol. 2013;25(2):218–24.
17. Ying L, et al. Clinical utility of endoscopic ultrasound elastography for identification of malignant pancreatic masses: a meta-analysis. J Gastroenterol Hepatol. 2013;28(9):1434–43.
18. Cui XW, et al. Endoscopic ultrasound elastography: current status and future perspectives. World J Gastroenterol. 2015;21(47):13212–24.
19. Giovannini M, et al. Endoscopic ultrasound elastography: the first step towards virtual biopsy? Preliminary results in 49 patients. Endoscopy. 2006;38(4):344–8.
20. Soares JB, et al. Interobserver agreement of EUS elastography in the evaluation of solid pancreatic lesions. Endosc Ultrasound. 2015;4(3):244–9.
21. Chantarojanasiri T, Kongkam P. Endoscopic ultrasound elastography for solid pancreatic lesions. World J Gastrointest Endosc. 2017;9(10):506–13.
22. Iglesias-Garcia J, et al. EUS elastography for the characterization of solid pancreatic masses. Gastrointest Endosc. 2009;70(6):1101–8.
23. Janssen J, Schlörer E, Greiner L. EUS elastography of the pancreas: feasibility and pattern description of the normal pancreas, chronic pancreatitis, and focal pancreatic lesions. Gastrointest Endosc. 2007;65(7):971–8.
24. Hirche TO, et al. Indications and limitations of endoscopic ultrasound elastography for evaluation of focal pancreatic lesions. Endoscopy. 2008;40(11):910–7.
25. Săftoiu A, et al. Neural network analysis of dynamic sequences of EUS elastography used for the differential diagnosis of chronic pancreatitis and pancreatic cancer. Gastrointest Endosc. 2008;68(6):1086–94.
26. Săftoiu A, et al. Accuracy of endoscopic ultrasound elastography used for differential diagnosis of focal pancreatic masses: a multicenter study. Endoscopy. 2011;43(7):596–603.
27. Schrader H, et al. Diagnostic value of quantitative EUS elastography for malignant pancreatic tumors: relationship with pancreatic fibrosis. Ultraschall Med. 2012;33(7):E196–e201.
28. Săftoiu A, et al. Combined contrast-enhanced power Doppler and real-time sonoelastography performed during EUS, used in the differential diagnosis of focal pancreatic masses (with videos). Gastrointest Endosc. 2010;72(4):739–47.
29. Hocke M, Ignee A, Dietrich CF. Advanced endosonographic diagnostic tools for discrimination of focal chronic pancreatitis and pancreatic carcinoma--elastography, contrast enhanced high mechanical index (CEHMI) and low mechanical index (CELMI) endosonography in direct comparison. Z Gastroenterol. 2012;50(2):199–203.
30. Chantarojanasiri T, et al. Endoscopic ultrasound in diagnosis of solid pancreatic lesions: elastography or contrast-enhanced harmonic alone versus the combination. Endosc Int Open. 2017;5(11):E1136–e1143.
31. Iglesias-Garcia J, et al. Differential diagnosis of solid pancreatic masses: contrast-enhanced harmonic (CEH-EUS), quantitative-elastography (QE-EUS), or both? United European Gastroenterol J. 2017;5(2):236–46.
32. Walczyk J, Sowa-Staszczak A. Diagnostic imaging of gastrointestinal neuroendocrine neoplasms with a focus on ultrasound. J Ultrason. 2019;19(78):228–35.
33. Jenssen C, et al. EFSUMB Guidelines on Interventional Ultrasound (INVUS), Part IV - EUS-guided Interventions: general aspects and EUS-guided sampling (long version). Ultraschall Med. 2016;37(2):E33–76.
34. Lee TH, Cha SW, Cho YD. EUS elastography: advances in diagnostic EUS of the pancreas. Korean J Radiol. 2012;13(Suppl 1):S12–6.
35. Hirota M, et al. The seventh nationwide epidemiological survey for chronic pancreatitis in Japan: clinical significance of smoking habit in Japanese patients. Pancreatology. 2014;14(6):490–6.

36. Catalano MF, et al. EUS-based criteria for the diagnosis of chronic pancreatitis: the Rosemont classification. Gastrointest Endosc. 2009;69(7):1251–61.
37. Kuwahara T, et al. Usefulness of shear wave elastography as a quantitative diagnosis of chronic pancreatitis. J Gastroenterol Hepatol. 2018;33(3):756–61.
38. Iglesias-Garcia J, et al. Quantitative elastography associated with endoscopic ultrasound for the diagnosis of chronic pancreatitis. Endoscopy. 2013;45(10):781–8.
39. Yamashita Y, et al. Utility of elastography with endoscopic ultrasonography shear-wave measurement for diagnosing chronic pancreatitis. Gut Liv. 2020;14:659.
40. Dominguez-Muñoz JE, et al. EUS elastography to predict pancreatic exocrine insufficiency in patients with chronic pancreatitis. Gastrointest Endosc. 2015;81(1):136–42.
41. Shimosegawa T, et al. International consensus diagnostic criteria for autoimmune pancreatitis: guidelines of the International Association of Pancreatology. Pancreas. 2011;40(3):352–8.
42. Church NI, et al. Autoimmune pancreatitis: clinical and radiological features and objective response to steroid therapy in a UK series. Am J Gastroenterol. 2007;102(11):2417–25.
43. Abraham SC, et al. Pancreaticoduodenectomy (Whipple resections) in patients without malignancy: are they all 'chronic pancreatitis'? Am J Surg Pathol. 2003;27(1):110–20.
44. Weber SM, et al. Lymphoplasmacytic sclerosing pancreatitis: inflammatory mimic of pancreatic carcinoma. J Gastrointest Surg. 2003;7(1):129–37; discussion 137–9.
45. Barone JE. Pancreaticoduodenectomy for presumed pancreatic cancer. Surg Oncol. 2008;17(2):139–44.
46. de Castro SM, et al. Incidence and characteristics of chronic and lymphoplasmacytic sclerosing pancreatitis in patients scheduled to undergo a pancreatoduodenectomy. HPB (Oxford). 2010;12(1):15–21.
47. van Heerde MJ, et al. Prevalence of autoimmune pancreatitis and other benign disorders in pancreatoduodenectomy for presumed malignancy of the pancreatic head. Dig Dis Sci. 2012;57(9):2458–65.
48. Ishikawa T, et al. Usefulness of endoscopic ultrasound elastography combined with the strain ratio in the estimation of treatment effect in autoimmune pancreatitis. Pancreas. 2020;49:e21–2.
49. Dietrich CF, et al. Real-time tissue elastography in the diagnosis of autoimmune pancreatitis. Endoscopy. 2009;41(8):718–20.

Part IV

Extrahepatic Diseases: Bowel

Application of Elastography in Patients with Inflammatory Bowel Diseases

15

Federica Branchi and Mirella Fraquelli

15.1 Introduction

Inflammatory bowel diseases are chronic inflammatory conditions that affect the gastrointestinal tract and are often associated with extra-intestinal conditions. Among them, Crohn's disease can involve every segment of the gastrointestinal tract, the small bowel being frequently affected [1]. According to the Montreal classification, Crohn's disease can manifest with a predominantly inflammatory, fistulizing, or stricturing pattern [2].

Among the most common complications affecting patients with Crohn's disease, intestinal fibrotic strictures are responsible for significant morbidity and need for surgical intervention [1]. The link between chronic inflammation and intestinal fibrogenesis in Crohn's disease is still far from being clearly understood, although recent data shows that bowel wall fibrosis results from extracellular matrix deposition and mesenchymal cell activation, which are both observed after release of pro-inflammatory mediators in the tissue [3, 4] (Fig. 15.1). This pathogenetic mechanism explains why Crohn's disease behavior may vary over time, from an initial inflammatory phenotype to the development of stricturing complications as chronic inflammation progressively damages and alters the structure of the bowel wall [5, 6].

The ability to discriminate between inflammatory and fibrotic strictures takes on a relevant meaning when it comes to the clinical management of patients with

Supplementary Information The online version of this chapter (https://doi.org/10.1007/978-3-030-74132-7_15) contains supplementary material, which is available to authorized users.

F. Branchi
Medical Department, Division of Gastroenterology, Infectious Diseases and Rheumatology, Campus Benjamin Franklin, Charité Universitätsmedizin Berlin, Berlin, Germany

M. Fraquelli (✉)
Gastroenterology and Endoscopy Unit, Fondazione IRCCS Ca' Granda Ospedale Maggiore Policlinico, Milan, Italy

© Springer Nature Switzerland AG 2021
M. Fraquelli (ed.), *Elastography of the Liver and Beyond*,
https://doi.org/10.1007/978-3-030-74132-7_15

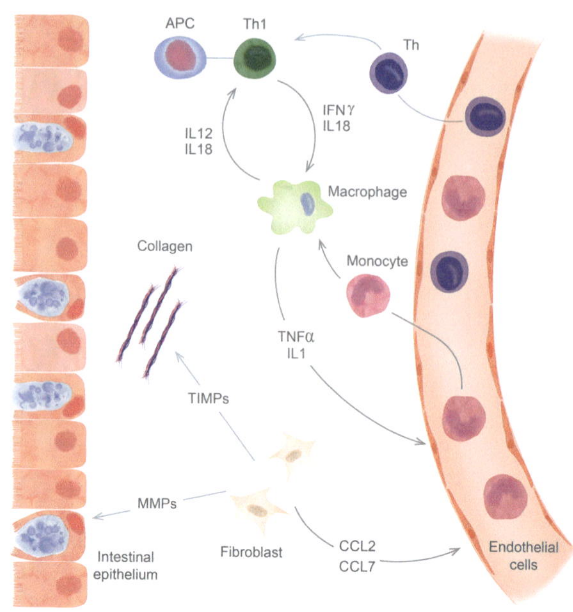

Fig. 15.1 Inflammation and fibrogenesis in inflammatory bowel diseases. The inflammatory process triggered by a Th immune response (involving APC, Th1 and macrophages) causes the activation of fibroblasts and the endothelial cells, which increases the production of inflammatory cytokines and the deposition of extracellular matrix, thus leading to the development of fibrosis. *Th* T helper lymphocytes, *APC* antigen-presenting cells, *TNF* tumor necrosis factor, *IL* interleukin, *TIMPs* tissue inhibitors of metalloproteinases, *MMPs* matrix metallopeptidases

Crohn's disease: inflammatory tissue will be likely to respond to currently available medical therapies and may also act as a disease modifier and prevent the development of fibrotic strictures [7, 8]. On the other hand, patients who have already developed fibrotic strictures will need endoscopic dilation or (in up to 60% of cases) will eventually require surgery [6, 8, 9].

Noninvasive imaging techniques have been widely used to discriminate between inflammatory and fibrotic tissue in bowel wall segments affected by inflammatory bowel diseases, including computed tomography [10], magnetic resonance imaging [11], and ultrasound with or without contrast enhancement [12, 13]. Elastography is the latest technique that has been studied as a mean of predicting intestinal fibrosis in the setting of inflammatory bowel diseases [14–16].

Thanks to its wide availability and applicability as an additional tool in ultrasound devices, elastography has shown its potential in the setting of Crohn's disease, where identifying inflammatory and fibrotic bowel segments and tracing their modifications over time are crucial for the correct management of these patients [17].

15.2 Elastography in Inflammatory Bowel Diseases: First Data from Animal Models and Surgical Series

Both strain elastography, acoustic radiation force impulse (ARFI) imaging, and shear wave elastography have been evaluated in the setting of inflammatory bowel diseases (see Table 15.1 for a summary of the technical characteristics of these different technologies) (Fig. 15.2).

With *strain elastography*, the compression exerted on a tissue with the ultrasound transducer generates a strain transmitted to the tissue along the transducer's axis, which can be calculated and then converted to an elastic modulus profile [18]. Harder/stiffer tissues have low compliance to stress thus low strain. The quantitative imaging of strain and elastic modulus distributions in soft tissues displayed along with real-time ultrasound images is called strain imaging or ultrasound elasticity imaging (UEI).

The first data on the potential application of strain elastography in gastrointestinal disorders were shown in an animal model of left-sided colitis and fibrosis: six rats treated with intra-rectal 2,4,6-trinitrobenzenesulfonic acid (TNBS) and five controls were evaluated with both strain measurement in vivo, with a transducer connected to a deformation device, and direct elastometry ex vivo, by means of a specific elastometer [14]. The association between the degree of chronic inflammation/fibrosis in a tissue and its stiffness was confirmed by the significant difference observed between the strain values of affected and healthy colon segments, as well as between the correspondent Young's modulus computed with direct elastometry. The good correlation between Young's modulus and strain suggested a good accuracy of the indirect assessment of tissue stiffness with strain elastography [14]. In this first study, the ability of strain elastography to discriminate between an inflammatory and a fibrotic process was not addressed; however, a second study by the

Table 15.1 Elastography techniques studied in the setting of inflammatory bowel diseases

Technique	Excitation method	Clinical applications proposed
Strain elastography or UEI	Physical characteristic measured: **Strain** Excitation method: *Manual compression*	Crohn's disease • Discrimination between inflammation and fibrosis • Assessment of fibrotic strictures Ulcerative colitis • Evaluation of disease activity (preliminary data)
ARFI imaging	Physical characteristic measured: **Strain** Excitation method: *Acoustic radiation force impulse*	Crohn's disease • Assessment of fibrotic strictures
Shear wave elastography	Physical characteristic measured: **Shear wave speed** – Point shear wave speed measurement – Shear wave speed imaging (real time) Excitation method: *Acoustic radiation force impulse*	Crohn's disease • Evaluation of inflammatory activity • Assessment of fibrotic strictures Ulcerative colitis • Evaluation of disease activity (preliminary data)

UEI ultrasound elasticity imaging, *ARFI* acoustic radiation force impulse

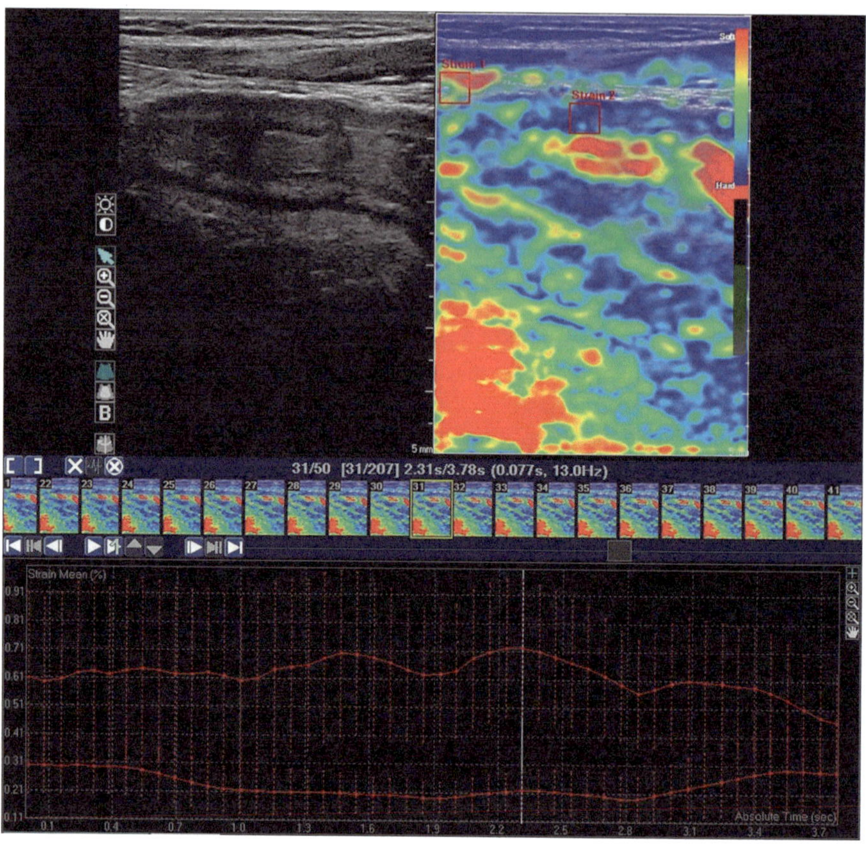

Fig. 15.2 Strain elastography in Crohn's disease: A thickened terminal ileum with focal alterations of the multi-layered pattern is shown with ultrasound (left) and strain elastography (right). In the lower half of the picture, strain values of the ileal wall and a control area (the surrounding mesenteric tissue) expressed as percentage are plotted over time for the calculation of the mean strain ratio

same group suggested that this technique could discriminate between inflammatory and fibrotic tissue based on the preliminary data from animal models [15].

In the same study, the first small group of patients with stricturing Crohn's disease tested with strain elastography underwent strain measurement of the affected bowel segment before surgery and the direct measurement of bowel wall stiffness after surgical resection [15]. The analysis showed a significant correlation between strain elastography and bowel wall stiffness, thus providing the first data on the ability of strain elastography to distinguish between healthy bowel and fibrotic tissue.

Strain elastography was evaluated in another preliminary study on resected surgical specimens (16 Crohn's disease bowel segments, 18 adenocarcinomas, and four adenomas) [19]. The tissue stiffness was expressed with different methods, including a visual analog scale (VAS) and the *strain ratio*, which is the ratio between the mean strain of reference surrounding tissue and the mean strain of the lesion/affected tissue. A significant difference in stiffness was observed between adenoma versus adenocarcinoma and Crohn's disease, while the differentiation between adenocarcinoma and Crohn's disease by means of strain elastography results was not possible, probably because of the relevant fibrosis degree in both lesions [19]. The reproducibility of strain elastography was assessed for the first time with two independent operators showing a good correlation for the VAS evaluation of tissue stiffness (Pearson's $r = 0.55$, $p = 0.002$), while the separate intra-observer strain ratio measurements showed moderate-to-good correlation (Spearman's rho 0.47–0.82).

Acoustic radiation force impulse (ARFI) uses ultrasound beam pulses to deform a chosen tissue area [20]. With *shear wave elastography*, a technique that uses ARFI technology, the deformation induced by the mechanical excitation of the tissue is measured as velocity of an induced shear wave and expressed as point shear wave speed measurement or shear wave speed imaging [20].

The first data from an animal model of colitis showed that the shear wave speed measurement was significantly higher in case of fibrosis than that of acute inflammation (0% and 30%, $p = 0.047$ and $p = 0.02$, respectively) [21]. With an AUROC of 0.971 for differentiating fibrotic from inflamed bowel, the shear wave velocity ratio (mean velocity/applied strain) emerged as a potential tool to be applied in the clinical setting [21]. Similarly, promising results were shown in a series of 17 human resected bowel specimens, where the application of shear wave elastography allowed to discriminate between tissue with high and low degree of fibrosis, but not between different degrees of inflammation [22].

15.3 Elastography and Crohn's Disease: Assessing Fibrotic Strictures

15.3.1 Strain Elastography

The potential ability of elastography to indirectly identify fibrotic tissue has prompted further investigation in the clinical setting of Crohn's disease, where the discrimination between inflammatory activity and fibrosis has major relevance especially when it comes to stricturing disease.

After the first preliminary studies, new data on the performances of strain elastography emerged (Table 15.2). Strain elastography was performed in ten patients with Crohn's disease elected for surgery and compared with results of direct tensiometry after surgery and histology [16]. As in previous studies, the strain measurement was performed with the aid of a press guide function in order to allow for the same amount of compression and to obtain values of the strain without the need to sample surrounding tissue to obtain a ratio. Bowel segments affected by Crohn's disease showed a significantly lower strain than those unaffected (mean ± standard deviation, 43.0 ± 25.9 versus 169.0 ± 27.9, $p < 0.001$). The comparison with histology showed a correlation between strain and collagen deposits or muscular fibers as

Table 15.2 Clinical studies addressing the role of strain elastography in Crohn's disease

	Subjects	Comparison	Elastography performance
Stidham (2011) [15]	Seven CD patients with stricturing disease	Direct mechanical measurement Histology	It discriminates between stenotic and unaffected bowel
Havre (2014) [19]	Human intestinal surgical specimens 16 CD 18 adenocarcinomas Four adenomas	Histology	It discriminates between adenoma and adenocarcinoma/CD, not between adenocarcinoma and CD
Baumgart (2015) [16]	Ten CD patients elected for surgery	Direct mechanical measurement Histology	It discriminates between unaffected and affected bowel; it correlates with higher fibrosis and muscular hypertrophy
Fraquelli (2015) [23]	23 CD patients elected for surgery 20 CD controls	Histology	It discriminates between inflammation and fibrosis and identifies severe fibrosis
Sconfienza (2016) [24]	16 CD patients	MRI	It potentially discriminates between fibrosis and inflammation
Serra (2017) [26]	26 CD patients elected for surgery	Histology	It does not seem to discriminate between fibrosis and inflammation
Quaia (2018) [25]	20 CD patients	Histology (17 biopsy, three surgery)	Potentially discriminates between fibrosis and inflammation
Ding (2019) [30]	25 CD patients	Histology (biopsy)	Seem not to discriminate between fibrosis and inflammation

CD Crohn's disease, *US* ultrasound, *MRI* magnetic resonance imaging

signs of fibrosis, although the role of inflammatory tissue changes in determining strain values was not fully explored [16].

The performance of strain elastography in predicting bowel fibrosis and discriminating between inflammation and fibrosis in vivo was addressed in another study, where strain elastography was performed on 23 Crohn's patients with ileal or ileocolonic disease, elected for surgical resection, and on 20 uncomplicated Crohn's disease patients serving as controls [23]. Tissue strain was assessed by means of both a semi-quantitative visual color scale and the strain ratio, as previously described [19], using the mesenchymal tissue surrounding the affected bowel wall as the reference. The results were compared to histology after resection, and a significant correlation between the strain ratio values and the severity of fibrosis at both semi-quantitative and quantitative histological image analysis was showed. The strain ratio was proven to have excellent discriminatory ability for severe bowel fibrosis (AUROC: 0.917; 95% CI 0.788–1.000), and for the first time, the issue of tissue inflammation as a possible confounder was explored, at multivariate analysis showing no influence of the histological degree of inflammation on strain ratio results [23]. Further data on the ability of strain elastography to distinguish between inflamed and fibrotic tissue was provided in a later study, which tested 16 patients with Crohn's disease of the terminal ileum, using magnetic resonance enterography as the reference standard for the detection of inflammation or fibrosis [24]. Elastography results, evaluated by two independent operators (with good inter-observer agreement) and expressed as a semi-quantitative score with higher scores corresponding to harder tissue, were significantly lower in patients with inflammatory than fibrotic strictures identified at magnetic resonance ($p = 0.003$) [24]. Moreover, a pilot study aimed at assessing the diagnostic performance of ultrasound techniques showed that the diagnostic performance of conventional ultrasound in discriminating inflammatory from fibrotic strictures was implemented by adding strain assessment and contrast enhancement ultrasound [25]. The data on the performance of strain elastography alone were not brilliant as compared to histology (accuracy 30–35%), but a visual classification of bowel wall appearance at real-time strain elastography was used to evaluate bowel wall stiffness instead of strain ratio [25].

Interestingly, a study questioned the previously promising observations on the potentiality of strain elastography [26]: 26 symptomatic Crohn's disease patients were evaluated with ultrasound, contrast-enhanced ultrasound, and strain elastography before surgery. The authors found no significant correlation between fibrosis at histology and mean strain ratio, attributing a possible confounding role to the presence of inflammation [26]. It is important to point out, though, that the mean strain ratio was obtained by selecting as a reference not the tissue surrounding the affected area but a dark red area in the deepest portion of the elastogram, representing the bottom of the color scale [26]. The "strain" represents the tissue deformation under a given pressure and has to be expressed as strain ratio during real-time elastography since the manual pressure applied by the operator cannot be measured—the ratio is calculated between two areas that receive roughly the same amount of stress and thus varies according to the specific stiffness of the tissue sampled as a region of interest (ROI). The use of an optical artifact like the bottom of the scale area as the reference tissue may have influenced the results since in that case the applied pressure of the operator has no influence on the value of the strain.

15.3.2 Acoustic Radiation Force Impulse: Shear Wave Elastography

The application of shear wave technology in the setting of Crohn's disease has been investigated in various studies (a summary is provided in Table 15.3).

The first clinical study on the subject enrolled 105 patients, 15 of whom underwent surgical resection during follow-up [27]. Point shear wave speed measurements for the evaluation of bowel wall stiffness were performed, and the results were compared between patients who underwent surgery and those who did not, as well as to the histological analysis of fibrosis, inflammation, and muscle hypertrophy. Interesting results were shown: first of all, the mean shear wave velocity was higher in patients who underwent surgery (2.8 ± 0.7 m/s vs. 2.2 ± 0.8 m/s, $p < 0.01$),

Table 15.3 Clinical studies investigating shear wave elastography techniques in Crohn's disease

	Subjects	Technique	Comparison	Elastography performance
Dillman (2014) [22]	17 human intestinal surgical specimens (from subjects with known or suspected IBD)	Point SW speed measurement and SW speed imaging	Histology	It discriminates between inflammation and fibrosis
Lu (2017) [27]	105 CD patients (15 elected for surgery)	Point SW speed measurement	Histology	It correlates with muscular hypertrophy of the bowel wall
Chen (2018) [28]	35 CD patients with strictures elected for surgery	SW speed imaging	Histology	It detects intestinal fibrosis; it potentially discriminates between fibrosis and inflammation
Goertz (2018) [36]	77 retrospective 21 prospective CD patients	Point SW speed measurement	Clinical data	It potentially identifies inflammatory activity
Ding (2019) [30]	25 CD patients	Point SW speed measurement (+ ARFI imaging and strain elastography)	Histology (biopsies)	Point SW speed measurement discriminates between fibrosis and inflammation

IBD inflammatory bowel diseases, *CD* Crohn's disease, *SW* shear wave

confirming the previous observations linking higher wall stiffness with the presence of a chronic/fibrotic process. A moderate correlation was found between shear wave velocity and muscular hypertrophy ($r = 0.59$, $p = 0.02$), but not with fibrosis. However, strictured bowel segments showed more muscular hypertrophy than fibrosis ($p < 0.001$). All in all, this study suggested that the dominant cause of bowel wall stiffness in chronic Crohn's strictures may not be fibrosis but muscle hypertrophy as a marker of chronic inflammation and that this feature could be detected by shear wave elastography.

A successive study on 35 Crohn's patients was able to refocus the attention on the role of elastographic techniques (in this case, real-time shear wave elastography or shear wave speed imaging) in assessing the presence of fibrosis [28]. Shear wave elastography was performed on the stenotic bowel wall of 35 Crohn's disease patients with ileal or ileocolonic strictures within a week before surgical resection. The results were compared to the degree of fibrosis and inflammation at histology, showing significantly different mean shear wave values (expressed in kPa) between severe, moderate, and mild fibrosis (23.0 ± 6.3 kPa vs. 7.4 ± 3.8 kPa vs. 14.4 ± 2.1 kPa, respectively, with $p = 0.008$), while no difference was observed between different degrees of inflammation. The authors established a 22.5 kPa for severe fibrosis, showing a sensitivity of 69.6% and specificity of 91.7% for shear-wave elastography in diagnosing severe fibrosis (AUROC 0.822). Although the 22.5 kPa cut-off value seems quite arbitrarily established, the study has shown promising results on the performance of shear wave elastography in identifying fibrotic strictures.

Another study performed shear wave velocity measurements on various segments of the intestinal tract of Crohn's patients in order to establish a possible correlation with inflammatory activity: not surprisingly, considering previous data contradicting this hypothesis, no significant correlation was found [29].

15.3.3 Comparison Between Elastographic Techniques

A comparison between the different elastographic techniques, including ARFI imaging, has been attempted in a recent study on 25 patients with Crohn's stenosis [30]. Between the semi-quantitative evaluation of strain elastography and ARFI imaging and point shear wave elastography, only the last technique seemed to achieve a satisfactory performance for the detection of fibrotic strictures, with a sensitivity of 75% and a specificity of 100% with a 2.73 m/s cut-off. However, both strain elastography and ARFI results were assessed by means of a semi-quantitative color scale, which—in the case of strain elastography—already proved less accurate than the strain ratio [23].

To date, some systematic reviews have shown that elastographic techniques seem to correlate with the presence of fibrosis in Crohn's disease; however, the heterogeneity of these studies as regards techniques as well as methods prevents from formulating conclusive statements on the accuracy of elastography [31, 32].

15.4 Elastography as a Predictor of Therapy Outcome in Crohn's Disease?

Considering the overall promising data available on the ability of elastography to predict the presence of fibrosis in Crohn's disease strictures, efforts have been made to establish whether elastography results could predict the response to anti-inflammatory therapy. Since inflammatory processes tend to respond to medical treatment, while fibrotic strictures usually require endoscopic dilation or surgery, the noninvasive assessment of the degree of fibrosis may possibly help identify which patients will benefit from treatment and which ones should be evaluated for surgery. In a recent study, 30 consecutive patients with ileal/ileocolonic Crohn's disease were evaluated by ultrasound and strain elastography before and after the beginning of anti-TNF treatment [17]. The bowel wall stiffness was assessed by calculating the strain ratio, with a ratio ≥ 2 as cut-off value for severe ileal fibrosis [23]. The bowel wall thickness measured by standard ultrasound was used to define transmural healing (cut-off: 3 mm) at 14 and 52 weeks after starting the treatment. In patients with a strain ratio ≥ 2 at baseline, subsequent surgery was performed more frequently ($p = 0.003$). Noteworthy, a significant inverse correlation between the strain ratio values at baseline and the reduction in bowel wall thickness following therapy was observed, while the patients who achieved transmural healing had a significantly lower baseline strain ratio ($p < 0.05$). All in all, evaluation by strain elastography, its accurately identifying severe fibrosis, seems to be able to predict therapeutic outcomes for Crohn's patients, although further studies are needed to confirm these promising results.

15.5   Other Applications of Elastography

15.5.1 Pediatric Crohn's Disease

Strain elastography in the setting of pediatric Crohn's disease may help widening the range of noninvasive methods in this group of patients. A specifically designed study examined 48 bowel segments of 14 pediatric Crohn's patients [33]. The development of a visual classification of bowel wall appearance at strain elastography (remission bowel, inflammatory wall, and fibrotic wall) and its correlation with clinical and imaging features was attempted. The results suggested a possible correlation between different visual patterns and signs of disease activity or complications. However, no comparison to histology or other reference standards was made, and, therefore, these preliminary results still require validation [33].

15.5.2 Ulcerative Colitis

Elastography has been tested as a potential diagnostic tool in another inflammatory bowel disease, ulcerative colitis. Preliminary data is available from murine [34] and human models [35, 36]. A single-center, retrospective, and prospective study conducted on 37 patients with ulcerative colitis compared real-time tissue elastography with endoscopic findings and disease activity [35]. Elastographic findings showed a significant correlation with endoscopic activity at colonoscopy, with individuals in the active phase of the disease more likely to show "abnormal" elastographic findings. However, no conclusive data can be drawn, at present, regarding the association between elastography results and disease activity.

A further study compared bowel wall stiffness measured by ARFI in ulcerative colitis patients and healthy volunteers, showing that ARFI elastography of the colonic bowel wall and the terminal ileum is feasible, but the results were scattered with high standard deviation [36]. According to the authors' experience, ARFI shear wave velocities appear to be slightly higher in patients with ulcerative colitis than in healthy volunteers, particularly in the sigmoid and transverse colon [36]. All in all, interesting preliminary data suggests that a role of elastographic techniques can be hypothesized in the management of patients with ulcerative colitis, but further larger prospective studies are needed before drawing any conclusions.

15.6   Summary

Elastography is an extremely promising technology that may develop to play a major role in the field of inflammatory diseases, particularly Crohn's disease. Its overall simplicity and availability allow to expect the validation of the available data on its accuracy with larger studies, as well as the broadening of its application in the near future. The current European recommendations for gastrointestinal ultrasound already state that elastography "can be used to evaluate the stiffness of a patient's pathological thickened bowel" [37].

Strain elastography has shown very promising results as a discriminator between fibrotic and inflammatory strictures and may acquire a role as a predictor of response to treatment. Contradictory results questioning its accuracy and reproducibility in this setting may derive from methodological differences in the small studies available. In particular, the measurement of the strain ratio, thanks to an easily available software, has been proven more reliable than visual or semi-quantitative color scales, as well as more accurately correlated with the degree of tissue fibrosis.

On the other hand, shear wave elastography may indeed prove a simpler and more reproducible technique in comparison to strain elastography with strain ratio calculation. However, there is still little and dispersed data pointing to the correlation between shear wave elastography results and both fibrosis and inflammation, still generating inconclusive inferences.

For all techniques, clear-cut quantitative cut-offs may be difficult to obtain but are needed to improve the clinical applicability of these techniques, as well as their ability to orient clinical decision-making. For the strain ratio measurement, a cut-off of 2 for the identification of severe fibrosis has shown good discriminatory ability and good performance [17]. A recent study on shear wave elastography proposes a cut-off of 22.5 kPa for the identification of severe fibrosis which shows good accuracy but certainly needs validation in bigger prospective studies before being introduced in routine clinical practice [28].

References

1. Peyrin-Biroulet L, Loftus EV, Colombel JF, Sandborn WJ. The natural history of adult Crohn's disease in population-based cohorts. Am J Gastroenterol. 2010;105(2):289–97.
2. Silverberg MS, Satsangi J, Ahmad T, Arnott ID, Bernstein CN, Brant SR, et al. Toward an integrated clinical, molecular and serological classification of inflammatory bowel disease: report of a Working Party of the 2005 Montreal World Congress of Gastroenterology. Can J Gastroenterol. 2005;19(Suppl A):5A–36A.
3. Rieder F, Kessler SP, West GA, Bhilocha S, de la Motte C, Sadler TM, et al. Inflammation-induced endothelial-to-mesenchymal transition: a novel mechanism of intestinal fibrosis. Am J Pathol. 2011;179(5):2660–73.
4. Rieder F, Georgieva M, Schirbel A, Artinger M, Zügner A, Blank M, et al. Prostaglandin E2 inhibits migration of colonic lamina propria fibroblasts. Inflamm Bowel Dis. 2010;16(9):1505–13.
5. Cosnes J, Cattan S, Blain A, Beaugerie L, Carbonnel F, Parc R, et al. Long-term evolution of disease behavior of Crohn's disease. Inflamm Bowel Dis. 2002;8(4):244–50.
6. Rieder F, Zimmermann EM, Remzi FH, Sandborn WJ. Crohn's disease complicated by strictures: a systematic review. Gut. 2013;62(7):1072–84.
7. Lichtenstein GR, Olson A, Travers S, Diamond RH, Chen DM, Pritchard ML, et al. Factors associated with the development of intestinal strictures or obstructions in patients with Crohn's disease. Am J Gastroenterol. 2006;101(5):1030–8.
8. Govani SM, Stidham RW, Higgins PD. How early to take arms against a sea of troubles? The case for aggressive early therapy in Crohn's disease to prevent fibrotic intestinal strictures. J Crohn Colit. 2013;7(11):923–7.

9. Dignass A, Van Assche G, Lindsay JO, Lémann M, Söderholm J, Colombel JF, et al. The second European evidence-based consensus on the diagnosis and management of Crohn's disease: current management. J Crohn Colit. 2010;4(1):28–62.

10. Chiorean MV, Sandrasegaran K, Saxena R, Maglinte DD, Nakeeb A, Johnson CS. Correlation of CT enteroclysis with surgical pathology in Crohn's disease. Am J Gastroenterol. 2007;102(11):2541–50.

11. Sinha R, Murphy P, Sanders S, Ramachandran I, Hawker P, Rawat S, et al. Diagnostic accuracy of high-resolution MR enterography in Crohn's disease: comparison with surgical and pathological specimen. Clin Radiol. 2013;68(9):917–27.

12. Maconi G, Carsana L, Fociani P, Sampietro GM, Ardizzone S, Cristaldi M, et al. Small bowel stenosis in Crohn's disease: clinical, biochemical and ultrasonographic evaluation of histological features. Aliment Pharmacol Ther. 2003;18(7):749–56.

13. Ripollés T, Rausell N, Paredes JM, Grau E, Martínez MJ, Vizuete J. Effectiveness of contrast-enhanced ultrasound for characterisation of intestinal inflammation in Crohn's disease: a comparison with surgical histopathology analysis. J Crohn Colit. 2013;7(2):120–8.

14. Kim K, Johnson LA, Jia C, Joyce JC, Rangwalla S, Higgins PD, et al. Noninvasive ultrasound elasticity imaging (UEI) of Crohn's disease: animal model. Ultrasound Med Biol. 2008;34(6):902–12.

15. Stidham RW, Xu J, Johnson LA, Kim K, Moons DS, McKenna BJ, et al. Ultrasound elasticity imaging for detecting intestinal fibrosis and inflammation in rats and humans with Crohn's disease. Gastroenterology. 2011;141(3):819–26.e1.

16. Baumgart DC, Müller HP, Grittner U, Metzke D, Fischer A, Guckelberger O, et al. US-based real-time elastography for the detection of fibrotic gut tissue in patients with stricturing Crohn disease. Radiology. 2015;275:889.

17. Orlando S, Fraquelli M, Coletta M, Branchi F, Magarotto A, Conti CB, et al. Ultrasound elasticity imaging predicts therapeutic outcomes of patients with Crohn's disease treated with anti-tumour necrosis factor antibodies. J Crohn Colit. 2018;12(1):63–70.

18. Ophir J, Céspedes I, Ponnekanti H, Yazdi Y, Li X. Elastography: a quantitative method for imaging the elasticity of biological tissues. Ultrason Imaging. 1991;13(2):111–34.

19. Havre RF, Leh S, Gilja OH, Ødegaard S, Waage JE, Baatrup G, et al. Strain assessment in surgically resected inflammatory and neoplastic bowel lesions. Ultraschall Med. 2014;35(2):149–58.

20. Shiina T, Nightingale KR, Palmeri ML, Hall TJ, Bamber JC, Barr RG, et al. WFUMB guidelines and recommendations for clinical use of ultrasound elastography: Part 1: Basic principles and terminology. Ultrasound Med Biol. 2015;41(5):1126–47.

21. Dillman JR, Stidham RW, Higgins PD, Moons DS, Johnson LA, Rubin JM. US elastography-derived shear wave velocity helps distinguish acutely inflamed from fibrotic bowel in a Crohn disease animal model. Radiology. 2013;267(3):757–66.

22. Dillman JR, Stidham RW, Higgins PD, Moons DS, Johnson LA, Keshavarzi NR, et al. Ultrasound shear wave elastography helps discriminate low-grade from high-grade bowel wall fibrosis in ex vivo human intestinal specimens. J Ultrasound Med. 2014;33(12):2115–23.

23. Fraquelli M, Branchi F, Cribiù FM, Orlando S, Casazza G, Magarotto A, et al. The role of ultrasound elasticity imaging in predicting ileal fibrosis in Crohn's disease patients. Inflamm Bowel Dis. 2015;21(11):2605–12.

24. Sconfienza LM, Cavallaro F, Colombi V, Pastorelli L, Tontini G, Pescatori L, et al. In-vivo axial-strain sonoelastography helps distinguish acutely-inflamed from fibrotic terminal ileum strictures in patients with Crohn's disease: preliminary results. Ultrasound Med Biol. 2016;42(4):855–63.

25. Quaia E, Gennari AG, Cova MA, van Beek EJR. Differentiation of inflammatory from fibrotic ileal strictures among patients with Crohn's disease based on visual analysis: feasibility study combining conventional B-mode ultrasound, contrast-enhanced ultrasound and strain elastography. Ultrasound Med Biol. 2018;44(4):762–70.

26. Serra C, Rizzello F, Pratico' C, Felicani C, Fiorini E, Brugnera R, et al. Real-time elastography for the detection of fibrotic and inflammatory tissue in patients with stricturing Crohn's disease. J Ultrasound. 2017;20(4):273–84.

27. Lu C, Gui X, Chen W, Fung T, Novak K, Wilson SR. Ultrasound shear wave elastography and contrast enhancement: effective biomarkers in Crohn's disease strictures. Inflamm Bowel Dis. 2017;23(3):421–30.
28. Chen YJ, Mao R, Li XH, Cao QH, Chen ZH, Liu BX, et al. Real-time shear wave ultrasound elastography differentiates fibrotic from inflammatory strictures in patients with Crohn's disease. Inflamm Bowel Dis. 2018;24(10):2183–90.
29. Goertz RS, Lueke C, Wildner D, Vitali F, Neurath MF, Strobel D. Acoustic radiation force impulse (ARFI) elastography of the bowel wall as a possible marker of inflammatory activity in patients with Crohn's disease. Clin Radiol. 2018;73(7):678.e1–5.
30. Ding SS, Fang Y, Wan J, Zhao CK, Xiang LH, Liu H, et al. Usefulness of strain elastography, ARFI imaging, and point shear wave elastography for the assessment of Crohn disease strictures. J Ultrasound Med. 2019;38(11):2861–70.
31. Pescatori LC, Mauri G, Savarino E, Pastorelli L, Vecchi M, Sconfienza LM. Bowel sonoelastography in patients with Crohn's disease: a systematic review. Ultrasound Med Biol. 2018;44(2):297–302.
32. Bettenworth D, Bokemeyer A, Baker M, Mao R, Parker CE, Nguyen T, et al. Assessment of Crohn's disease-associated small bowel strictures and fibrosis on cross-sectional imaging: a systematic review. Gut. 2019;68(6):1115–26.
33. Fufezan O, Asavoaie C, Tamas A, Farcau D, Serban D. Bowel elastography - a pilot study for developing an elastographic scoring system to evaluate disease activity in pediatric Crohn's disease. Med Ultrason. 2015;17(4):422–30.
34. Nair A, Liu CH, Singh M, Das S, Le T, Du Y, et al. Assessing colitis. Quant Imag Med Surg. 2019;9(8):1429–40.
35. Ishikawa D, Ando T, Watanabe O, Ishiguro K, Maeda O, Miyake N, et al. Images of colonic real-time tissue sonoelastography correlate with those of colonoscopy and may predict response to therapy in patients with ulcerative colitis. BMC Gastroenterol. 2011;11:29.
36. Goertz RS, Lueke C, Schellhaas B, Pfeifer L, Wildner D, Neurath MF, et al. Acoustic radiation force impulse (ARFI) shear wave elastography of the bowel wall in healthy volunteers and in ulcerative colitis. Acta Radiol Open. 2019;8(4):2058460119840969.
37. Nylund K, Maconi G, Hollerweger A, Ripolles T, Pallotta N, Higginson A, et al. EFSUMB recommendations and guidelines for gastrointestinal ultrasound - Part 1: Examination techniques and normal findings (long version). Ultraschall Med. 2017;38:e1.

Part V

Spleen Involvement in Liver and Non-Liver Diseases

Liver and Spleen Stiffness in Vascular Liver Disease

16

Federico Ravaioli, Elton Dajti, Luigina V. Alemanni, and Antonio Colecchia

16.1 Introduction

Vascular liver disease related to portal hypertension is an exciting and not completely studied issue that includes the most common manifestations of non-cirrhotic portal hypertension, acute non-cirrhotic portal vein thrombosis (NCPVT), extrahepatic portal vein obstruction (EHPVO), and idiopathic non-cirrhotic portal hypertension (INCPH).

These entities though diverse and undergoing to periodic update not infrequently are present in hepatological departments, and very often their recognition is a diagnostic challenge because the shared clinical manifestations are due to portal hypertension (ascites, esophageal varices, splenomegaly, etc.). Their correct diagnosis involves different expertise, as hepatologists, radiologists, hematologists, and experts in coagulation; thus, often a multidisciplinary approach should be necessary. Firstly, the presence of liver cirrhosis should be ruled out through non-invasive tools useful for fibrosis staging and portal hypertension to avoid misclassifications. Imaging techniques like color duplex ultrasound or MRI/CT scan are considered as modality of choice for these diseases; however, in the long term, there could be some difficulty in differentiating between portal vein thrombosis due to cirrhosis or EHPVO.

Correct diagnosis is critical, as the evaluation, prognosis, and treatment can be different. In the last decade, a new non-invasive tool, elastographic ultrasound, born to assess fibrosis staging, and in time also portal hypertension, has deeply modified the clinical diagnosis and management of liver diseases. In fact, international

F. Ravaioli · E. Dajti · L. V. Alemanni
Department of Medical and Surgical Sciences (DIMEC), S. Orsola-Malpighi Hospital, University of Bologna, Bologna, Italy

A. Colecchia (✉)
Gastroenterology Unit, Borgo Trento, University Hospital, Verona, Italy
e-mail: antonio.colecchia@aovr.veneto.it

© Springer Nature Switzerland AG 2021
M. Fraquelli (ed.), *Elastography of the Liver and Beyond*,
https://doi.org/10.1007/978-3-030-74132-7_16

235

guidelines included elastographic ultrasound in almost all diagnostic flow chart and clinical decision-making.

In this chapter, we describe the role of the measurement of liver and spleen stiffness in the different vascular liver conditions. In diseases such as pre-hepatic portal hypertension, the simultaneous elastographic assessment of the liver and the spleen stiffness represents the unique approach to reach quickly and non-invasively a diagnosis. Likewise, in Budd-Chiari syndrome, it could help the hepatologists making the best clinical decision since during follow-up it can identify the timing for interventional treatments or liver transplantation. In others, as hepatic veno-occlusive disease, liver stiffness measurement can allow a pre-clinical diagnosis, anticipating the treatment and leading to a reduction of the overall mortality.

16.2 Part I: Liver and Spleen Stiffness in Patients with Budd-Chiari Syndrome

The Budd-Chiari syndrome (BCS) is a rare vascular disease of the liver, defined as the obstruction of hepatic venous outflow that can be located from the small hepatic venules up to the entrance of inferior vena cava (IVC) into the right atrium [1]. In Western countries, thrombosis of the hepatic veins is the most frequent site of obstruction, whereas in Asian countries, IVC thrombosis is the more predominant form [2]. The most common clinical presentation is that of hepatic decompensation, with ascites, hepatomegaly, and abdominal pain being the most frequent signs and symptoms [3]. However, one must bear in mind that its manifestation can be highly variable, ranging from asymptomatic to fulminant disease. Of consequence, the prognosis of BCS patients is also variable, and, despite significant advances in the medical management of these patients, still, 49–64% require endovascular and/or surgical derivative treatments, 12–17% liver transplantation (LT), and 20–22% die [4, 5]. Therefore, the availability of accurate prognostic models able to stratify the risk of complications and to identify the patients with a more severe course of the disease would be of tremendous help for the clinician. To date, this represents an unmet clinical need for patients with BCS. Standard prognostic scores used in hepatology, such as model for end-stage liver disease (MELD), are suboptimal in these patients because liver function might be preserved despite complications due to severe portal hypertension [6]. Many authors have tried to develop and validate specific scores for BCS [5, 7, 8]; these models present moderate overall accuracy in predicting clinical outcomes such as the need for invasive therapies (c-statistic = 0.697–0.797) or LT (c-statistic 0.619–0.693) [4] and are suboptimal for individual patients in day-to-day clinical practice [1].

Liver stiffness measurement (LSM) has been extensively validated as a useful diagnostic and prognostic tool in hepatology, especially in the context of viral hepatitis [9]. Its values correlate well with the degree of fibrosis [10] and indirectly with that of portal hypertension [11, 12]. However, LSM may also reflect other conditions, such as cholestasis, inflammation, and congestion [13]. While these components might interfere with the accuracy of LSM incorrectly identifying the fibrosis stage in patients with chronic liver disease, the fact that LSM reflects hepatic congestion [14, 15] is precisely the reason why LSM can help in assessing the degree of the outflow obstruction and the severity of the disease in patients with BCS. Spleen stiffness, on the other hand, is a more recently described non-invasive test that is to be considered a direct surrogate of portal hypertension [16]. Therefore, it correlates better with the hepatic venous pressure gradient (HVPG) [16], is more accurate for the diagnosis of clinically significant hypertension [17, 18] or esophageal varices [19, 20], and generally reflects better the degree of portal hypertension despite its cause (i.e., pre-, post-, or intrasinusoidal) [11].

Despite these premises, data on elastosonography in BCS is still minimal (Table 16.1). The most extensive series focuses on LSM values in the setting of severe BCS requiring endovascular interventional procedures (i.e., TIPS placement or angioplasty) and its changes after treatment [21, 24, 27]. For the first time, Mukund et al. reported high LSM values (range 20.5–75 kPa, mean 62.8 kPa), as evaluated by transient elastography (TE), in 25 BCS patients before endovascular procedures; these values were reduced significantly at 24 h after treatment (mean 26.3 kPa, $p < 0.001$) and then again slightly after 3 months (21 kPa, $p = 0.003$), suggesting for the first time that LSM was predominantly determined by hepatic congestion in BCS patients. Similar findings were reported later by Wang et al. [27], who assess LSM by two-dimensional shear wave elastography in 32 patients with BCS before and after angioplasty. The authors found that LSM progressively and significantly decreased at +2 days and +3 months, but no significant changes were found between the measurements at +3 months vs. +6 months after angioplasty. Noteworthy, the authors reported a significant correlation between hepatic venous pressure and LSM before angioplasty ($r = 0.701$, $p < 0.001$), but not between LSM and fibrosis stage at liver specimen (not even after the intervention). Xu et al. recently confirmed these results [24] in 23 BCS patients undergoing magnetic resonance elastography (MRE) before and after endovascular treatment, as the authors found a significant correlation between changes in LSM and those in pressure gradient before and after treatment ($r = 0.651$, $p = 0.009$). Importantly, given the heterogeneity of BCS, the authors evaluated LSM in three liver regions (right posterior, right anterior, and left medial) and found no significant difference among the different evaluations, with an excellent intra- and inter-observer agreement for LSM determination by MRE in all three segments.

Long-term data on LSM after endovascular treatments are very scarce. We recently reported two cases in which LSM was low (<10 kPa) [12] at 1 and 10 years after TIPS placement, in patients who indeed had responded well to TIPS and had remained compensated throughout this period [23]. Oppositely, a sudden increase in LSM during follow-up was associated with a recurrence of BCS [25, 27] or TIPS obstruction [23], suggesting that LSM could play a role in the non-invasive assessment of response to endovascular treatments, alongside with routine Doppler ultrasound.

As mentioned above, BCS is very heterogeneous, and not all patients present severe cases requiring endovascular derivative therapies. In fact, in many patients, medical management of ascites and/or varices, as well as anticoagulation with

Table 16.1 Main papers reporting liver and/or spleen stiffness in patients with Budd-Chiari syndrome

Nr.	Citation	N. of patients	Inclusion criteria	Elastometry technique	Main result
1.	Mukund et al. [21]	25	TIPS, PTA	TE	Progressive LSM reduction after 24 h and after 3 months after treatment
					No difference in ΔLSM across fibrosis stages (Metavir >2 vs. ≤2)
					No correlation between ΔLSM and Δ in pressure gradient
2.	Wang et al. [22]	32	PTA	2D-SWE	Progressive LSM reduction after 2 days and 3 months, but not at 6 months
					LSM correlates with hepatic venous pressure, but not with fibrosis stage
					ΔLSM significantly lower in patients with fibrosis stage >2
3.	Dajti et al. [23]	7	Mixed	TE	The first description of SSM in BCS patients
					LSM reduces <10 kPa a long time after TIPS
4.	Xu et al. [24]	23	Endovascular treatment	MRE	LSM was reduced after endovascular treatment
					Changes in LSM correlate with changes in portal pressure
5.	Nakatsuka et al. [25]	2	PTA	TE	LSM can monitor response to PTA and can detect early restenosis
6.	Mancuso et al. [26]	3	Medical therapy	TE	Reduction in LSM corresponded with a compensated state of the disease after anticoagulation

2D-SWE two-dimensional shear wave elastography, *PTA* percutaneous transluminal angioplasty, *LSM* liver stiffness measurement, *MRE* magnetic resonance elastography, *SSM* spleen stiffness measurement, *TE* transient elastography, *TIPS* transjugular intrahepatic portosystemic shunt

eventual etiological therapy, might be sufficient, as suggested by a stepwise approach to BCS treatment according to the last European guidelines [1]. However, no prognostic tools are available today to identify which patients could safely undergo only medical therapy and which could benefit from early endovascular intervention. In this view, although data on LSM and BCS patients undergoing only medical therapy are limited, it can be hypothesized that elastography could play a role in stratification of venous outflow obstruction degree, disease severity assessment, and response to medical therapy. We previously reported that LSM decreased after anticoagulation in two young patients [23]. More recently, Mancuso et al. [26] showed that lower, or at least stable, LSM values after anticoagulation correlated with stable liver disease in two patients. In contrast, an increase in LSM despite medical therapy in one patient was associated with the development of refractory ascites and referral for liver transplantation. Both works suggest the role of elastosonography also in the assessment of the response to medical therapy.

Last but not least, only one paper by our group reported SSM measurement in patients with BCS [23]. In our experience, LSM and SSM values are incredibly high (both up to 75 kPa) in patients with severe BCS; these findings are very unusual for cirrhotic patients. Therefore near-upper-limit LSM and SSM values might help to direct the diagnosis towards BCS in patients manifesting as decompensated cirrhosis. Moreover, SSM decreases slower than LSM after TIPS placement. For instance, in one young female undergoing TIPS placement, LSM and SSM were both 75 kPa. At 1 year after TIPS, LSM, but not SSM value, was significantly reduced (LSM and SSM, respectively, 8 kPa and 65.2 kPa); the following year LSM was 11.2 kPa, and SSM had decreased to 23.8 kPa. This pragmatic case suggests that LSM reflects the immediate resolution of the outflow obstruction and hepatic congestion after TIPS, but SSM reflects the long-term structural changes due to portal hypertension and eventually its improvement. Finally, our data suggest that SSM reflected better than LSM the progression of the disease in patients undergoing solely medical therapy for BCS.

In conclusion, there is increasing evidence that elastosonography techniques can provide insights on the outcomes of interventional therapy in patients with BCS and could be used as surveillance tools to assess its benefits longitudinally over time and transplantation-free survival in these patients. The reported results were consistent among the different elastography techniques. The combination of LSM and SSM, both at diagnosis and after medical therapy, should be further evaluated in order to identify BCS with a better prognosis than do not require interventional treatments or liver transplantation.

16.3   Part II: Liver and Spleen Stiffness in Patients Non-cirrhotic Portal Hypertension

The most common manifestations of non-cirrhotic portal hypertension that will be discussed in this chapter are acute non-cirrhotic portal vein thrombosis (NCPVT), extrahepatic portal vein obstruction (EHPVO), and idiopathic non-cirrhotic portal hypertension (INCPH). The nomenclature of these conditions is ambiguous in current literature, but, according to the last European guidelines [1], acute PVT is the recent formation of a thrombus within the portal vein and/or intrahepatic branches, in the absence of cirrhosis or malignancy. After the acute thrombus formation, if no recanalization occurs, the portal venous lumen is obliterated, and numerous porto-portal collaterals develop through a process caused cavernomatous transformation, defining thus EHPVO. Idiopathic non-cirrhotic portal hypertension, on the other hand, is often defined also as hepatoportal sclerosis, non-cirrhotic portal fibrosis, and incomplete septal cirrhosis of nodular regenerative hyperplasia (NRH). The diagnosis of idiopathic non-cirrhotic portal hypertension can be made only if known causes of non-cirrhotic portal hypertension, such as infiltrative diseases, sarcoidosis, congenital hepatic fibrosis, cystic fibrosis, etc., can be excluded. More recently, the term porto-sinusoidal vascular disease was proposed for this condition by a group of experts [28], with a focus on the histopathological findings in these patients. In this paper, new diagnostic criteria were proposed, aiming to promote earlier diagnosis of this condition, before overt clinical manifestations such as variceal bleeding or ascites develop.

Since all these conditions require that cirrhosis is ruled out, non-invasive surrogates of fibrosis staging and portal hypertension can be very helpful to raise suspicion and diagnose these forms of PH. The main studies reporting LSM and/or SSM in non-cirrhotic portal hypertension are summarized in Table 16.2.

One of the most important papers on the role of elastography in patients with EHPVO is that of Sharma et al. [35], who described that LSM values are slightly higher than those seen in healthy controls (mean 6.7 kPa vs. 4.6 kPa, respectively) but lower than those of cirrhotic patients (median 44.2 kPa). SSM values, on the other hand, were higher than those seen in controls (51.7 kPa vs. 16 kPa, respectively) and could accurately distinguish between patients with and without a history of variceal bleeding at multivariate analysis. In this view, the most common findings in patients with EHPVO are normal [54] or slightly elevated LSM values [35], high SSM, and therefore high SSM/LSM ratio [35, 52, 55]. The SSM values could reflect the degree of obstruction and severity of PH directly, as higher values were associated with the grade of varices [52, 56], and history of bleeding [35], although these results were not always confirmed [43]. The prognostic role of LSM, on the other hand, is not clear. Although less common than in INCPH (see below), LSM in patients with EHPVO can be high (>10 kPa) and overlap with those seen in patients with advanced chronic liver disease (ACLD). Whether these values express a certain degree of fibrosis or intrahepatic thrombosis due to chronic obstruction [35, 57] or reflect a "misdiagnosed" INCPH complicated later on by PVT, it is not known [58]. The facts that up to 30% of INCPH are complicated by PVT during follow-up [59] and that the two conditions share many etiological and risk factors [1] make it very difficult to establish which condition came first.

The interpretation of elastography values in patients with INCPH is more complicated. Since the very first papers reporting LSM in patients with human immunodeficiency virus (HIV) that had developed PH in the absence of known causes of liver disease, it was shown that LSM was high and overlapped with cirrhotic values in 30–60% of the cases [60–62]. In a large cohort of patients with NRH [63], the range of LSM values was 2.5–16.8 kPa; 17 (63%) and 11 (41%) patients had values >7.1 kPa and 10 kPa, compatible with significant fibrosis and ACLD, respectively. Moreover, LSM did not correlate with fibrosis stage at liver biopsy, nor with the presence of varices, ascites, or splenomegaly. Seijo et al. [64] measured both LSM and HVPG in 30 patients with biopsy-proven INCPH, 24 patients with NCPVT, and 39 patients with liver cirrhosis. The authors reported that LSM was significantly

Table 16.2 Main papers reporting liver and/or spleen stiffness in patients with non-cirrhotic portal hypertension

Nr.	Citation	N. of patients	Etiology	Elastometry technique	LSM or SSM value (median, range)	Comment on diagnosis or results
1.	Chang et al. [29]	5	INCPH in HIV	TE	LSM: 8.9 kPa (6.8–14.9 kPa)	Diagnosis with liver biopsy
2.	Panos et al. [30]	5	INCPH in HIV	TE	LSM: 11.8 kPa (9.9–21.1) 3/5 pts >10 kPa	Liver biopsy, high LSM (>10 kPa) in patients without cirrhosis
3.	Cesari et al. [31]	11	INCPH in HIV	TE	LSM: 8.1 kPa (2.5–11 kPa) 3/11 pts >10 kPa	Signs of portal hypertension at imaging/endoscopy, 5/11 liver biopsy
4.	Laharie et al. [32]	27/30	INCPH	TE	LSM: 7.9 kPa (3.5–16.8 kPa) 11/27 pts >10 kPa	Liver biopsy in patients with NRH
5.	Scourfield et al. [33]	11/17	INCPH in HIV	TE	LSM: 6/11 >9.6 kPa, of whom 4/6 >21 kPa	Liver biopsy in HIV patients without liver disease
6.	Jackson et al. [34]	4/5	INCPH in HIV	TE	LSM: 11 kPa (6.3–13.3 kPa) 3/4 >10 kPa	Radiological or endoscopic signs of PH, 4/5 liver biopsy
7.	Sharma et al. [35]	65	NCPVT	TE	LSM: 6.7 kPa (3.4–14.6 kPa) SSM: 51.7 kPa (11.7–75 kPa)	Higher SSM in patients with previous variceal bleeding
8.	Seijo et al. [36]	30/39	INCPH	TE	LSM: 8.4 ± 3.6 kPa 14/30 pts >7.8 kPa, 2/30 >13.6 kPa	Signs of PH and absence of cirrhosis at liver biopsy
		24/39	NCPVT	TE	LSM: 6.4 ± 2.2 kPa	PVT and absence of cirrhosis at liver biopsy

(continued)

Table 16.2 (continued)

Nr.	Citation	N. of patients	Etiology	Elastometry technique	LSM or SSM value (median, range)	Comment on diagnosis or results
9.	Furuichi et al. [37]	17	INCPH	pSWE, ARFI	LSM: 1.56 m/s (0.98–2.37 m/s)	Liver biopsy in all patients
					SSM: 3.88 m/s (2.69–4.79 m/s)	SSM/LSM ratio: AUROC 0.933
10.	Logan et al. [38]	2/81	INCPH in HIV	TE	LSM: 8 and 10 kPa	Abnormal TE, ultrasound or liver enzymes => liver biopsy, 2 confirmed INCPH
11.	Scherpbier et al. [39]	7	INCPH in HIV	TE	LSM: 8.3 kPa (5.6–9.5 kPa)	
12.	Madhusudhan et al. [40]	50	NCPVT	2D-SWE	LSM: 5.96 kPa (4.27–8.63 kPa)	No difference with LSM in healthy controls
13.	Sood et al. [41]	19	INCPH, children	TE	LSM: 10.6 kPa (7.6–13.5 kPa)	Clinical, imaging, and endoscopic findings
14.	Sharma et al. [42]	20	INCPH	TE	LSM: 6.8 kPa (2.9–11.9 kPa)	Liver biopsy, HVPG
15.	Madhusudhan et al. [43]	21	NCPVT	2D-SWE	SSM: 46.04 ± 8 kPa	SSM did not correlate with portal pressure (intra-operative) or esophageal varices
16.	Chougule et al. [44]	66	INCPH	TE	LSM: 9.2 kPa (4.4–26.3 kPa)	Liver biopsy; no correlation with periportal fibrosis
17.	Vuppalanchi et al. [45]	22	INCPH	TE	LSM: range 4.4–22 kPa	A high rate of patients with LSM >10 kPa (cACLD) in patients with NCPVT and INCPH
					11/22 pts >10 kPa	
		13	NCPVT	TE	LSM: range 3.6–18.8 kPa	
					4/13 pts >10 kPa	
		8	Other NCPH	TE	LSM: 7.4–67.8 kPa	
					6/8 pts >10 kPa	

18.	Madhusudhan et al. [46]	52	NCPVT	2D-SWE	SSM: 44.92 kPa (25.3–75.6 kPa)	*Poor AUROC for HRV diagnosis** *Almost all had varices, LRV vs. HRV*
19.	Sutton et al. [47]	15/67	NCPVT, children	TE	LSM: 19.4 kPa vs. 8.7 kPa (no EV) / SSM: 62.8 kPa vs. 13.2 kPa (no EV)	SSM was accurate to predict varices
20.	Cunningham et al. [48]	44	NCPH, mixed	TE	LSM: 8.7 kPa (6.7–11.5 kPa)	LSM not useful for HRV diagnosis
22.	Navin et al. [49]	41	NCPH, mixed	MRE	LSM: 3.4 ± 1 kPa (56% >3 kPa, F2) / SSM: 8.2 ± 4.9	LSM 4.7 kPa AUROC 0.99 for NCPH diagnosis (vs. cirrhosis)
23.	Ahmad et al. [50]	11	INCPH in HIV	pSWE	LSM: 6.8 kPa (5–12 kPa) / SSM: 76.3 kPa (18–197 kPa)	SSM is more accurate that LSM
24.	Cannella et al. [51]	37	INCPH	MRE	LSM: 3.56 ± 1.10 kPa	Liver biopsy as the reference
25.	Yuldashev et al. [52]	34	NCPVT	2D-SWE	SSM: 47.23 (16.3–104.5 kPa)	SSM correlated with EV grade, decreased after surgical shunt
26.	Gupta et al. [53]	53	NCPVT	pSWE	LSM: 1.2 m/s (1–1.9 m/s)	LSM higher in INCPH vs. NCPVT
		63	INCPH		LSM: 1.5 m/s (0.9–2.8 m/s)	

2D-SWE two-dimensional shear wave elastography, *EV* esophageal varices, *HIV* human immunodeficiency virus, *INCPH* idiopathic non-cirrhotic portal hypertension, *LSM* liver stiffness measurement, *MRE* magnetic resonance elastography, *NCPVT* non-cirrhotic portal vein thrombosis, *NCPH* non-cirrhotic portal hypertension, *SWE* point shear wave elastography, *SSM* spleen stiffness measurement, *TE* transient elastography
SEARCH STRING: (("non-cirrhotic" OR "noncirrhotic" OR "idiopathic") AND ("portal hypertension" OR "portal vein thrombosis") OR "portal vein obstruction" OR "nodular regenerative hyperplasia") AND ("liver stiffness" OR "spleen stiffness" OR "elastography" OR "elastometry")

higher in patients with INCPH than in patients with NCPVT (8.4 ± 3.6 kPa vs. 6.4 ± 2.2 kPa) but much lower than the one seen in cirrhotic patients. Moreover, no correlation was found between LSM, HVPG, and variceal bleeding. These results were later confirmed also by other authors [44, 65].

Similar to what reported for EHPVO, spleen stiffness, a direct surrogate of PH, is high in patients with INCPH, and once again, the combination of LSM and SSM can be extremely helpful in distinguishing between cirrhosis and INCPH. In a famous study by Furuichi et al. [66], both LSM and SSM were measured in patients with INCPH and control groups of patients with liver cirrhosis, chronic hepatitis, and healthy subjects. The SSM/LSM ratio was elevated in INCPH patients, and with a cut-off of 1.71, the AUROC of the ratio was excellent (0.933), higher than that of LSM or SSM alone. Similar findings were recently reported also by Ahmad et al. [50] and Navin et al. [67], measuring LSM and SSM with point shear wave elastography and MRE, respectively.

In conclusion, LSM should be routinely evaluated in patients with suspected non-cirrhotic portal hypertension, as low values can rule out cirrhosis and help to establish the diagnosis. In patients with NCPVT, slightly high LSM values (7.1–10 kPa) could suggest hepatic involvement or INCPH and therefore might be used to select patients that should undergo liver biopsy. Moreover, since an overlap with LSM values in cirrhotic patients, especially for INCPH, has been consistently reported in the literature, LSM alone is not reliable to exclude a pre-sinusoidal cause of PH. In this view, the combination of LSM and SSM has shown promising results in improving the accuracy of the non-invasive diagnosis of NCPH. Further studies are required to evaluate the prognostic role of LSM and SSM, in terms of risk stratification and prediction of variceal bleeding, need for TIPS, and transplantation. Finally, we believe that the evaluation of both liver and spleen stiffness, alongside with a careful examination of patient history, exclusion of other causes of liver disease, evaluation of risk factors, and histopathologic findings, should help the clinician to suspect and make an early diagnosis of non-cirrhotic portal hypertension, or porto-sinusoidal disease, even before dreadful complications such as variceal bleeding occur.

16.4　Part III: Liver Stiffness in Patients with Sinusoidal Obstruction Syndrome (SOS/VOD)

Sinusoidal obstruction syndrome, also known as hepatic veno-occlusive disease (hereafter as SOS/VOD), is a clinical syndrome occurring after high-dose chemotherapy and hematopoietic stem cell transplantation (HSCT) [68] and, less commonly, after ingestion of toxic alkaloids (toxic injury) [69] and after high doses of radiotherapy [70] or liver transplantation [71]. According to SOS/VOD pathogenesis, the syndrome has been classified as a (sinusoidal) portal hypertension [72, 73]. Indeed, hepatotoxic agents (HSCT, alkaloids, radiotherapy, etc.) exerting their action on sinusoidal endothelial cells lead to a loss of integrity of the sinusoidal wall, detachment of endothelium, and embolization of the hepatic acinus. These events result in an obstacle to the outflow of liver blood, with sinusoidal obstruction and consequent congestion and increase in portal pressures, thus generating the status of portal hypertension (PH) [74, 75]. Although this condition is rather rare in other clinical contexts, after HSCT the syndrome has a clinically relevant incidence (from 5% to >30% in high-risk populations) with a high mortality rate in severe forms (>80%) [76]. To date, the diagnostic systems of SOS/VOD are based on the combination of clinical and biochemical scores [77]; the definitive and confirmatory diagnosis would remain determined by liver biopsy and/or measurement of the hepatic venous pressure gradient (HVPG) [78]. In the last 10 years, as more detailed in the Chap. 11 of this book, many efforts have been taken in place to determine the role of LSM for the assessment of PH degree and PH-related conditions concluding that LSM is a very accurate surrogate of PH measure [11, 72, 79]. Since a timely SOS/VOD diagnosis is of critical importance, due to improving the survival rate and given the availability of therapeutic options with favorable outcome, the clinical research has been recently focused on this "niche" condition investigating the role of LSM (Table 16.3) [68, 77, 92].

Recently, data from the animal model have published showing the elevation of LSM in SOS/VOD murine models [93–95]. Park et al. have achieved the first proof of concept on the elastography usefulness in SOS/VOD assessment. The authors induced SOS/VOD with different severity stages in rat models, by monocrotaline gavage or by intraperitoneal injection of 5-fluorouracil, leucovorin, and oxaliplatin. Liver shear wave velocity (SWV), assessed by ARFI imaging in the median lobe, was higher in the SOS/VOD rat models than the matched control group [94]. This year J. Shin et al. have achieved similar results determining the effectiveness of supersonic shear wave imaging (SSI) and dual-energy computed tomography (DECT) for diagnosing hepatic SOS using a rabbit model. Indeed, SSI and DECT were significantly increased in the livers of a rabbit SOS model [95].

The first cases reported of modification in LSM in patients with SOS/VOD date back to 2011 when a Madrid group reported increased shear wave velocity, assessed by ARFI, in two patients who developed VOD/SOS after HSCT [96]. Later on, Auberger et al. suggested that a pre-transplant LSM cut-off of 8 kPa could predict and differentiate patients that developed liver toxicity (defined as increased bilirubin values) after HSCT [81].

Thanks to Karlas and colleagues, an extensive commitment to study the role of ultrasound elastography in post-HSCT complications has been done [97]. In 2014, the authors prospectively enrolled 59 patients; among them, major complications occurred in seven patients (grade 4 Common Terminology Criteria (CTC) for adverse events): four with acute GvHD and/or severe liver toxicity, two with VOD/SOS development, and one case of transplant rejection. The authors showed that baseline liver and spleen size, liver perfusion, TE, and right lobe LSM (R-ARFI) did not differ significantly between patients with and without severe liver complications. The only baseline left lobe LSM (L-ARFI) values were significantly increased in the group with complications. In general, these authors found a slight increase in LSM values in almost all patients throughout the post-HSCT period, probably due to edema and hepatic inflammation caused by the high number of drugs

Table 16.3 Main papers reporting liver stiffness in patients with sinusoidal obstruction syndrome/veno-occlusive disease (SOS/VOD)

Author (year)	Study type	Methods	Cohort size	Main findings	Further commentary	Human or animal
Fontanilla et al. (2011) [80]	Case series	Point shear wave elastography (pSWE), serial measurements	Two adult patients with SOS	Increased shear wave velocities at diagnosis normalized after successful treatment	Comprehensive diagnostic workup including contrast-enhanced and Doppler ultrasound	Human
Auberger et al. (2013) [81]	Single-center analysis with pre-transplant non-invasive transient elastography	LSM assessed with transient elastography (TE)	67 post-HCT	Maximal total serum bilirubin after HCT was significantly higher in patients with pre-transplant LS values >8.0 kPa than with values <8.0 kPa		Human
Karlas et al. (2014) [82]	A monocentric prospective study with systematic follow-up examinations at 2–3 weeks, 4–8 weeks, and 12–20 weeks after SCT	LSM assessed with transient elastography (TE) and right and left liver lobe ARFI (r-ARFI; 1-ARFI)	59 before and after HCT	Baseline l-ARFI was significantly elevated in patients who subsequently developed severe complications and continued to be elevated post-HCT Transient elastography showed increasing LS in patients with complications	TE and r-ARFI baseline assessments not significantly different between patients with and without severe complications during post-HCT follow-up	Human
Colecchia et al. (2017) [83]	Interim analysis of a monocentric prospective study with systematic follow-up for 30 days after allogeneic	LSM assessed with transient elastography (TE) prior HCT and on Days +7 to 10, +17 to 20, and +27 to 30	22 pediatric patients; 4 patients developed SOS	A sudden increase of LSM was a note in SOS patients before the appearance of SOS		Human

So Hyun Park et al. (2018) [84]	An animal case-control study, evaluate on Days 2, 4, 7, 10 the liver shear wave velocity	Liver shear wave velocity (SWV) measured with acoustic radiation force impulse (ARFI) elastography	Rat SOS models of various severities were created by monocrotaline gavage ($N = 40$) or by intraperitoneal injection of 5-fluorouracil, leucovorin and oxaliplatin (FOLFOX) ($N = 16$)	The liver SWV was significantly elevated in the SOS models compared with that of the matched control rats		Rat
Reddivalla et al. (2018) [85]	A monocentric prospective study with systematic follow-up for 24 days after allogeneic SCT	2D shear wave elastography (SWE) was performed at three predefined time points	25 pediatric patients; 5 patients developed SOS	SOS patients had a marked increase of LSM between Day 10 and 20 after SCT	LSM changes occurred before further observations in imaging and laboratory tests	Human
Hao Han et al. (2019) [86]	The animal case-control study evaluates on Days 3 and 5 liver SWV in the low- and high-dose groups	Liver shear wave velocity (SWV) by virtual touch tissue imaging quantification	70 rats were randomly divided into a control group ($n = 10$), a low-dose monocrotaline group ($n = 30$), and a high-dose monocrotaline group ($n = 30$).	Liver SWV in the low- and high-dose groups were elevated; the portal vein velocity (PVV) of these groups was decreased compared with the control group	The liver SWV values had significant correlations with the histologic score and PVV	Rat

(continued)

Table 16.3 (continued)

Author (year)	Study type	Methods	Cohort size	Main findings	Further commentary	Human or animal
Karlas et al. (2019) [87]	A monocentric prospective study with systematic follow-up for 3 months	LSM assessed with TE and pSWE including spleen pSWE. Evaluation before allogeneic SCT and at the onset of hepatic symptoms	Total cohort = 106; 9 developed SOS	Patients with confirmed SOS and/or severe other hepatic complications had elevated LSM compared to those without confirmed liver event	No specific stratification between liver GvHD, drug-induced liver injury, and SOS	Human
Colecchia A. Ravaioli F. et al. (2019) [88]	A monocentric prospective study with systematic follow-up for 24 days after allogeneic SCT	LSM assessed with transient elastography (TE) prior HCT and on Days +9/10, +15/17, and +23/24	Total cohort = 78 patient; 4 developed SOS	A sudden increase of LSM was observed in all SOS patients 2–12 days prior to the onset of clinical symptoms	LSM increase was only observed in SOS cases, but not in other types of hepatobiliary complications	Human
Lazzari et al. (2019) [89]	Case report	TE and 2D-SWE at SOS diagnosis, serial LSM during treatment	Adult patient	Maximum LSM values were measured at SOS diagnosis	Normalized LSM values within 100 days after SCT	Human
Zama et al. (2019) [90]	Case series	Serial measurements with TE and 2D-SWE	Three pediatric patients	SOS was associated with a significant increase in LSM.	LSM normalized within 2 weeks after successful treatment	Human
Jaeseung Shin et al. (2020) [91]	Animal case-control study	Liver stiffness was measured using supersonic shear wave imaging (SSI) and dual-energy computed tomography (DECT) on Days 0, 3, 10, and 20	Nine New Zealand white rabbits, three in the control group	Significant stiffness changes measured by SSI were observed starting on Day 10, with no apparent morphologic change even with contrast-enhanced CT throughout the test days	Compared to Day 0, liver stiffness and perfusion parameters were higher on Day 20 in the SOS group	Rabbit

administered in this context. On the other hand, in just five patients who developed severe hepatic complications, LSM by TE was significantly higher in comparison with the whole population cohort [97]. Later on, in 2019, the same research group, enlarging the previous cohort and prospectively enrolled 106 consecutive patients undergoing allogeneic HSCT, evaluated the impact of LSM, assessed both by TE and pSWE, on liver event-free survival and all-cause mortality at 1 year. They observed 33 life-threatening events (14 died), including 16 liver complications (9 SOS/VOD) at 100 days. The hazard ratios for liver-related complications at 100 days were 3.2 (95% CI: 1.8–14.6, $p = 0.0022$) and 4.4 (95% CI: 1.6–11.9, $p = 0.0042$) for elevated TE values ($n = 11$) and pSWE values ($n = 31$), respectively. Results were analogous for all-cause mortality at 1 year. The authors concluded that TE and pSWE are promising for predicting the risk of free survival from hepatic events and all-cause mortality to 1 year [87].

Our research group has worked intensely on the role of LSM change, assessed by different elastographic techniques in SOS/VOD development after HSCT [88, 98]. Our first observation was investigating the predictive role of LSM changes, assessed by TE, in SOS/VOD development after HSCT in a cohort of 22 pediatric patients [98]. Five of those developed SOS/VOD after HSCT. LSMs were carried out at baseline (before HSCT) and subsequently at the bedside at Days 7–10, 17–20, and 27–30 after HSCT. Even though none significant differences were observed at baseline LSM between patients that developed SOS/VOD and those that did not, in patients that developed SOS/VOD, LSM values increased markedly compared to the previous measurement. This LSM increment was observed from 3 to 6 days before clinical VOD/SOS diagnosis based on Seattle/Baltimore criteria. Based on these preliminary results, a national multicenter, multi-elastographic technique, prospective study in Italy ("ElastoVOD Study" ClinicalTrials.gov: NCT03426358, ongoing) was set up, aimed at confirming the prognostic role of LSM. With similar results, later on, Reddivalla et al. [99] evaluated SWV by 2D-SWE in 25 pediatrics patients at baseline and Days +5 and +14 after HSCT. The incidence of SOS/VOD clinical diagnosis was 5 out of 25 (20%), observing no differences in pre-conditioning SWV between VOD/SOS and the control group. Analogously, a significant increase in SWV velocity was observed in patients that developed SOS/VOD, and the SWV increase generally preceded a clinical and US-based VOD/SOS diagnosis by 9 and 11 days. D. Zama et al. [100] reported the role of LSM in the management of three pediatric patients after the diagnosis of VOD/SOS. The authors showed that after a specific SOS/VOD treatment (i.e., defibrotide), liver stiffness values showed a progressive reduction pattern in all three patients, with normalization after 2 weeks leading to a speculative conclusion of being able to monitor the therapeutic response with subsequent LSM assessments.

From the perspective of adult patients' cohort, we recently published the first monocentric study on 78 adult patients undergoing HSCT. We confirmed what we observed in little patients that LSM increases, here also assessed by TE, occurred from +2 to +12 days before clinical SOS/VOD appearance and gradually decreased following successful SOS/VOD specific treatment. Moreover, for the first time, we observed that LSM values did not significantly increase in patients experiencing hepatobiliary complications other than VOD/SOS [100].

These results need to be further validated by extensive prospective studies to define the most suitable application of LSM in clinical practice. Currently, based on quite a large number of patients in real-life HSCT practice, and suggests that LSM by all the elastography techniques available could be considered a promising method to perform an early, pre-clinical diagnosis and predict SOS/VOD after HSCT. Besides, it could be further used to assess treatment response in adult patients undergoing HSCT and developing SOS/VOD. Since the elastographic techniques are non-invasive, bedside method, very well tolerated by patients and easily reproducible, the LSM will find a great space as non-invasive evaluations of SOS/VOD diagnosis. LSM could be helping the clinician to a more prompt and accurate clinical diagnosis of SOS/VOD in the HSCT context and to differentiate this condition to the other liver-related HSCT complications [92].

References

1. Association E. EASL Clinical Practice Guidelines: vascular diseases of the liver. J Hepatol. 2016;64:179–202.
2. Plessier A, Valla DC. Budd-Chiari syndrome. Semin Liver Dis. 2008;28:259–69.
3. Darwish Murad S, Plessier A, Hernandez-Guerra M, et al. Etiology, management, and outcome of the Budd-Chiari syndrome. Ann Intern Med. 2009;151:167–75.
4. Rautou P-E, Moucari R, Escolano S, et al. Prognostic indices for Budd–Chiari syndrome: valid for clinical studies but insufficient for individual management. Am J Gastroenterol. 2009;104:1140–6.
5. Murad SD, Valla DC, De Groen PC, Zeitoun G, Hopmans JAM, Haagsma EB, Van Hoek B, Hansen BE, Rosendaal FR, Janssen HLA. Determinants of survival and the effect of portosystemic shunting in patients with Budd-Chiari syndrome. Hepatology. 2004;39:500–8.
6. Murad SD, Kim WR, de Groen PC, Kamath PS, Malinchoc M, Valla DC, Janssen HLA. Can the model for end-stage liver disease be used to predict the prognosis in patients with Budd-Chiari syndrome? Liver Transpl. 2007;13:867–74.
7. Zeitoun G, Escolano S, Hadengue A, et al. Outcome of Budd-Chiari syndrome: a multivariate analysis of factors related to survival including surgical portosystemic shunting. Hepatology. 1999;30:84–9.
8. Langlet P, Escolano S, Valla D, et al. Clinicopathological forms and prognostic index in Budd-Chiari syndrome. J Hepatol. 2003;39:496–501.
9. Castera L, Yuen Chan HL, Arrese M, Afdhal N, Bedossa P, Friedrich-Rust M, Han KH, Pinzani M. EASL-ALEH Clinical Practice Guidelines: non-invasive tests for evaluation of liver disease severity and prognosis. J Hepatol. 2015;63:237–64.
10. Castera L. Non-invasive tests for liver fibrosis progression and regression. J Hepatol. 2016;64:232–3.
11. Berzigotti A. Non-invasive evaluation of portal hypertension using ultrasound elastography. J Hepatol. 2017;67:399–411. https://doi.org/10.1016/j.jhep.2017.02.003.
12. de Franchis R, Baveno VI Faculty. Expanding consensus in portal hypertension: report of the Baveno VI Consensus Workshop: stratifying risk and individualising care for portal hypertension. J Hepatol. 2015;63:743–52.
13. Dietrich C, Bamber J, Berzigotti A, et al. EFSUMB Guidelines and Recommendations on the clinical use of liver ultrasound elastography, update 2017 (long version). Ultraschall Med. 2017;38:e16. https://doi.org/10.1055/s-0043-103952.

14. Simonetto DA, Yang H, Yin M, et al. Chronic passive venous congestion drives hepatic fibrogenesis via sinusoidal thrombosis and mechanical forces. Hepatology. 2015;61:648–59.

15. Colli A, Pozzoni P, Berzuini A, Gerosa A, Canovi C, Molteni EE, Barbarini M, Bonino F, Prati D. Decompensated chronic heart failure: increased liver stiffness measured by means of transient elastography. Radiology. 2010;257:872–8.

16. Colecchia A, Montrone L, Scaioli E, et al. Measurement of spleen stiffness to evaluate portal hypertension and the presence of esophageal varices in patients with HCV-related cirrhosis. Gastroenterology. 2012;143:646–54.

17. Song J, Huang J, Huang H, Liu S, Luo Y. Performance of spleen stiffness measurement in prediction of clinical significant portal hypertension: a meta-analysis. Clin Res Hepatol Gastroenterol. 2018;42:216–26.

18. Singh R, Wilson MP, Katlariwala P, Murad MH, McInnes MDF, Low G. Accuracy of liver and spleen stiffness on magnetic resonance elastography for detecting portal hypertension: a systematic review and meta-analysis. Eur J Gastroenterol Hepatol. 2021;32:237. https://doi.org/10.1097/MEG.0000000000001724.

19. Colecchia A, Ravaioli F, Marasco G, Colli A, Dajti E, Di Biase AR, Bacchi Reggiani ML, Berzigotti A, Pinzani M, Festi D. A combined model based on spleen stiffness measurement and Baveno VI criteria to rule out high-risk varices in advanced chronic liver disease. J Hepatol. 2018;69:308. https://doi.org/10.1016/j.jhep.2018.04.023.

20. Ma X, Wang L, Wu H, Feng Y, Han X, Bu H, Zhu Q. Spleen stiffness is superior to liver stiffness for predicting esophageal varices in chronic liver disease: a meta-analysis. PLoS One. 2016;11:e0165786.

21. Mukund A, Pargewar SS, Desai SN, Rajesh S, Sarin SK. Changes in liver congestion in patients with Budd–Chiari syndrome following endovascular interventions: assessment with transient elastography. J Vasc Interv Radiol. 2017;28:683–7. https://doi.org/10.1016/j.jvir.2016.11.091.

22. Wang H-W, Shi H-N, Cheng J, Xie F, Luo Y-K, Tang J. Real-time shear wave elastography (SWE) assessment of short- and long-term treatment outcome in Budd-Chiari syndrome: a pilot study. Strnad P, ed. PLoS One. 2018;13(5):e0197550. https://doi.org/10.1371/journal.pone.0197550.

23. Dajti E, Ravaioli F, Colecchia A, Marasco G, Vestito A, Festi D. Liver and spleen stiffness measurements for assessment of portal hypertension severity in patients with Budd Chiari syndrome. Can J Gastroenterol Hepatol. 2019;2019:1673197. https://doi.org/10.1155/2019/1673197.

24. Xu P, Lyu L, Ge H, Sami MU, Liu P, Xu K. Segmental liver stiffness evaluated with magnetic resonance elastography is responsive to endovascular intervention in patients with Budd-Chiari syndrome. Korean J Radiol. 2019;20:773–80. https://doi.org/10.3348/kjr.2018.0767.

25. Nakatsuka T, Soroida Y, Nakagawa H, et al. Utility of hepatic vein waveform and transient elastography in patients with Budd-Chiari syndrome who require angioplasty: two case reports. Medicine (Baltimore). 2019;98(45):e17877. https://doi.org/10.1097/MD.0000000000017877.

26. Mancuso A, Amata M, Politi F, Mitra M, Marsala MGL, Maringhini A. Controversies in Budd-Chiari syndrome management: potential role of liver stiffness. Am J Gastroenterol. 2020;115(6):952–3. https://doi.org/10.14309/ajg.0000000000000586.

27. Wang H-W, Shi H-N, Cheng J, Xie F, Luo Y-K, Tang J. Real-time shear wave elastography (SWE) assessment of short- and long-term treatment outcome in Budd-Chiari syndrome: a pilot study. PLoS One. 2018;13:e0197550.

28. De Gottardi A, Rautou P-E, Schouten J, et al. Porto-sinusoidal vascular disease: proposal and description of a novel entity. Lancet Gastroenterol Hepatol. 2019;4:399–411.

29. Chang P-E, Miquel R, Blanco J-L, et al. Idiopathic portal hypertension in patients with HIV infection treated with highly active antiretroviral therapy. Am J Gastroenterol. 2009;104(7):1707–14. https://doi.org/10.1038/ajg.2009.165.

30. Panos G, Farouk L, Stebbing J, et al. Cryptogenic pseudocirrhosis: a new clinical syndrome of noncirrhotic portal hypertension (unassociated with advanced fibrosis) that can

be detected by transient elastography in patients with HIV. J Acquir Immune Defic Syndr. 2009;52(4):525–7. https://doi.org/10.1097/QAI.0b013e3181bb27b1.

31. Cesari M, Schiavini M, Marchetti G, et al. Noncirrhotic portal hypertension in HIV-infected patients: a case control evaluation and review of the literature. AIDS Patient Care STDs. 2010;24(11):697–703. https://doi.org/10.1089/apc.2010.0160.

32. Laharie D, Vergniol J, Bioulac-Sage P, et al. Usefulness of non-invasive tests in nodular regenerative hyperplasia of the liver. Eur J Gastroenterol Hepatol. 2010;22(4):487–93. https://doi.org/10.1097/MEG.0b013e328334098f.

33. Scourfield A, Waters L, Holmes P, et al. Non-cirrhotic portal hypertension in HIV-infected individuals. Int J STD AIDS. 2011;22(6):324–8. https://doi.org/10.1258/ijsa.2010.010396.

34. Jackson BD, Doyle JS, Hoy JF, et al. Non-cirrhotic portal hypertension in HIV mono-infected patients. J Gastroenterol Hepatol. 2012;27(9):1512–9. https://doi.org/10.1111/j.1440-1746.2012.07148.x.

35. Sharma P, Mishra SR, Kumar M, Sharma BC, Sarin SK. Liver and spleen stiffness in patients with extrahepatic portal vein obstruction. Radiology. 2012;263(3):893–9. https://doi.org/10.1148/radiol.12111046.

36. Seijo S, Reverter E, Miquel R, et al. Role of hepatic vein catheterisation and transient elastography in the diagnosis of idiopathic portal hypertension. Dig Liver Dis. 2012;44(10):855–60. https://doi.org/10.1016/j.dld.2012.05.005.

37. Furuichi Y, Moriyasu F, Taira J, et al. Non-invasive diagnostic method for idiopathic portal hypertension based on measurements of liver and spleen stiffness by ARFI elastography. J Gastroenterol. 2013;48(9):1061–8. https://doi.org/10.1007/s00535-012-0703-z.

38. Logan S, Rodger A, Maynard-Smith L, et al. Prevalence of significant liver disease in human immunodeficiency virus-infected patients exposed to Didanosine: a cross sectional study. World J Hepatol. 2016;8(36):1623–8. https://doi.org/10.4254/wjh.v8.i36.1623.

39. Scherpbier HJ, Terpstra V, Pajkrt D, et al. Noncirrhotic portal hypertension in perinatally HIV-infected adolescents treated with didanosine-containing antiretroviral regimens in childhood. Pediatr Infect Dis J. 2016;35(8):e248–52. https://doi.org/10.1097/INF.0000000000001202.

40. Madhusudhan KS, Sharma R, Kilambi R, et al. 2D Shear Wave Elastography of Liver in Patients with Primary Extrahepatic Portal Vein Obstruction. J Clin Exp Hepatol. 2017;7(1):23–7. https://doi.org/10.1016/j.jceh.2016.12.001.

41. Sood V, Lal BB, Khanna R, Rawat D, Bihari C, Alam S. Noncirrhotic portal fibrosis in pediatric population. J Pediatr Gastroenterol Nutr. 2017;64(5):748–53. https://doi.org/10.1097/MPG.0000000000001485.

42. Sharma P, Agarwal R, Dhawan S, et al. Transient elastography (fibroscan) in patients with non-cirrhotic portal fibrosis. J Clin Exp Hepatol. 2017;7(3):230–4. https://doi.org/10.1016/j.jceh.2017.03.002.

43. Madhusudhan KS, Kilambi R, Shalimar, Pal S, Sharma R, Srivastava DN. Evaluation of splenic stiffness in patients of extrahepatic portal vein obstruction using 2D shear wave elastography: comparison with intra-operative portal pressure. J Clin Exp Hepatol. 2018;8(3):250–5. https://doi.org/10.1016/j.jceh.2017.12.002.

44. Chougule A, Rastogi A, Maiwall R, Bihari C, Sood V, Sarin SK. Spectrum of histopathological changes in patients with non-cirrhotic portal fibrosis. Hepatol Int. 2018;12(2):158–66. https://doi.org/10.1007/s12072-018-9857-y.

45. Vuppalanchi R, Mathur K, Pyko M, Samala N, Chalasani N. Liver stiffness measurements in patients with noncirrhotic portal hypertension—the devil is in the details. Hepatology. 2018;68(6):2438–40. https://doi.org/10.1002/hep.30167.

46. Madhusudhan KS, Kilambi R, Shalimar, et al. Measurement of splenic stiffness by 2D-shear wave elastography in patients with extrahepatic portal vein obstruction. Br J Radiol. 2018;91(1092):20180401. https://doi.org/10.1259/bjr.20180401.

47. Sutton H, Fitzpatrick E, Davenport M, et al. Transient elastography measurements of spleen stiffness as a predictor of clinically significant varices in children. J Pediatr Gastroenterol Nutr. 2018;67(4):446–51. https://doi.org/10.1097/MPG.0000000000002069.

48. Cunningham ME, Parastandeh-Chehr G, Cerocchi O, Wong DK, Patel K. Noninvasive predictors of high-risk varices in patients with non-cirrhotic portal hypertension. Can J Gastroenterol Hepatol. 2019;2019:1–7. https://doi.org/10.1155/2019/1808797.

49. Navin PJ, Gidener T, Allen AM, et al. The role of magnetic resonance elastography in the diagnosis of noncirrhotic portal hypertension. Clin Gastroenterol Hepatol. 2020;18:3051. https://doi.org/10.1016/j.cgh.2019.10.018.

50. Ahmad AK, Atzori S, Taylor-Robinson SD, Maurice JB, Cooke GS, Garvey L. Spleen stiffness measurements using point shear wave elastography detects noncirrhotic portal hypertension in human immunodeficiency virus. Medicine (Baltimore). 2019;98(47):e17961. https://doi.org/10.1097/MD.0000000000017961.

51. Cannella R, Minervini MI, Rachakonda V, Bollino G, Furlan A. Liver stiffness measurement in patients with nodular regenerative hyperplasia undergoing magnetic resonance elastography. Abdom Radiol. 2020;45(2):373–83. https://doi.org/10.1007/s00261-019-02367-8.

52. Yuldashev RZ, Aliev MM, Shokhaydarov SI, Tursunova DB. Spleen stiffness measurement as a non-invasive test to evaluate and monitor portal hypertension in children with extrahepatic portal vein obstruction. Pediatr Surg Int. 2020;36(5):637–41. https://doi.org/10.1007/s00383-020-04648-6.

53. Gupta S, Pottakkat B, Verma SK, Kalayarasan R, Chandrasekar AS, Pillai AA. Pathological abnormalities in splenic vasculature in non-cirrhotic portal hypertension: its relevance in the management of portal hypertension. World J Gastrointest Surg. 2020;12(1):1–8. https://doi.org/10.4240/wjgs.v12.i1.1.

54. Madhusudhan KS, Sharma R, Kilambi R, Shylendran S, Shalimar, Sahni P, Gupta AK. 2D shear wave elastography of liver in patients with primary extrahepatic portal vein obstruction. J Clin Exp Hepatol. 2017;7:23–7.

55. Madhusudhan KS, Kilambi R, Shalimar, Sahni P, Sharma R, Srivastava DN, Gupta AK. Measurement of splenic stiffness by 2D-shear wave elastography in patients with extrahepatic portal vein obstruction. Br J Radiol. 2018;91:20180401. https://doi.org/10.1259/bjr.20180401.

56. Sutton H, Fitzpatrick E, Davenport M, Burford C, Alexander E, Dhawan A, Grammatikopoulos T. Transient elastography measurements of spleen stiffness as a predictor of clinically significant varices in children. J Pediatr Gastroenterol Nutr. 2018;67:446–51.

57. Verheij J, Schouten JNL, Komuta M, Nevens F, Hansen BE, Janssen HLA, Roskams T. Histological features in western patients with idiopathic non-cirrhotic portal hypertension. Histopathology. 2013;62:1083–91.

58. Gioia S, Nardelli S, Riggio O. Letter to the editor: liver stiffness in noncirrhotic portal hypertension: the devil is in the diagnosis. Hepatology. 2019;70:444–5.

59. Gioia S, Nardelli S, Pasquale C, Pentassuglio I, Nicoletti V, Aprile F, Merli M, Riggio O. Natural history of patients with non cirrhotic portal hypertension: comparison with patients with compensated cirrhosis. Dig Liver Dis. 2018;50:839–44.

60. Chang P-E, Miquel R, Blanco J-L, Laguno M, Bruguera M, Abraldes J-G, Bosch J, Garcia-Pagan J-C. Idiopathic portal hypertension in patients with HIV infection treated with highly active antiretroviral therapy. Am J Gastroenterol. 2009;104:1707–14.

61. Panos G, Farouk L, Stebbing J, Holmes P, Valero S, Randell P, Bower M, Gazzard B, Anderson M, Nelson M. Cryptogenic pseudocirrhosis: a new clinical syndrome of noncirrhotic portal hypertension (unassociated with advanced fibrosis) that can be detected by transient elastography in patients with HIV. J Acquir Immune Defic Syndr. 2009;52:525–7.

62. Cesari M, Schiavini M, Marchetti G, Caramma I, Ortu M, Franzetti F, Galli M, Antinori S, Milazzo L. Noncirrhotic portal hypertension in HIV-infected patients: a case control evaluation and review of the literature. AIDS Patient Care STDs. 2010;24:697–703.

63. Laharie D, Vergniol J, Bioulac-Sage P, Diris B, Poli J, Foucher J, Couzigou P, Drouillard J, De Lédinghen V. Usefulness of non-invasive tests in nodular regenerative hyperplasia of the liver. Eur J Gastroenterol Hepatol. 2010;22:487–93.

64. Seijo S, Reverter E, Miquel R, Berzigotti A, Abraldes JG, Bosch J, García-Pagán JC. Role of hepatic vein catheterisation and transient elastography in the diagnosis of idiopathic portal hypertension. Dig Liver Dis. 2012;44:855–60.

65. Sharma P, Agarwal R, Dhawan S, Bansal N. Transient elastography in patients with non-cirrhotic portal fibrosis. J Clin Exp Hepatol. 2017;XX:1–5.

66. Furuichi Y, Moriyasu F, Taira J, Sugimoto K, Sano T, Ichimura S, Miyata Y, Imai Y. Non-invasive diagnostic method for idiopathic portal hypertension based on measurements of liver and spleen stiffness by ARFI elastography. J Gastroenterol. 2013;48:1061–8.

67. Navin PJ, Gidener T, Allen AM, Yin M, Takahashi N, Torbenson MS, Kamath PS, Ehman RL, Venkatesh SK. The role of magnetic resonance elastography in the diagnosis of noncirrhotic portal hypertension. Clin Gastroenterol Hepatol. 2020;18:3051. https://doi.org/10.1016/j.cgh.2019.10.018.

68. Ravaioli F, Colecchia A, Alemanni LV, Vestito A, Dajti E, Marasco G, Sessa M, Pession A, Bonifazi F, Festi D. Role of imaging techniques in liver veno-occlusive disease diagnosis: recent advances and literature review. Expert Rev Gastroenterol Hepatol. 2019;13:463–84.

69. Lin G, Wang JY, Li N, et al. Hepatic sinusoidal obstruction syndrome associated with consumption of Gynura segetum. J Hepatol. 2011;54:666–73.

70. Reed GB Jr, Cox AJ Jr. The human liver after radiation injury. A form of veno-occlusive disease. Am J Pathol. 1966;48:597–611.

71. Rosen HR, Martin P, Schiller GJ, Territo M, Lewin DN, Shackleton CR, Busuttil RW. Orthotopic liver transplantation for bone-marrow transplant-associated veno-occlusive disease and graft-versus-host disease of the liver. Liver Transpl Surg. 1996;2:225–32.

72. Ravaioli F, Montagnani M, Lisotti A, Festi D, Mazzella G, Azzaroli F. Noninvasive assessment of portal hypertension in advanced chronic liver disease: an update. Gastroenterol Res Pract. 2018;2018:1–11.

73. Association for the Study of the Liver E. EASL Clinical Practice Guidelines: vascular diseases of the liver. J Hepatol. 2016;64:179–202.

74. Jones RJ, Lee KS, Beschorner WE, Vogel VG, Grochow LB, Braine HG, Vogelsang GB, Sensenbrenner LL, Santos GW, Saral R. Venoocclusive disease of the liver following bone marrow transplantation. Transplantation. 1987;44:778–83.

75. Carreras E, Granena A, Navasa M, Bruguera M, Marco V, Sierra J, Tassies MD, Garcia-Pagan JC, Marti JM, Bosch J. On the reliability of clinical criteria for the diagnosis of hepatic veno-occlusive disease. Ann Hematol. 1993;66:77–80.

76. Carreras E, Diaz-Beya M, Rosinol L, Martinez C, Fernandez-Aviles F, Rovira M. The incidence of veno-occlusive disease following allogeneic hematopoietic stem cell transplantation has diminished and the outcome improved over the last decade. Biol Blood Marrow Transplant. 2011;17:1713–20.

77. Bonifazi F, Barbato F, Ravaioli F, Sessa M, Defrancesco I, Arpinati M, Cavo M, Colecchia A. Diagnosis and treatment of VOD/SOS after allogeneic hematopoietic stem cell transplantation. Front Immunol. 2020;11:489.

78. Shulman HM, Gooley T, Dudley MD, Kofler T, Feldman R, Dwyer D, McDonald GB. Utility of transvenous liver biopsies and wedged hepatic venous pressure measurements in sixty marrow transplant recipients. Transplantation. 1995;59:1015–22.

79. Colecchia A, Ravaioli F, Marasco G, Festi D. Spleen stiffness by ultrasound elastography. In: Diagnostic methods for cirrhosis and portal hypertension. New York, NY: Springer; 2018. https://doi.org/10.1007/978-3-319-72628-1_8.

80. Fontanilla T, Hernando CG, Claros JCV, et al. Acoustic radiation force impulse elastography and contrast-enhanced sonography of sinusoidal obstructive syndrome (Veno-occlusive disease): preliminary results. J Ultrasound Med. 2011;30(11):1593–8. https://doi.org/10.7863/jum.2011.30.11.1593.

81. Auberger J, Graziadei I, Clausen J, Vogel W, Nachbaur D. Non-invasive transient elastography for the prediction of liver toxicity following hematopoietic SCT. Bone Marrow Transplant. 2013;48(1):159–60. https://doi.org/10.1038/bmt.2012.113.

82. Karlas T, Weber J, Nehring C, et al. Value of liver elastography and abdominal ultrasound for detection of complications of allogeneic hemopoietic SCT. Bone Marrow Transplant. 2014;49:806–11. https://doi.org/10.1038/bmt.2014.61.

83. Colecchia A, Marasco G, Ravaioli F, et al. Usefulness of liver stiffness measurement in predicting hepatic veno-occlusive disease development in patients who undergo HSCT. Bone Marrow Transplant. 2017;52(3):494–7. https://doi.org/10.1038/bmt.2016.320.

84. Park SH, Lee SS, Sung JY, et al. Non-invasive assessment of hepatic sinusoidal obstructive syndrome using acoustic radiation force impulse elastography imaging: a proof-of-concept study in rat models. Eur Radiol. 2018;28(5):2096–106. https://doi.org/10.1007/s00330-017-5179-z.

85. Reddivalla N, Robinson AL, Reid KJ, et al. Using liver elastography to diagnose sinusoidal obstruction syndrome in pediatric patients undergoing hematopoetic stem cell transplant. Bone Marrow Transplant. 2020;55(3):523–30. https://doi.org/10.1038/s41409-017-0064-6.

86. Han H, Yang J, Li X, et al. Role of virtual touch tissue imaging quantification in the assessment of hepatic sinusoidal obstruction syndrome in a rat model. J Ultrasound Med. 2019;38(8):2039–46. https://doi.org/10.1002/jum.14893.

87. Karlas T, Weiße T, Petroff D, et al. Predicting hepatic complications of allogeneic hematopoietic stem cell transplantation using liver stiffness measurement. Bone Marrow Transplant. 2019;54(11):1738–46. https://doi.org/10.1038/s41409-019-0464-x.

88. Colecchia A, Ravaioli F, Sessa M, et al. Liver stiffness measurement allows early diagnosis of veno-occlusive disease/sinusoidal obstruction syndrome in adult patients who undergo hematopoietic stem cell transplantation: results from a monocentric prospective study. Biol Blood Marrow Transplant. 2019;25(5):995–1003. https://doi.org/10.1016/j.bbmt.2019.01.019.

89. Lazzari L, Marra P, Greco R, et al. Ultrasound elastography techniques for diagnosis and follow-up of hepatic veno-occlusive disease. Bone Marrow Transplant. 2019;54(7):1145–7. https://doi.org/10.1038/s41409-019-0432-5.

90. Zama D, Bossù G, Ravaioli F, et al. Longitudinal evaluation of liver stiffness in three pediatric patients with veno-occlusive disease. Pediatr Transplant. 2019;23(5):e13456. https://doi.org/10.1111/petr.13456.

91. Shin J, Yoon H, Cha YJ, et al. Liver stiffness and perfusion changes for hepatic sinusoidal obstruction syndrome in rabbit model. World J Gastroenterol. 2020;26(8):706–16. https://doi.org/10.3748/wjg.v26.i7.706.

92. Chan SS, Colecchia A, Duarte RF, Bonifazi F, Ravaioli F, Bourhis JH. Imaging in hepatic veno-occlusive disease/sinusoidal obstruction syndrome. Biol Blood Marrow Transplant. 2020;26:1770. https://doi.org/10.1016/j.bbmt.2020.06.016.

93. Han H, Yang J, Li X, Zhuge Y, Zhu C, Chen J, Fu Y, Wu M. Role of virtual touch tissue imaging quantification in the assessment of hepatic sinusoidal obstruction syndrome in a rat model. J Ultrasound Med. 2019;38:2039–46.

94. Park SH, Lee SS, Sung J-Y, Na K, Kim HJ, Kim SY, Park BJ, Byun JH. Non-invasive assessment of hepatic sinusoidal obstructive syndrome using acoustic radiation force impulse elastography imaging: a proof-of-concept study in rat models. Eur Radiol. 2018;28:2096. https://doi.org/10.1007/s00330-017-5179-z.

95. Shin J, Yoon H, Cha YJ, Han K, Lee MJ, Kim MJ, Shin HJ. Liver stiffness and perfusion changes for hepatic sinusoidal obstruction syndrome in rabbit model. World J Gastroenterol. 2020;26:706–16.

96. Fontanilla T, Hernando CG, Claros JCV, Bautista G, Minaya J, Del Carmen VM, Piazza A, Mendez S, Rodriguez C, Aranguena RP. Acoustic radiation force impulse elastography and contrast-enhanced sonography of sinusoidal obstructive syndrome (Veno-occlusive Disease): preliminary results. J Ultrasound Med. 2011;30:1593–8.

97. Karlas T, Weber J, Nehring C, Kronenberger R, Tenckhoff H, Mössner J, Niederwieser D, Tröltzsch M, Lange T, Keim V. Value of liver elastography and abdominal ultrasound for detection of complications of allogeneic hemopoietic SCT. Bone Marrow Transplant. 2014;49:806–11.

98. Colecchia A, Marasco G, Ravaioli F, Kleinschmidt K, Masetti R, Prete A, Pession A, Festi D. Usefulness of liver stiffness measurement in predicting hepatic veno-occlusive disease development in patients who undergo HSCT. Bone Marrow Transplant. 2017;52:494–7.

99. Reddivalla N, Robinson AL, Reid KJ, Radhi MA, Dalal J, Opfer EK, Chan SS. Using liver elastography to diagnose sinusoidal obstruction syndrome in pediatric patients undergoing hematopoetic stem cell transplant. Bone Marrow Transplant. 2018;55:523–30.

100. Zama D, Bossù G, Ravaioli F, Masetti R, Prete A, Festi D, Pession A. Longitudinal evaluation of liver stiffness in three pediatric patients with veno-occlusive disease. Pediatr Transplant. 2019;23:c13456.

Liver and Spleen Stiffness in Hematological Diseases

17

Mariangela Giunta and Mirella Fraquelli

Elastographic techniques are non-invasive user-friendly tests to measure the tissue stiffness of parenchymal organs. In hepatology the main initial target of elastographic measurements has been the liver, using transient elastography (TE, FibroScan®). Liver stiffness (LS) is now a widely accepted and validated method to predict the severity and prognosis of chronic liver diseases [1–3], it being an accurate marker of hepatic fibrosis.

Because of the strict relationship between the severity of chronic liver diseases and splenic modifications with a progressive splenomegaly related to congestion, hypertrophy, and hyperplasia of the spleen parenchyma, spleen stiffness (SS) too was subsequently investigated in these patients, it becoming particularly attractive as compared to liver stiffness, especially in more advanced phases of hepatic involvement. In fact, spleen modifications appear to better represent the dynamic changes occurring in the advanced stages of liver cirrhosis and to provide useful diagnostic information towards the assessment and staging of portal hypertension.

The spleen is also frequently involved in hematological disorders, where the degree of splenomegaly is often related to disease prognosis. Following the favorable results obtained in hepatology, some researchers and physicians have been more recently investigating how liver elasticity and spleen elasticity change in patients affected by hematological disorders.

According to the literature to date, elastography comes with two main potential and promising uses in patients affected by hematological diseases:

M. Giunta (✉)
Division of Endoscopy, IEO, European Institute of Oncology IRCCS, Milan, Italy
e-mail: mariangela.giunta@ieo.it

M. Fraquelli
Gastroenterology and Endoscopy Division, Fondazione IRCCS Ca' Granda Ospedale Maggiore Policlinico, Milan, Italy

M. Fraquelli (ed.), *Elastography of the Liver and Beyond*,
https://doi.org/10.1007/978-3-030-74132-7_17

1. Liver stiffness measurement to assess the severity of liver damage, in hematological diseases characterized by secondary hepatic involvement, mainly in beta-thalassemia patients and in patients affected by sickle cell disease, presenting with liver injury correlated to hepatic fibrosis and/or siderosis, due to iron overload and sometimes concomitant viral hepatitis (especially HCV infection).
2. Spleen stiffness measurement to assess the severity of the hematological disease itself, in the case of diseases occurring with splenomegaly without hepatic involvement, mainly in myeloproliferative disorders. Studies conducted in these set of patients have investigated the relationship between the splenic stiffness and some prominent parameters of hematological disease severity, such as bone marrow fibrosis or some prognostic scoring systems.

The present chapter aimed to offer a comprehensive review of the current knowledge and of the available results achieved on this topic.

17.1 Liver Elastography in Hematological Diseases

Beta-thalassemia (in its forms major and intermedia) is the most common genetic disorder worldwide, with a remarkable impact and burden on a patient's health especially in the Mediterranean region. Even if the survival of beta-thalassemia major (TM) and intermedia (TI) patients has significantly improved over the past few decades, as better treatment and follow-up have been made available, complications are still common and affect patients' quality of life. In particular, iron overload is the major concern for these patients as it happens through regular blood transfusions and increased intestinal iron absorption. It affects particularly the liver, heart, and endocrine organs and continues to be the main contributor to severe morbidity and early mortality for these patients.

Inappropriate therapy or no iron chelation therapy (ICT) causes life-threatening morbidities and early death. In addition, adult patients with TM and TI represent a population with a high prevalence of hepatitis C due to transfusions of HCV-infected blood units prior to the introduction of HCV screening [4–9].

The potential use of liver elastography as a non-invasive test of liver damage in TM and IT patients has been extensively investigated. The first goal with these patients is to assess the liver fibrosis stage. Actually, liver biopsy is still considered the reference standard for the evaluation of hepatic fibrosis [10]. However, the use of non-invasive tools such as liver elastography is very attractive, since patients affected by MT and IT (especially those with concomitant HCV infection) are at higher risk of liver biopsy-related complications, as compared to other chronically HCV-infected patients, and because they need continuous revaluation during their follow-up.

A further important goal in these patients is to quantify the amount of iron overload. The reference standard to determine hepatic iron content is the tissue determination of liver iron concentration (LIC) in a liver specimen. However, more recently

T2* magnetic resonance imaging (MRI) of the liver has been taken as the standard non-invasive technique in use to quantify and monitor the degree of hepatic iron overload.

To improve on the non-invasive management of thalassemia patients, some studies have aimed at assessing the diagnostic accuracy of LS, for both predicting the degree of liver fibrosis (mainly to help the decision on antiviral treatment in HCV-infected patients and to define the prognosis and the appropriate conditioning regimen in patients that are candidates for hematopoietic stem cell transplantation) and assessing the amount of iron overload, in order to tailor iron chelation therapy.

Several studies have demonstrated that TE is a reliable tool for assessing liver fibrosis in thalassemia patients (Table 17.1).

In fact, the relationship between liver stiffness and liver fibrosis is significant and reliable. In a study performed by our group [11], 14 out of 115 adult patients with beta-thalassemia major ($n = 59$) or intermedia ($n = 56$) underwent liver biopsy. The histological stage of liver fibrosis was significantly related to TE results ($r = 0.73$, $p = 0.003$), whereas the histological score did not correlate with LIC values. A TE cut-off value of 12 kPa diagnosed cirrhosis with 100% sensitivity (95% CI 23–100) and 92% specificity (95% CI 62–99), LR+ 12 and LR− 0.1, respectively. Despite the small size of the histological data set, which is the main limit of this study, the result achieved suggests that LS is, as measured by TE, a reliable tool for assessing liver fibrosis in patients with thalassemia. Also, in the prospective study by Di Marco et al. [12] who dealt with 56 consecutive transfusion-dependent thalassemic patients undergoing liver biopsy and TE, LS was found highly accurate in identifying patients with cirrhosis (F4 vs. F1–F3), whereas it performed less well at lower stages of fibrosis. The AUROC for prediction of cirrhosis was 0.997 (95% CI 92.5–100). At a cut-off value of 13 kPa, the sensitivity of LS for cirrhosis was 100% (95% CI 69.0–100) and specificity 95.3% (95% CI 84.2–99.3). The positive and negative predictive values for the diagnosis of cirrhosis were respectively 83.3% and 100%. In another study by Poustchi et al. [13], 76 patients with beta-thalassemia and chronic hepatitis C underwent liver TE, liver biopsy, and T2* MRI, and the results showed that, regardless of liver iron concentration (LIC), TE alone or in combination with Fibrosis 4 test (FIB-4) or the aspartate aminotransferase to platelet ratio index (APRI) shows moderate to high accuracy for the evaluation of liver fibrosis: the area under the receiver operating characteristic curve (AUROC) for predicting cirrhosis was 80% (95% CI 59–100), and using a cut-off value of 11 kPa, LS showed 78% sensitivity and 88.1% specificity in diagnosing cirrhosis. Also, a study involving 83 pediatric transplantation candidates affected by MT (no one with concomitant viral hepatitis) [14] supports these results: all the patients were investigated by liver TE and liver biopsy, and the results revealed that TE increases proportionally to the Metavir fibrosis stages ($p < 0.001$) and necroinflammatory grade ($p < 0.001$) and the TE score also correlated to liver iron content measure by liver biopsy ($p < 0.001$).

One study in the literature has investigated the possibility to use a different elastographic technique, which is real-time elastography (RTE) [15], for assessing liver fibrosis in 50 patients affected by TM ($n = 37$) and TI ($n = 13$) with iron overload

Table 17.1 Summary of findings from the studies assessing the role of electrographic techniques in staging hepatic fibrosis in thalassemia patients

Study	Population (n)	Fibrosis stage	Technique (cut-off, kPa)	Liver biopsy	Sens	Spec	LR+	LR−	Variables associated to LS
[12]	56	F = 4	TE 13	56	100	95	20	0.001	Stage of fibrosis ($p = 0.002$), AST ($p = 0.006$)
[11]	59 TM	F ≥ 3	TE 10.3	14	60	89	5.4	0.4	ALT ($p = 0.01$), GGT ($p = 0.001$), bilirubin levels ($p = 0.01$), and HCV-RNA positivity ($p = 0.03$)
		F = 4	TE 12.0		100	92	12	0.1	
	56 TI								ALT ($p = 0.007$), GGT ($p = 0.01$), bilirubin levels ($p = 0.04$), previous cholecystectomy ($p = 0.011$), and splenectomy ($p = 0.018$)
[13]	76 TM	F = 4	TE 11	76	78	88.1	6.5	0.2	NA
[14]	83	F ≥ 1	TE 3.2	83	87.5	46.2	1.6	0.3	Stage of fibrosis ($p = 0.023$), necroinflammatory grade ($p = 0.029$)

Sens sensitivity, *Spec* specificity, *LR+* positive likelihood ratio, *LR−* negative likelihood ratio, *LS* liver stiffness, *TM* thalassemia major, *TI* thalassemia intermedia, *LB* liver biopsy

documented by MRI. The results showed that RTE values significantly correlate with TE values ($r = 0.645$, $p < 0.0001$), the diagnostic accuracy of RTE in the range of $F \geq 2$ represented by AUROC was 0.798 (95% CI 0.674–0.890), and the diagnostic accuracy of RTE for $F \geq 3$ was 0.909 (95% CI 0.806–0.968). No studies have confirmed the correlation of RTE measurements and histological data, but, on consideration of the consistent results which support the accuracy of TE, it is reasonable to think that LS values too, as measured using other electrographic techniques, could be reliable for assessing liver fibrosis.

On the other hand, conflicting results have been reported regarding the relationship of LS and the amount of iron overload (Table 17.2). Most studies were unable to show any significant correlation between LS and LIC obtained by T2* MRI, suggesting that liver elastography may not be sensitive enough to detect subtle changes in hepatic parenchymal stiffness associated with liver iron deposition [11, 12, 16, 17]. In the study by Fraquelli et al. [11] on 115 patients affected by thalassemia major ($n = 59$) and thalassemia intermedia ($n = 56$), who underwent T2* MRI and liver TE, both groups showed no correlation between LIC, measured by T2* MRI, and TE results ($r = -0.14257$ and $r = 0.09$). At multivariate analysis the variables independently associated with TE values were ALT, GGT, and bilirubin levels in both groups and, in patients with TM, HCV-RNA positivity but not LIC measured by T2* MRI.

Similar results were obtained by Ferraioli et al. [17] in their study involving 119 patients with TM and 183 healthy controls and by Ou et al. [16], whose study observed no significant correlation between TE reading and LIC values, based on T2* MRI (pooled estimate of correlation was -0.06). In the study by Di Marco et al. [12], involving 56 consecutive transfusion-dependent thalassemic patients (45 adults and 11 children) assessed by TE, atomic absorption spectrometry, and liver biopsy, LS increased proportionally to the METAVIR stage, with a highly significant relationship with fibrosis ($r = 0.70$; $p < 0.001$), independently of LIC values

Table 17.2 Correlation between liver stiffness and iron overload (mainly LIC measured by T2* MRI) in patients affected by thalassemia major (TM) or thalassemia intermedia (TI)

Authors	Year	Patients (n)	Correlation coefficient (r)	p
Di Marco et al.	2010	56	0.01	0.932
Fraquelli et al.	2010	59 TM	−0.14	0.876
		56 TI	0.09	
Hamidieh et al.	2014	83	0.42	<0.001
Ferraioli et al.	2016	119	−0.04	0.7
Pipaliya et al.	2017	154	0.85	<0.001
Al-Khabori et al.	2019	94	LIC was higher in patients with significant LSM (median LIC: 7.2 g/g dw) than in patients without significant LSM (median LIC: 5.4 g/g dw)	0.02

($r = 0.01$; $p = 0.932$). It is interesting to note that in all those studies, where no correlation between LS and LIC was found, the proportion of HCV-infected viremic patients was high, ranging between 35% and 49%. Liver stiffness in thalassemic patients could be influenced by different factors. Probably, HCV infection and iron overload interact reciprocally in the progression of liver fibrosis, and the possible presence of cardiac insufficiency can act as a further confounding factor, as increased venous pressure levels [18] can also decrease liver parenchyma elasticity. To support this hypothesis, in other studies conducted on different series of thalassemic patients without or with very low percentage of HCV-RNA positivity [19–21], liver stiffness values were significantly related to LIC values. For example, Al-Khabori et al. studied 94 patients with TM who underwent hepatic 2D shear wave elastography and T2* MRI. In this study the authors found higher LIC values in patients with LS values within the range of significant fibrosis ($p = 0.0225$). The study by Maira et al. [22] on 99 transfusion-dependent thalassemia patients found a significant reduction in LS (6.6 ± 3.2 kPa, $p = 0.017$) and hepatic siderosis measured by LIC (3.65 ± 3.45 mg/g dw, $p = 0.001$) after 4 years on chelation therapy. However, in this study as well, in a subset of HCV-RNA-positive patients on anti-HCV treatment, there was no correlation with LIC despite the improvement in LS: the authors speculated that this circumstance could be due to the increased transfusion requirement during HCV treatment. In another study [23], conducted on 154 pediatric thalassemia patients undergoing TE and T2* MRI, LS measurements correlated with T2* MRI values ($r = 0.85$; $p < 0.001$), and TE results were useful to stratify patients according to the degree (severe, moderate, and mild) of iron overload with AUROC values of 94.8%, 84.5%, and 84.7%, respectively, using LS cut-off values of 13.5 kPa, 7.8 kPa, and 5.5 kPa. In another pediatric study [14] with no cases of HCV coinfection, TE values correlated with liver iron content measured by liver biopsy ($p < 0.001$). Thus, to date, the evidence is still not strong enough to recommend liver elastography as a reliable tool to assess the iron overload in thalassemia patients: in the current guidelines, the combination of serum ferritin and T2* MRI data is reported as the preferred strategy [10] to pursue during the management of patients affected by beta-thalassemia.

Sickle cell disease (SCD) is another common hematological disorder, where various forms of acute and chronic hepatic damage can occur. It is characterized by deformation of red blood cells, thereby vaso-occlusion, ischemia/infarction, and hemolysis involving different organs. The main reasons of liver damage are acute vaso-occlusive crisis (VOC) involving the liver, with a frequency ranging from 10% to 39% [24], iron overload, and concomitant viral hepatitis infection, due to chronic transfusion therapy [25]. Liver serum biomarkers poorly correlate with hepatic involvement during acute VOC, and a precise diagnostic definition and strategy of hepatic involvement during VOC are not available. Thus in 2013 Koh et al. [26] investigated TE as a marker of hepatic involvement during VOC: 23 patients affected by SCD underwent laboratory tests and TE at steady state, and during acute VOC, 15 of them had a liver biopsy at steady state, and all the patients underwent transthoracic echocardiogram to measure tricuspid regurgitation velocity. The results showed that TE at steady state correlated with liver fibrosis ($p = 0.01$) and tricuspid regurgitation velocity ($p = 0.0063$) but not with hepatic iron concentration. In this small population, according to histological results, none of the patients had cirrhosis (Ishak's score 5–6), 14 had no fibrosis or portal fibrosis (Ishak's score 0–2), and only one patient had bridging fibrosis (Ishak's score 3–4). Furthermore, the mean TE measurements increased during acute VOC (6.2–12.3 kPa, $p = 0.003$) paralleling the concomitant increase of alanine aminotransferase (ALT) and alkaline phosphatase ($p = 0.009$ and $p = 0.01$). The authors concluded that TE can be a useful tool during VOC, even if the low number of patients, the lack of a reference standard to diagnose hepatic damage during VOC, and such possible confounding factors as hepatic and systemic necroinflammation and right-heart dysfunction impose further studies to confirm these results.

In the study of Bortolotti et al. [27], that enrolled 68 adult sickle cell patients (17 with sickle cell anemia (SCA), 38 with sickle cell thalassemia (HbS/β-Thal), and 13 with HbSC disease), structural liver abnormalities, defined by abdominal ultrasound and liver stiffness values, resulted more severe in SCA and HbS/β-Thal than HbSC patients. In addition, a statistically significant correlation was found between liver structure at ultrasound and liver stiffness.

As regards the correlation between liver stiffness and liver fibrosis, another study [28] has demonstrated a positive correlation between LS and Ishak's score ($r = 0.068$, $p \leq 0.0001$) in a total of 50 patients with SCD, suggesting how LS could be a reliable non-invasive tool to assess hepatic fibrosis.

Finally, a few studies have investigated the correlation between LS and iron overload with conflicting results. For their prospective study, Delicou et al. [29] enrolled 15 patients affected by SCD and investigated them by TE and T2* MRI at baseline and after 12 months on chelation therapy (deferasirox). The results showed a significant improvement in liver stiffness values, from 9.7 to 6.7 kPa ($p = 0.001$), and in LIC values, from 7.86 to 5.62 mg Fe/g dry weight ($p = 0.043$) after 12 months on deferasirox. Furthermore, a correlation between LIC and LS at baseline ($r = 0.6344$) and at the end of the study ($r = 0.6075$) was found. Also in the prospective study by Drasar et al. [30] on 139 patients affected by SCD, there was a weak but significant correlation between TE values and markers of iron overload (ferritin $r = 0.24$, $p = 0.006$; total blood unit transfused $r = 0.2$, $p = 0.02$; and LIC $r = 0.18$ and $p = 0.04$) even if LIC measured by MRI was available only for 35 patients. On the contrary, in the retrospective study by Pinto et al. [31], no significant correlation was found between mean liver stiffness (measured by FibroScan) and liver iron concentration (measured by MRI), and no significant correlation was documented between liver stiffness and ALT at baseline or at follow-up in 37 patients with SCD. Also, the study by Costa et al. [32] on a pediatric population has showed no correlation between iron quantification (measured by MRI) and LS ($r = -0.077$, $p = 0.769$).

Overall, in the setting of patients with SCD, only a few studies are available; they are based on small size samples and are highly heterogeneous in terms of aims and study design formats. Thus, despite some promising results, no definitive data can be obtained, and further investigation should be conducted.

Hemophilia is a genetic disorder characterized by spontaneous or provoked, often uncontrolled, bleeding into joints, muscles, and other soft tissues. Chronic infection with hepatitis C virus (HCV) has long been the dominant complication of substitution therapy in patients with inherited blood disorders and the cause of anticipated death due to end-stage liver disease. In fact, the prevalence of HCV infection, until a few years ago, has been quite high, because viral inactivation procedures and viral screening of plasma products were not available before 1992. Liver biopsies are generally not performed in these patients because of increased bleeding risk; thus, the search for non-invasive approaches, such as elastography, for the assessment of liver fibrosis is particularly attractive as regards patients with hemophilia and other congenital bleeding disorders. In 2006, Posthouer et al. [33] enrolled 124 patients affected by bleeding disorders and chronic hepatitis C and, using TE to assess LS, found severe fibrosis in 18% and cirrhosis in 17% of them. In the study by Maor et al. [34], 57 hepatitis C-infected patients with hemophilia were evaluated by FibroTest and TE: the results showed that the corresponding concordance rates and κ score for fibrosis stage $\geq$F2, $\geq$F3, or =F4 between FibroTest and TE were 62%, 69%, and 85% and 0.24, 0.32, and 0.44 respectively. Later, Moessner et al. [35] found that among 73 patients with hemophilia A or B and chronic or past hepatitis C, there was significant fibrosis in 17.1% and cirrhosis in 2.9% by LS $\geq$8 and $\geq$12 kPa. It is necessary to underline that all these studies are limited by the lack of liver biopsy as the reference standard and the authors speculate that, knowing the strong correlation of LS with histological results in patients without bleeding disorders, there is no a priori reason to assume that LS would be less reliable in patients with bleeding disorders. Anyway, there are no strict guidelines at present regarding the best method to assess liver fibrosis in hemophilic patients, and the combination of different non-invasive tests (including TE) seems a reliable strategy to apply in most cases.

17.2 Spleen Elastography in Hematological Diseases

To date, a few studies have investigated the potential use of spleen stiffness for evaluating the severity of hematological diseases and to predict prognosis.

In 2015 Webb et al. conducted a small study [36] on nine patients with myelofibrosis, 11 patients with cirrhosis, and eight healthy volunteers, showing that, as determined by TE and shear wave elastography, SS has little ability to distinguish between patients with myelofibrosis and those with cirrhosis, but it allows to differentiate both patient groups from the healthy volunteers. More interestingly, in 2013 Fraquelli et al. [37], for the first time, showed that SS could be clinically useful in patients with myeloproliferative disorders. During an investigation on the diagnostic accuracy of combining LS and SS in order to predict liver fibrosis and portal hypertension in patients with chronic viral hepatitis, the authors evaluated LS and SS in a cohort of 48 patients with hematological malignancies, used as controls without significant hepatic comorbidity. All the patients were characterized according to the WHO histological classification of bone marrow fibrosis, and none of them had splanchnic vessel thrombosis. The most interesting result found in these patients was a correlation between SS and bone marrow fibrosis ($r = 0.64, p < 0.01$), which was more pronounced in patients with primary myelofibrosis (PMF) than in those with other hematological malignancies. In addition, SS values significantly correlated with the longitudinal diameter and volume of the spleen ($r = 0.39$ and $r = 0.66, p < 0.001$), and liver TE and spleen TE did not correlate with each other or with age, gender, and BMI.

Following these results and given the critical association between bone marrow fibrosis and spleen status in PMF patients, Iurlo et al. conducted a study [38] with the aim to assess whether SS measured by TE can be used as a marker of the bone marrow fibrosis and as a predictor of clinical prognosis. Liver and spleen TE were successfully performed in 81.5% of the 108 consecutive PMF patients. Besides, bone marrow fibrosis grade and clinical and laboratory features were collected. The results showed a significant correlation, at univariate analysis, between SS and LS with the severity of bone marrow fibrosis ($p < 0.001$ and $p < 0.007$, respectively), with the values of Hb and LDH ($p < 0.001$ and $p < 0.001$) and with the three different main prognostic scoring systems. More importantly, multivariate analysis has shown that only SS, LDH, and International Prognostic Scoring System (IPSS) maintained a significant correlation with bone marrow fibrosis, with the area under the receiver operating characteristic curve being 0.909 (95% CI 0.850–0.968). These parameters were incorporated in a diagnostic algorithm that allowed to classify 40% of the patients as being at pre-fibrotic/early fibrotic stage and 22% at advanced fibrotic stage. An interesting small data set was also to show that in three patients treated with ruxolitinib, the improvements in constitutional symptoms were paralleled by reduction in SS.

References

1. Vergniol J, Foucher J, Terrebonne E, Bernard PH, le Bail B, Merrouche W, et al. Noninvasive tests for fibrosis and liver stiffness predict 5-year outcomes of patients with chronic hepatitis C. Gastroenterology. 2011;140(7):1970–9. https://doi.org/10.1053/j.gastro.2011.02.058, 1979.e1–3.
2. de Lédinghen V, Vergniol J, Barthe C, Foucher J, Chermak F, Le Bail B, et al. Non-invasive tests for fibrosis and liver stiffness predict 5-year survival of patients chronically infected with hepatitis B virus. Aliment Pharmacol Ther. 2013;37(10):979–88. https://doi.org/10.1111/apt.12307.
3. Vergniol J, Boursier J, Coutzac C, Bertrais S, Foucher J, Angel C, et al. Hepatology. 2014;60(1):65–76. https://doi.org/10.1002/hep.27069.
4. Elalfy MS, Esmat G, Matter RM, Abdel Aziz HE, Massoud WA. Liver fibrosis in young Egyptian beta-thalassemia major patients: relation to hepatitis C virus and compliance with chelation. Ann Hepatol. 2013;12(1):54–61.
5. Musallam KM, Motta I, Salvatori M, Fraquelli M, Marcon A, Taher AT, et al. Longitudinal changes in serum ferritin levels correlate with measures of hepatic stiffness in

transfusion-independent patients with β-thalassemia intermedia. Blood Cells Mol Dis. 2012;49(3–4):136–9. https://doi.org/10.1016/j.bcmd.2012.06.001.

6. Elalfy MS, Adly AA, Attia AA, Ibrahim FA, Mohammed AS, Sayed AM. Effect of antioxidant therapy on hepatic fibrosis and liver iron concentrations in β-thalassemia major patients. Hemoglobin. 2013;37(3):257–76. https://doi.org/10.3109/03630269.2013.778866.

7. Kamal S, Abdelhakam S, Ghoraba D, Mohsen MA, Salam AA, Hassan H, et al. The course of hepatitis C infection and response to anti-viral therapy in patients with thalassemia major and hepatitis C infection: a longitudinal, prospective study. Mediterr J Hematol Infect Dis. 2019;11(1):e2019060. https://doi.org/10.4084/MJHID.2019.060.

8. Allegra S, Cusato J, De Francia S, Longo F, Pirro E, Massano D, et al. The effect of vitamin D pathway genes and deferasirox pharmacogenetics on liver iron in thalassaemia major patients. Pharm J. 2019;19(5):417–27. https://doi.org/10.1038/s41397-019-0071-7.

9. Cassinerio E, Orofino N, Roghi A, Duca L, Poggiali E, Fraquelli M, et al. Combination of deferasirox and deferoxamine in clinical practice: an alternative scheme of chelation in thalassemia major patients. Blood Cells Mol Dis. 2014;53(3):164–7. https://doi.org/10.1016/j.bcmd.2014.04.006.

10. Cappellini MD, Cohen A, Porter J, Taher A, Viprakasit V, editors. Guidelines for the management of Transfusion Dependent Thalassaemia (TDT). 3rd ed. Nicosia: Thalassaemia International Federation; 2014. PMID: 25610943.

11. Fraquelli M, Cassinerio E, Roghi A, Rigamonti C, Casazza G, Colombo M, et al. Transient elastography in the assessment of liver fibrosis in adult thalassemia patients. Am J Hematol. 2010;85(8):564–8. https://doi.org/10.1002/ajh.21752.

12. Di Marco V, Bronte F, Cabibi D, Calvaruso V, Alaimo G, Borsellino Z, et al. Noninvasive assessment of liver fibrosis in thalassaemia major patients by transient elastography (TE) - lack of interference by iron deposition. Br J Haematol. 2010;148(3):476–9. https://doi.org/10.1111/j.1365-2141.2009.07996.x.

13. Poustchi H, Eslami M, Ostovaneh MR, Modabbernia A, Saeedian FS, Taslimi S, et al. Transient elastography in hepatitis C virus-infected patients with beta-thalassemia for assessment of fibrosis. Hepatol Res. 2013;43(12):1276–83. https://doi.org/10.1111/hepr.12088.

14. Hamidieh AA, Shazad B, Ostovaneh MR, Behfar M, Tayebi S, Malekzadeh R, et al. Noninvasive measurement of liver fibrosis using transient elastography in pediatric patients with major thalassemia who are candidates for hematopoietic stem cell transplantation. Biol Blood Marrow Transplant. 2014;20(12):1912–7. https://doi.org/10.1016/j.bbmt.2014.07.025.

15. Paparo F, Cevasco L, Zefiro D, Biscaldi E, Bacigalupo L, Balocco M, et al. Diagnostic value of real-time elastography in the assessment of hepatic fibrosis in patients with liver iron overload. Eur J Radiol. 2013;82(12):e755–61. https://doi.org/10.1016/j.ejrad.2013.08.038.

16. Ou G, Ko HH, Tiwari P, Sandhu N, Galorport C, Lee T, et al. Utility of transient elastography in estimating hepatic iron concentration in comparison to magnetic resonance imaging in patients who are transfusion-dependent: a Canadian center experience. Hemoglobin. 2017;41(1):21–5. https://doi.org/10.1080/03630269.2017.1307763.

17. Ferraioli G, Lissandrin R, Tinelli C, Scudeller L, Bonetti F, Zicchetti M, et al. Liver stiffness assessed by transient elastography in patients with β thalassaemia major. Ann Hepatol. 2016;15(3):410–7. https://doi.org/10.5604/16652681.1198817.

18. Millonig G, Friedrich S, Adolf S, Fonouni H, Golriz M, Mehrabi A, et al. Liver stiffness is directly influenced by central venous pressure. J Hepatol. 2010;52(2):206–10. https://doi.org/10.1016/j.jhep.2009.11.018.

19. Al-Khabori M, Daar S, Al-Busafi SA, Al-Dhuhli H, Alumairi AA, Hassan M, et al. Noninvasive assessment and risk factors of liver fibrosis in patients with thalassemia major using shear wave elastography. Hematology. 2019;24(1):183–8. https://doi.org/10.1080/10245332.2018.1540518.

20. Sinakos E, Perifanis V, Vlachaki E, Tsatra I, Raptopoulou-Gigi M. Is liver stiffness really unrelated to liver iron concentration? Br J Haematol. 2010;150(2):247–8. https://doi.org/10.1111/j.1365-2141.2010.08183.x.

21. Sousos N, Sinakos E, Klonizakis P, Adamidou D, Daniilidis A, Gigi E, et al. Deferasirox improves liver fibrosis in beta-thalassaemia major patients. A five-year longitudinal study from a single thalassaemia centre. Br J Haematol. 2018;181(1):140–2. https://doi.org/10.1111/bjh.14509.
22. Maira D, Cassinerio E, Marcon A, Mancarella M, Fraquelli M, Pedrotti P, et al. Progression of liver fibrosis can be controlled by adequate chelation in transfusion-dependent thalassemia (TDT). Ann Hematol. 2017;96(11):1931–6. https://doi.org/10.1007/s00277-017-3120-9.
23. Pipaliya N, Solanke D, Parikh P, Ingle M, Sharma R, Sharma S, et al. Comparison of tissue elastography with magnetic resonance imaging T2* and serum ferritin quantification in detecting liver iron overload in patients with thalassemia major. Clin Gastroenterol Hepatol. 2017;15(2):292–298.e1. https://doi.org/10.1016/j.cgh.2016.08.046.
24. Koskinas J, Manesis EK, Zacharakis GH, Galiatsatos N, Sevastos N, Archimandritis AJ. Liver involvement in acute vaso-occlusive crisis of sickle cell disease: prevalence and predisposing factors. Scand J Gastroenterol. 2007;42(4):499–507.
25. Chaturvedi S, DeBaun MR. Evolution of sickle cell disease from a life-threatening disease of children to a chronic disease of adults: the last 40 years. Am J Hematol. 2016;91(1):5–14. https://doi.org/10.1002/ajh.24235.
26. Koh C, Turner T, Zhao X, Minniti CP, Feld JJ, Simpson J, et al. Liver stiffness increases acutely during sickle cell vaso-occlusive crisis. Am J Hematol. 2013;88(11):E250–4. https://doi.org/10.1002/ajh.23532.
27. Bortolotti M, D'Ambrosio R, Fraquelli M, Pedrotti P, Consonni D, Migone De Amicis M, Scaramellini N, Di Pierro E, Graziadei G. Liver damage and sickle cell disease: genotype relationship. Ann Hematol. 2020;99:2065. https://doi.org/10.1007/s00277-020-04113-3.
28. Ben Yakov G, Sharma D, Alao H, Surana P, Kapuria D, Etzion O, et al. Vibration controlled transient elastography (FibroScan®) in sickle cell liver disease - could we strike while the liver is hard? Br J Haematol. 2019;187(1):117–23. https://doi.org/10.1111/bjh.16047.
29. Delicou S, Maragkos K, Tambaki M, Kountouras D, Koskinas J. Transient Elastography (TE) is a useful tool for assessing the response of liver iron chelation in sickle cell disease patients. Mediterr J Hematol Infect Dis. 2018;10(1):e2018049. https://doi.org/10.4084/MJHID.2018.049.
30. Drasar E, Fitzpatrick E, Gardner K, Awogbade M, Dhawan A, Bomford A, et al. Interim assessment of liver damage in patients with sickle cell disease using new non-invasive techniques. Br J Haematol. 2017;176(4):643–50. https://doi.org/10.1111/bjh.14462.
31. Pinto VM, Gianesin B, Balocco M, Bacigalupo L, Forni GL. Noninvasive monitoring of liver fibrosis in sickle cell disease: longitudinal observation of a cohort of adult patients. Am J Hematol. 2017;92(12):E666–8. https://doi.org/10.1002/ajh.24918.
32. Costa P, Rudolph B, Kogan-Liberman D, Manwani D, Silver EJ, Ovchinsky N. Liver stiffness measurement by vibration controlled transient elastography does not correlate to hepatic iron overload in children with sickle cell disease. J Pediatr Hematol Oncol. 2020;42(3):214–7. https://doi.org/10.1097/MPH.0000000000001726.
33. Posthouwer D, Mauser-Bunschoten EP, Fischer K, VAN Erpecum KJ, DE Knegt RJ. Significant liver damage in patients with bleeding disorders and chronic hepatitis C: non-invasive assessment of liver fibrosis using transient elastography. J Thromb Haemost. 2007;5(1):25–30. https://doi.org/10.1111/j.1538-7836.2006.02272.x.
34. Maor Y, Halfon P, Bashari D, Pénaranda G, Morali G, Klar R, et al. Fibrotest or Fibroscan for evaluation of liver fibrosis in haemophilia patients infected with hepatitis C. Haemophilia. 2010;16(1):148–54. https://doi.org/10.1111/j.1365-2516.2009.02092.x.
35. Moessner BK, Andersen ES, Weis N, Laursen AL, Ingerslev J, Lethagen S, et al. Previously unrecognized advanced liver disease unveiled by transient elastography in patients with Haemophilia and chronic hepatitis C. Haemophilia. 2011;17(6):938–43. https://doi.org/10.1111/j.1365-2516.2011.02520.x.
36. Webb M, Shibolet O, Halpern Z, Nagar M, Amariglio N, Levit S, et al. Assessment of liver and spleen stiffness in patients with myelofibrosis using fibroscan and shear wave elastography. Ultras Q. 2015;31(3):166–9. https://doi.org/10.1097/RUQ.0000000000000139.

37. Fraquelli M, Giunta M, Pozzi R, Rigamonti C, Della Valle S, Massironi S, et al. Feasibility and reproducibility of spleen transient elastography and its role in combination with liver transient elastography for predicting the severity of chronic viral hepatitis. J Viral Hepat. 2014;21(2):90–8. https://doi.org/10.1111/jvh.12119.
38. Iurlo A, Cattaneo D, Giunta M, Gianelli U, Consonni D, Fraquelli M, et al. Transient elastography spleen stiffness measurements in primary myelofibrosis patients: a pilot study in a single centre. Br J Haematol. 2015;170(6):890–2. https://doi.org/10.1111/bjh.13343.

Part VI

Case Studies

Case 1: Unexpected High Liver Stiffness as a Warning Sign

18

Ilaria Fanetti and Elisabetta Degasperi

18.1 Case Report

We report here on the case of an 80 year old patient, E.F., with a long-term history of chronic hepatitis C virus (HCV) infection.

E.F. presented to the Hepatology Unit of our Hospital in 1996, just after evidence of anti-HCV positivity at routine tests prescribed by his General Practitioner. The patient's medical history was not significant except for previous dental surgery and appendicectomy, which he had undergone when he was 20 years old. He had a normal body mass index (BMI 23) and denied any significant smoking or alcohol consumption, any prior blood transfusion, or use of intravenous drugs.

At admission he underwent complete blood testing: transaminases were slightly above the upper normal limit, without alteration of the other liver function tests (LFTs), while glucose, lipid panel, autoimmunity, and iron load were unremarkable and the patient's HBV profile was consistent with a previous exposure. HCV infection, genotype 1b, was confirmed. Abdominal ultrasound was normal and concomitant causes of liver damage were considered unlikely. In order to assess the severity of the disease, liver biopsy was performed and it showed a mild activity of disease with low fibrotic changes according to Ishak's staging. Therefore, by taking into account the unfavorable HCV genotype, the transaminases pattern, and the low

Supplementary Information The online version of this chapter (https://doi.org/10.1007/978-3-030-74132-7_18) contains supplementary material, which is available to authorized users.

I. Fanetti (✉)
Gastroenterology and Endoscopy Unit, Fondazione IRCCS Ca' Granda, Ospedale Maggiore Policlinico, Milan, Italy

E. Degasperi
Gastroenterology and Hepatology Unit, Fondazione IRCCS Ca' Granda, Ospedale Maggiore Policlinico, Milan, Italy

© Springer Nature Switzerland AG 2021
M. Fraquelli (ed.), *Elastography of the Liver and Beyond*,
https://doi.org/10.1007/978-3-030-74132-7_18

degree of fibrosis, he was not considered for IFN-based regimen and was regularly followed up at the Center with no antiviral treatment.

In 2018, after the availability of IFN-free regimens, the patient was proposed for HCV treatment with direct-acting antivirals (DAA) and he underwent a liver disease re-assessment. The blood tests still showed a slight elevation in transaminases and a mild increase in gGT level (83 U/L, nl <50 U/L); platelets were normal and HCV-RNA viral load was 12,644 UI/ml. Physical examination and abdominal ultrasound were normal, revealing a normal liver parenchyma, with smooth margins, and without any indirect sign of portal hypertension (the spleen longitudinal diameter was 9 cm, the portal diameter was 1 cm); liver stiffness assessed by transient elastography (Fibroscan®) resulted 6.1 kPa (IQR 1.2 kPa, SR 100%), consistent with a F0–F1 degree of fibrosis. Overall, the presence of advanced liver disease was deemed unlikely.

The patient was treated with elbasvir/grazoprevir for 12 weeks: HCV-RNA became undetectable at on-treatment week 4 and remained undetectable for 12 weeks after the end of treatment (EOT), resulting in the achievement of a sustained virological response (SVR). Other blood exams were unremarkable.

Transient elastography was performed 6 months after EOT and, unexpectedly, the liver stiffness value was 22.3 kPa (IQR 5.6 kPa, SR 100%). The blood tests, especially LFTs, were stable but a new abdomen ultrasound investigation revealed partial portal vein thrombosis (Fig. 18.1) and a focal hypoechoic lesion 12 mm wide in segment VII. Alpha-fetoprotein (aFP) was 414 ng/ml and a subsequent abdominal CT scan revealed multiple nodular lesions with arterial enhancement and portal

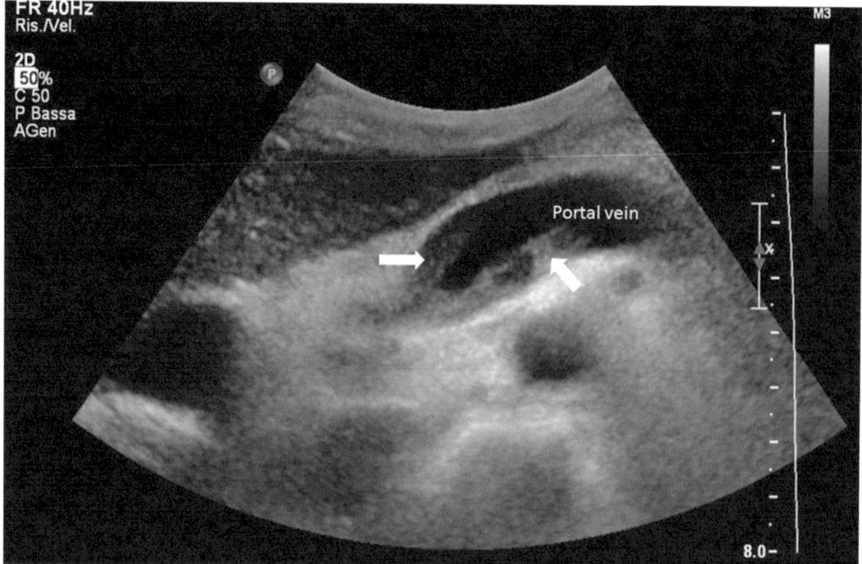

Fig. 18.1 Ultrasound image showing partial portal vein thrombosis represented by the presence of echogenic material inside the portal vein (arrows)

wash-out, which were consistent with a multi-focal hepatocellular carcinoma (HCC). Portal vein thrombosis (PVT) appeared to be neoplastic and multiple abdominal adenopathies were found at the hepatic hilum and close to the Inferior vena cava (IVC). Liver biopsy confirmed the HCC diagnosis. A complete stadiation was performed; thoracic computed tomography (CT) scan and scintigraphy were negative, but the evidence of abdominal distant adenopathies was consistent with BCLC stage C. Gastroscopy revealed F1 blue varices, without red signs. Therefore, the patient was proposed for sorafenib but eventually died shortly after disease progression.

18.2   Comments

The present case report refers to a patient with a long history of HCV infection, probably over more than 60 years; he develops a multi-focal HCC and neoplastic portal vein thrombosis (PVT) after the achievement of SVR, despite the evidence of persistently low-degree hepatic fibrosis. Transient elastography (TE) performed before DAA treatment was consistent with F0-F1 disease and appeared to remain stable for approximately 22 years, confirming the histological evaluation performed at HCV diagnosis.

The patient achieved SVR, but his liver stiffness assessed by transient elastography remarkably worsened shortly after treatment, significantly increasing from 6.1 to 22.3 kPa. However, subsequent imaging revealed PVT and the presence of a multi-focal HCC, giving out a clue for the unpredicted liver stiffness increase, possibly being a "false positive" of transient elastography and not associated with any "true worsening" of the liver fibrosis. Other causes of false-positive increase of TE are extrahepatic cholestasis, vascular congestion secondary to cardiac insufficiency, as well as liver damage due to acute hepatitis or transaminases flare and recent food intake: these factors can reversibly increase liver stiffness and lead to the misdiagnosis of severe liver fibrosis [1]. In this case, a possible explanation of stiffness increase, as hypothesized by Valla et al. [2], is the compensatory arterial buffer response to the PVT that can happen in the hepatic vasculature, similarly to what happens post-prandially because of the increased portal vein flow.

A similar case of increased liver stiffness and portal vein thrombosis was described by Huang et al. [3], where a non-cirrhotic patient with a previous diagnosis of PVT was found to have an abnormal TE value (17.3 kPa). However, as they reported, PVT was non-neoplastic and the patient was treated with antiretrovirals for HIV; both these conditions might represent confounding factors since an additional vascular mechanism might have been associated. Also, no previous elastography assessment was available.

Concerning HCC development, our patient showed a mild fibrosis stage and did not present with any significant comorbidity (irrelevant alcohol consumption and no metabolic syndrome associated), all accounting for a very low risk of HCC development. Also, he had no clinical or radiological evidence of any advanced liver disease and underwent abdominal ultrasounds on a 12-month interval, in agreement with the available guidelines for non-cirrhotic patients [4]. However, the possibility of

HCC development in non-cirrhotic patients has been reported and the long history of HCV infection might have played a role in this patient. HCC development in patients without cirrhosis may be associated with different pathogenic pathways and biochemical features [5]. Prospective studies on patients with eradicated HCV infection are needed in order to identify subgroups of patients who still are at risk of HCC development and who might still need active surveillance in spite of low fibrosis, the absence of comorbidities, and HCV eradication. In this setting, the role and accuracy of such noninvasive methods as liver stiffness measurement need further investigation.

References

1. Petitclerc L, Sebastiani G, Gilbert G, Cloutier G, Tang A. Liver fibrosis: review of current imaging and MRI quantification techniques. J Magn Reson Imaging. 2017;45:1276–95.
2. Valla DC, Condat B. Portal vein thrombosis in adults: pathophysiology, pathogenesis and management. J Hepatol. 2000;32:865–71.
3. Huang R, Zu-Hua G, Tang A, Sebastiani G, Deschenes M. Transient elastography is an unreliable marker of liver fibrosis in patients with portal vein thrombosis. Hepatology. 2018;68(2):783–5.
4. EASL Clinical Practice Guidelines: management of hepatocellular carcinoma. J Hepatol. 2018;69:182–236.
5. Gaddikeri S, McNeeley MF, Wang CL, Bhargava P, Dighe MK, Yeh MMC, et al. Hepatocellular carcinoma in the non-cirrhotic liver. Am J Roentgenol. 2014;203:34–47.

Case 2: Liver and Spleen Stiffness After TIPS

19

Simone Segato

19.1 Case Report

C.A., a 57 years old male, was first admitted to our hospital in October 2017 for the occurrence of ascites. During hospitalization he was diagnosed with decompensated liver cirrhosis with a double etiology: hepatitis C virus infection (HCV, genotype I) and chronic alcohol abuse. He was treated with large-volume paracentesis, albumin supplementation, and diuretic therapy with clinical benefit. He also underwent esophagogastroduodenoscopy, which showed the presence of esophageal varices (F2).

After discharge he stopped alcohol consumption and started chronic diuretic treatment.

Therapy with nonselective betablockers was also recommended for the primary prevention of variceal bleeding, but because of patient reported intolerance (fatigue), the treatment was stopped.

He was also treated with direct antiviral agents (sofosbuvir/velpatasvir + ribavirin) over 12 weeks for chronic HCV infection obtaining sustained viral response (SVR).

Despite these therapies, he progressively developed a condition of refractory ascites, with the need for weekly large-volume paracentesis.

For this reason, in July 2019 he was put forward for trans-jugular intrahepatic portosystemic shunt (TIPS) placement.

Supplementary Information The online version of this chapter (https://doi.org/10.1007/978-3-030-74132-7_19) contains supplementary material, which is available to authorized users.

S. Segato (✉)
Gastroenterology and Endoscopy Unit, Fondazione IRCCS Ca' Granda Ospedale Maggiore Policlinico, Milan, Italy
e-mail: simone.segato@unimi.it

© Springer Nature Switzerland AG 2021
M. Fraquelli (ed.), *Elastography of the Liver and Beyond*,
https://doi.org/10.1007/978-3-030-74132-7_19

Table 19.1 The patient's parameters measured by elastography and intravascular manometry before and after TIPS placement

| | TE (kPa) | | pSWE (kPa) | | Intravascular manometry (mmHg) | | |
	LS	SS	LS	SS	Portal	Caval	Gradient
Before tips	32 (IQR 12.2)	47 (IQR 14)	33.2 (IQR 4.7)	49.8 (IQR 11.8)	33	11	22
After tips	28 (IQR 6)	36 (IQR 7.5)	35.4 (IQR 6.7)	36.5 (IQR 10.1)	20	12	8

kPa kilo-Pascal, *IQR* inter-quartile range, *SR* success rate, *SD* standard deviation

Table 19.2 The patient's parameters measured by color-*Doppler* ultrasound (CDUS)

	Portal vein (flow direction)	Portal vein flow velocity (cm/sec)	Shunt flow velocity (cm/sec)	Intrahepatic portal vein branches (flow direction)
Before tips	Hepatopetal	17	–	–
After tips	Hepatopetal	35	95	Hepatofugal

According to our internal protocols, he underwent color-Doppler ultrasound (CDUS) examination, and liver and splenic measurement by transient elastography (TE, with Fibroscan by Echosens, Paris, France) and point shear-wave elastography (pSWE, with ElastPQ, iU22 by Philips, Bothell, Washington DC, USA) before and after TIPS placement.

Tables 19.1 and 19.2 provide the main measurements obtained by CDUS examination and elastography (both TE and pSWE) before and after TIPS placement.

19.2 Comments

The role of TIPS in the treatment of complications of portal hypertension is well established.

Despite that, since TIPS dysfunction is often asymptomatic, an accurate screening test is required to confirm shunt patency. The reference standard for assessing TIPS function is venography with portosystemic pressure gradient measurement: evidence of a reduction of PPG to less than 12 mmHg is considered the pressure target especially in those patients for whom bleeding was the indication for the shunt [1].

CDUS has been extensively studied for measuring intra-stent and main portal vein flow velocities and flow direction in the intrahepatic portal vein branches; CDUS has shown to be a reliable qualitative indicator of TIPS malfunction [1] (Fig. 19.1).

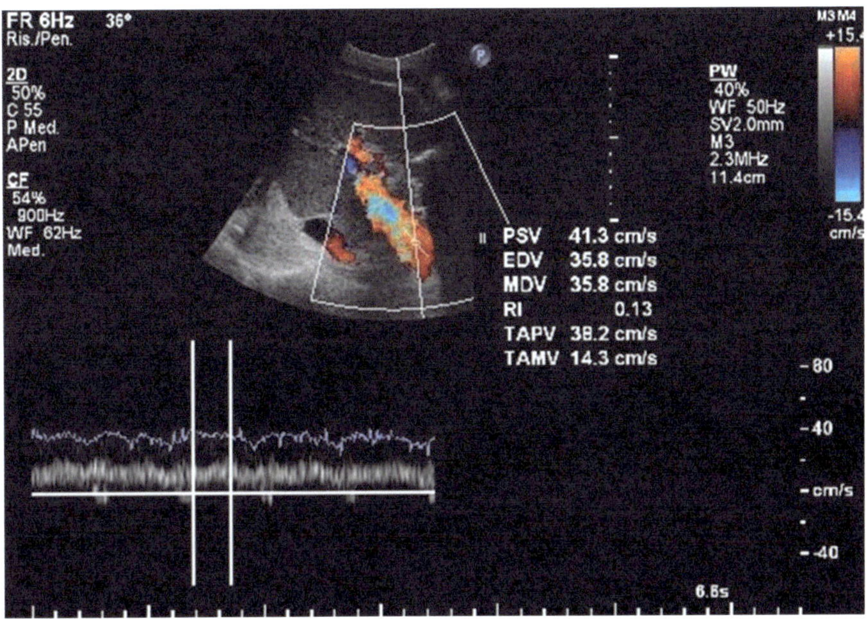

Fig. 19.1 Echo-Doppler ultrasound scan with portal vein velocity measurement

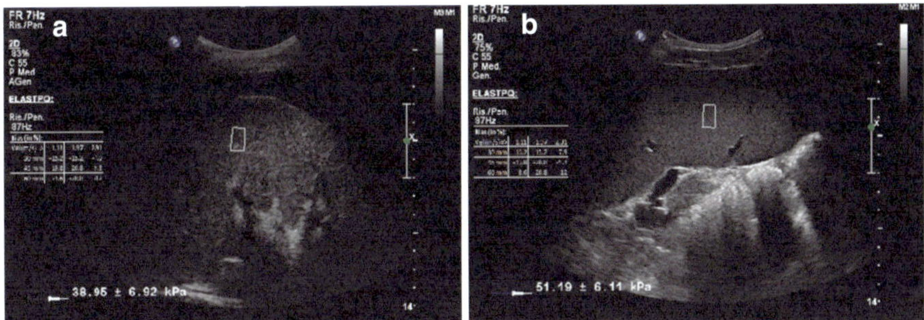

Fig. 19.2 Liver (**a**) and spleen (**b**) stiffness measurement with ARFI technique (ElastPQ)

In addition, recent data has indicated the promising role of liver and especially spleen stiffness (SS) in the assessment of portal hypertension thanks to its good correlation with HVPG values (Fig. 19.2a and b). Several studies have demonstrated the good diagnostic accuracy of SS, particularly in ruling the presence of esophageal varices out [2–6].

More recently, several preliminary studies [7–11] have shown a progressive significant reduction of SS values after successful TIPS implantation.

In a recent study Giunta et al. [12] have evaluated 24 patients undergoing TIPS placement and suggested that spleen point shear-wave elastography (with a 25-kPa cut off) and the assessment of blood flow direction in the intrahepatic portal vein branches (considering hepatopetal flow as pathologic) are good predictors of TIPS dysfunction.

In this clinical case, TIPS placement achieved good reduction of portal hypertension, with final pressures under the threshold of clinical significance (12 mmHg).

It must be noted that elastography values obtained with both methods (transient elastography and point shear-wave elastography) decrease in parallel with the degree of portal hypertension. In particular, spleen stiffness seems to have good rapid reduction in response to portal hypertension changes, considering the fact that the values reported were measured the day after TIPS placement. As concerns the CDUS parameters, the finding of hepatofugal blood flow direction within the intrahepatic portal vein branches suggests good TIPS function.

Further studies are needed to confirm the role of these techniques for the noninvasive evaluation of portal hypertension especially in the setting of portosystemic shunt function, which remains an important clinical challenge. However, the current knowledge on elastography and ultrasound parameters seems useful and reproducible.

References

1. Fagiuoli S, Bruno R, Debernardi Venon W, et al. Consensus conference on TIPS management: techniques, indications, contraindications. Dig Liver Dis. 2017;49(2):121–37. https://doi.org/10.1016/j.dld.2016.10.011.
2. Calvaruso V, Bronte F, Conte E, Simone F, Craxì A, Di Marco V. Modified spleen stiffness measurement by transient elastography is associated with presence of large oesophageal varices in patients with compensated hepatitis C virus cirrhosis. J Viral Hepat. 2013;20(12):867–74. https://doi.org/10.1111/jvh.12114.
3. Colecchia A, Montrone L, Scaioli E, et al. Measurement of spleen stiffness to evaluate portal hypertension and the presence of esophageal varices in patients with HCV-related cirrhosis. Gastroenterology. 2012;143(3):646–54. https://doi.org/10.1053/j.gastro.2012.05.035.
4. Sharma P, Kirnake V, Tyagi P, et al. Spleen stiffness in patients with cirrhosis in predicting esophageal varices. Am J Gastroenterol. 2013;108(7):1101–7. https://doi.org/10.1038/ajg.2013.119.
5. Fraquelli M, Giunta M, Pozzi R, et al. Feasibility and reproducibility of spleen transient elastography and its role in combination with liver transient elastography for predicting the severity of chronic viral hepatitis. J Viral Hepat. 2014;21(2):90–8. https://doi.org/10.1111/jvh.12119.
6. Boyer TD, Haskal ZJ. American Association for the Study of Liver Diseases Practice Guidelines: the role of transjugular intrahepatic portosystemic shunt creation in the management of portal hypertension. J Vasc Interv Radiol. 2005;16(5):615–29. https://doi.org/10.1097/01.RVI.0000157297.91510.21.
7. Gao J, Zheng X, Zheng Y-Y, et al. Shear wave elastography of the spleen for monitoring transjugular intrahepatic portosystemic shunt function: a pilot study. J Ultrasound Med. 2016;35(5):951–8. https://doi.org/10.7863/ultra.15.07009.
8. Ran HT, Ye XP, Zheng YY, et al. Spleen stiffness and splenoportal venous flow: assessment before and after transjugular intrahepatic portosystemic shunt placement. J Ultrasound Med. 2013;32(2):221–8. https://doi.org/10.7863/jum.2013.32.2.221.
9. Novelli PM, Cho K, Rubin JM. Sonographic assessment of spleen stiffness before and after transjugular intrahepatic portosystemic shunt placement with or without concurrent emboliza-

tion of portal systemic collateral veins in patients with cirrhosis and portal hypertension: a feasibility study. J Ultrasound Med. 2015;34(3):443–9. https://doi.org/10.7863/ultra.34.3.443.
10. De Santis A, Nardelli S, Bassanelli C, et al. Modification of splenic stiffness on acoustic radiation force impulse parallels the variation of portal pressure induced by transjugular intrahepatic portosystemic shunt. J Gastroenterol Hepatol. 2018;33(3):704–9. https://doi.org/10.1111/jgh.13907.
11. Buechter M, Manka P, Theysohn JM, Reinboldt M, Canbay A, Kahraman A. Spleen stiffness is positively correlated with HVPG and decreases significantly after TIPS implantation. Dig Liver Dis. 2018;50(1):54–60. https://doi.org/10.1016/j.dld.2017.09.138.
12. Giunta M, La Mura V, Conti CB, Casazza G, Tosetti G, Gridavilla D, Segato S, Nicolini A, Primignani M, Lampertico P, Fraquelli M. The role of spleen and liver elastography and color-Doppler ultrasound in the assessment of transjugular intrahepatic portosystemic shunt function. Ultrasound Med Biol. 2020; S0301-5629(20)30180-0.

Case 3: Congestive Hepatopathy with High Liver and Spleen Stiffness in a 17 Years Old Male Patient

Andrea Costantino, Mirella Fraquelli, Massimo Chessa, and Vincenzo La Mura

20.1 Case Report

We hereby report on the case of F.C., a 17 years old male patient, who was initially referred to our Unit on the advice of his cardiologist at a tertiary referral center. He presented with an anatomic single ventricle, also known as univentricular heart, a condition known since birth. The univentricular heart is defined as the presence of only one well-developed ventricle and the other rudimentary ventricle (if present) with less than 30% of its expected volume. The patient underwent a first surgical procedure by Glenn in 2005, followed by Fontan surgery in 2008. The Fontan procedure, firstly described as a surgical palliation for a single ventricle with tricuspid atresia, has become the standard operation for all patients with single-ventricle physiology (*e.g.*, hypoplastic left-heart syndrome, pulmonary atresia, unbalanced atrio-ventricular canal defects) [1–4].

The Fontan operation is a palliative surgical procedure aimed at diverting the systemic venous return to the lungs without a pump. The pulmonary blood flow is

Supplementary Information The online version of this chapter (https://doi.org/10.1007/ 978-3-030-74132-7_20) contains supplementary material, which is available to authorized users.

A. Costantino (✉) · M. Fraquelli
Gastroenterology and Endoscopy Unit, Fondazione IRCCS Ca' Granda Ospedale Maggiore Policlinico, Milan, Italy

M. Chessa
IRCCS Policlinico San Donato, ACHD Unit – Pediatric and Adult Congenital Heart Centre, San Donato M.se, Milan, Italy

V. La Mura
Fondazione IRCCS Ca' Granda Ospedale Maggiore Policlinico, "Angelo Bianchi Bonomi" Haemophilia and Thrombosis Center, Fondazione Luigi Villa, CRC "A. M. and A. Migliavacca" Center for Liver Diseases, Milan, Italy

Department of Biomedical Sciences for Health, Università degli Studi di Milano, Milan, Italy

M. Fraquelli (ed.), *Elastography of the Liver and Beyond*,
https://doi.org/10.1007/978-3-030-74132-7_20

driven by central venous pressure and is augmented by changes in the intra-thoracic pressure, active relaxation of the systemic ventricle (drawing blood forward), and the peripheral skeletal muscle pump [5].

The first surgical step (called Glenn procedure) is performed at the age of 1 year and consists of a direct anastomosis between the superior caval vein and the right pulmonary artery. The Fontan operation is regularly carried out as a second surgical step when the child is around 4 years old. It consists in a connection between the inferior systemic vein drainage and the pulmonary branches. This connection is achieved with an intra- or extracardiac prosthetic conduit of different sizes.

Following the Fontan procedure, patients can take morbidity and mortality risks and require lifelong follow-up by cardiologists experienced in the care of patients with complex congenital heart diseases.

F.C was diagnosed to have a univentricular heart already at prenatal age and since birth he has received specialist support. He was operated by Fontan procedure in May 2008. Since then he has been followed at the cardiological referral center without specific problems, but a very mild progressive desaturation.

The patient underwent regular cognitive and neuropsychological development assessments as well as all the mandatory immunization schedules for infants and children plus antipneumococcal immunization.

As regards family history, his 50 years old father was in good health and his 50 years old mother presented congenital nystagmus. The patient was the elder of two children, his 11-year-old brother being in good health.

The patient has been taking aspirin from childhood, except for a period of about 1.5 years on coumadin, interrupted on specialist indication with no history of drug mismanagement. He has completely abstained from alcohol and drugs.

On first referral to our Hepatology Outpatient Clinic, he was asymptomatic and had been conducting a normal lifestyle consistent with his age group. He only reported a tendency to muscle exhaustion during physical education and his cardiologist outlined the mild desaturation without other pathological signs.

Recent blood tests had revealed slightly increased hemoglobin levels (18.2 g/dL), gamma glutamyl transpeptidase (GGT) levels (69 U/L; n.v. <55 U/L in men) and alanine transaminases (ALT) levels (48 U/L, n.v. 5–40 U/L), and bilirubin 1.6 mg/dL (direct 1.1) with normal aspartate transaminases (AST) levels (31; n.v. 29–38 U/L). ProBNP levels resulted within the normal range (72 pg/mL, n.v. 100 pg/ml).

At physical examination the parameters were: blood pressure 130/75, heart rate 91 beats/min, BMI 20.8 kg/m^2. On inspection the patient's abdomen was flat, painless at deep palpation, and the peristalsis was normal. The liver and spleen edges were not palpable. A first reinforced sound (S1) could be heard at cardiac auscultation with no cardiac murmurs and peripheral bruits.

We performed an abdomen ultrasound scan (Epiq, Philips Ultrasound Inc., Bothell, WA) with shear-wave elastography and transient elastography (TE) (Echosens, Paris, France).

The abdominal ultrasound test revealed a normal-sized liver with a normal echotexture with no focal liver lesions. The liver margins were regular without surface nodularity when assessed by high-frequency transducer. There were regular patent hepatic veins with regular triphasic flow, a regular-sized portal vein (1 cm), hepato-petal biphasic flow with average speed at 14 cm/s, and normal intrahepatic biliary and main biliary tracts. The gallbladder was normally distended with no gallstones.

The patient's spleen size was within normal values (bipolar diameter 11.7 cm, area 49 cm²), with homogeneous echo-texture. The pancreas and kidneys showed normal findings. There was no abdominal effusion.

The patient's liver stiffness, as measured by TE, resulted 19.7 kPa, IQR/median 14% and spleen stiffness 50 kPa (IQR/median 7%).

These results were discussed with the patient's cardiologist and in January 2019 a right catheterization was performed showing a normal low mean pressure in all the "Fontan" system (inferior vena cava, prosthetic conduit, pulmonary branches) and a telediastolic pressure of the systemic ventricle. The only anomalous finding was the evidence of veno-venous fistulas, which were embolized. The veno-venous fistulas are the aftermath of the pressure increase in the hemodynamic Fontan system as an attempt of the vascular system to reduce the systemic venous pressure.

20.2 Comments

The different elastographic techniques applied showed increased liver and spleen stiffness, likely to be due to an impaired venous outflow.

Hepatic congestion may develop if the venous outflow from the liver is obstructed. Disorders leading to hepatic congestion that result in hepatomegaly and a firm tender liver edge include: Budd-Chiari syndrome, hepatic sinusoidal obstruction syndrome (SOS), previously termed veno-occlusive disease, and right-sided heart failure.

Any cause of right-sided heart failure can result in hepatic congestion, including constrictive pericarditis, mitral stenosis, tricuspid regurgitation, *cor pulmonale*, and cardiomyopathy. Tricuspid regurgitation in particular can be associated with severe hepatic congestion because of the transmission of right ventricular pressure directly into the hepatic veins. Liver dysfunction and passive congestion are common in patients with congenital heart disease and single-ventricle physiology who have undergone the Fontan intervention.

Patients with hepatic congestion are usually asymptomatic. In such patients, hepatic congestion may be suggested only by abnormal liver biochemical tests during routine evaluation. Symptomatic patients may present with jaundice, which may be mistaken for biliary obstruction.

The most common liver biochemical abnormality of Fontan-associated liver disease (FALD) is a mild elevation in the serum bilirubin level, which occurs in up to 70% of patients. The total serum bilirubin is usually less than 3 mg/dL, most of which is unconjugated [6].

The precise cause of the hyper-bilirubinemia is uncertain. Contributing factors may include: hepatocellular dysfunction, hemolysis, pulmonary infarction, canalicular obstruction due to distended hepatic veins, medications, and super-imposed sepsis.

Imaging studies to apply in such cases are: right-upper quadrant ultrasonography with Doppler studies of the portal and hepatic veins and hepatic artery, electrocardiogram, and echocardiography.

Other imaging approaches to identify hepatic congestion and assess fibrosis, including diffusion-weighted magnetic resonance imaging and magnetic resonance elastography, are under investigation at present [7–10].

As regards the possible role of elastography techniques in these patients some studies have reported high liver stiffness values [10, 11]. Whether the increased stiffness depends on flow congestion or initial fibrosis is an important issue to be ascertained and has been preliminary investigated. A recent review has underlined that noninvasive liver stiffness measurements are of minimal utility as all patients with congestive hepatopathy have elevated values, which cannot currently differentiate between congestion and fibrosis. In addition, fibrosis staging by liver biopsy is difficult to standardize because of heterogeneous collagen deposition in this disease [10].

In the Liver Adult-Pediatric-Congenital-Heart-Disease Dysfunction Study (LADS) hepatic stiffness and vascular Doppler indices using ultrasound (US) and liver stiffness measured by SWE were measured in a cohort of patients who had undergone Fontan surgery.

In that study patients with Fontan physiology had significantly higher hepatic stiffness (15.6 kPa *vs.* 5.5 kPa, $p < 0.0001$) as compared to the control group [11]. In fact, the elevated hepatic afterload in Fontan, manifested by high ventricular end-diastolic pressures and pulmonary arterial wedge pressures, is associated with remarkably increased hepatic stiffness, abnormal vascular flow patterns, and fibrotic histologic changes. Correlation was explored between SWE, US, hemodynamic and histopathologic data, obtained in a subset of patients, and greater stiffness correlated with greater degrees of histopathologic fibrosis [11].

A prospective multicenter observational study enrolled 152 patients who had undergone Fontan surgery [12]. The primary outcome was liver nodules detection at US and magnetic resonance (MRI) or computer tomography (CT) scan. Liver nodule prevalence was 29.6% on US and 47.7% (95% CI 39–56%) on MRI/CT. The sensitivity and specificity of US were 50% (95% CI 38–62%) and 85.3% (95% CI 75–92%), respectively. Hepatocellular carcinoma was histologically diagnosed in 2 of the 8 patients with hypervascular liver nodules displaying washout. While liver nodules are frequent in Fontan patients, they may go unnoticed at US. Liver nodules are usually hyperechoic, hypervascular, and predominantly peripheral. This population is at risk of hepatocellular carcinoma, the diagnosis of which requires confirmatory biopsy.

It is worth noting that, in a recent study involving 145 patients [13], the severity of FALD has significantly correlated with Fontan duration and impaired Fontan hemodynamics and that in the majority of patients hepatic abnormalities suggestive of FALD have been detectable by liver ultrasound, transient elastography, and laboratory analysis. At multivariate analysis Fontan duration has shown the only variable independently associated with FALD development.

In conclusion, FALD is increasingly recognized as more patients survive into adulthood and it is considered a significant prognostic factor.

The availability of reliable noninvasive markers of liver disease in these patients would be of great value, and liver stiffness as measured by elastography technique is very promising in association with imaging techniques to predict disease severity. Liver stiffness increases can be related either to hepatic congestion or, later on, to subsequent hepatic fibrosis. Therefore, liver stiffness deserves not only a role to identify the severity of a potential fibrogenic disease of the liver, but it also deserves potential interest as a noninvasive diagnostic tool to identify Fontan circuit dysfunction in a preclinical phase. Along this line, the evaluation of splenic stiffness is a further interesting issue to account for and that may be added in the clinical management of these patients. Further studies are required to confirm the possible prognostic role of these noninvasive tools in stratifying patients according to their risk of more severe disease.

References

1. Rychik J, Atz AM, Celermajer DS, Gatzoulis MA, Gewillig MH, Hsia MA, et al. Evaluation and management of the child and adult with Fontan circulation: a scientific statement from the american heart association. Circulation. 2019; CIR0000000000000696.
2. Stout KK, Daniels CJ, Aboulhosn JA, Bozkurt B, Broberg CS, Colman JM, et al. 2018 AHA/ACC Guideline for the Management of Adults With Congenital Heart Disease: A Report of the American College of Cardiology/American Heart Association Task Force on Clinical Practice Guidelines. J Am Coll Cardiol. 2019;73:e81.
3. Driscoll DJ. Long-term results of the Fontan operation. Pediatr Cardiol. 2007;28:438.
4. Fontan F, Baudet E. Surgical repair of tricuspid atresia. Thorax. 1971;26:240.
5. Shafer KM, Garcia JA, Babb TG, et al. The importance of the muscle and ventilatory blood pumps during exercise in patients without a subpulmonary ventricle (Fontan operation). J Am Coll Cardiol. 2012;60:2115.
6. Dunn GD, Hayes P, Breen KJ, Schenker S. The liver in congestive heart failure: a review. Am J Med Sci. 1973;265:174.
7. Wells ML, Fenstad ER, Poterucha JT, Hough DM, Young PM, Araoz PA, et al. Imaging findings of congestive hepatopathy. Radiographics. 2016;36:1024.
8. Dogan Y, Soylu A, Kilickesmez O, Demirtas T, Kilickesmez TA, Dogan SN, et al. The value of hepatic diffusion-weighted MR imaging in demonstrating hepatic congestion secondary to pulmonary hypertension. Cardiovasc Ultrasound. 2010;8:28.
9. Elsayes KM, Shaaban AM, Rothan SM, Javadi BL, Castillo RP, et al. A comprehensive approach to hepatic vascular disease. Radiographics. 2017;37:813.
10. Lemmer A, Van Wagner LB, Ganger D. Assessment of advanced liver fibrosis and the risk for hepatic decompensation in Patients with Congestive Hepatopathy. Hepatology. 2018;68:1633.
11. Kutty S, Peng Q, Danford D, Fletcher SE, Perry D, Talmon GA, et al. Increased hepatic stiffness as consequence of high hepatic afterload in the fontan circulation: a vascular doppler and elastography study. Hepatology. 2014;59:251–60.
12. Téllez L, Rodríguez de Santiago E, Minguez B, Payance A, Clemente A, Baiges A, et al. Prevalence, features and predictive factors of liver nodules in Fontan surgery patients: The VALDIG Fonliver prospective cohort. J Hepatol. 2020;72(4):702–10.
13. Schleiger A, Salzmann M, Kramer P, Danne F, Schubert S, Bassir C, et al. Severity of Fontan-associated liver disease correlates with fontan hemodynamics. Pediatr Cardiol. 2020;41(4):736–46.

Case 4: To Operate or Not to Operate? A Case of Crohn's Disease When Elastography Helped

Stefano Mazza and Mirella Fraquelli

21.1 Case Report

D.S., a 45 years old man, was diagnosed with ileal Crohn's disease when he was 36 years old. At his first presentation in July 2011, the patient complained of a 6-month history of diarrhea with 3–4 bowel movements per day, recurrent abdominal pain mainly located at the right flank/iliac fossa, and some episodes of food vomiting.

Ileo-colonoscopy revealed aphthous ileitis for a 10-cm (at least) length of the distal ileum, a rigid and ulcerated ileocecal valve, and a normal colonic and rectal mucosa.

The histological examination of the ileal biopsies was suggestive of Crohn's disease.

The patient was initially treated with azathioprine (2 mg/kg/die) with improvement of bowel habits, but persistence of recurrent abdominal pain and nausea. After 2–3 years, during 2014 the frequency of the pain episodes increased (about 5–6 occurrences per year), so in March 2015 the patient was started on biological therapy with anti-TNF-alfa (infliximab 5 mg/kg). Symptoms subsequently improved and the patient was well for about a year. However, in February 2016 he experienced a subocclusive episode with intense abdominal pain and repeated vomiting, which resolved spontaneously with fasting. At this point, the choices were: to optimize the infliximab treatment (i.e., to shorten the infusion frequency from 8 down to 4 weeks), to change the drug, or to proceed to surgery. In order to differentiate between a prevalent inflammatory disease activity that would benefit from therapy enhancement, and a fibrotic disease in which surgery would be the only effective approach, both bowel ultrasound (US) with ultrasound strain elasticity imaging (UEI) and

S. Mazza · M. Fraquelli (✉)
Gastroenterology and Endoscopy Unit, Fondazione IRCCS Ca' Granda Ospedale Maggiore Policlinico, Milan, Italy
e-mail: mirella.fraquelli@policlinico.mi.it

© Springer Nature Switzerland AG 2021
M. Fraquelli (ed.), *Elastography of the Liver and Beyond*,
https://doi.org/10.1007/978-3-030-74132-7_21

magnetic resonance enterography (MRE) were performed. US revealed a distal ileum involvement for at least 10 cm, with a thickened bowel wall (max 9–10 mm), slight wall hypervascularity at color-Doppler, and prevalently hypoechogenic pattern (Fig. 21.1a). Elastographic examination showed a predominantly hard (blue) pattern at the color scale (Fig. 21.1b), and a strain ratio of 2.4 at post-examination analysis (Fig. 21.1c). This strain ratio value was considered as indicative of severe ileal fibrosis, as reported [1, 2]. MRE, performed a week later, was basically in agreement with US: it showed a 9-cm segment of the distal ileum with wall thickening up to 12 mm and contrast hyperenhancement. Moreover, at delayed enhancement study the wall appeared stratified at the early phase (70 s, Fig. 21.2a) and homogeneous at the late phase (7 min, Fig. 21.2b), with enhancement progression over time. This contrast medium behavior has been reported as indicative of severe intestinal fibrosis at MRE [3]. Thus, the conclusion was that the patient had a fibrotic disease and in June 2016 he underwent surgery with a "classic" ileocecal resection

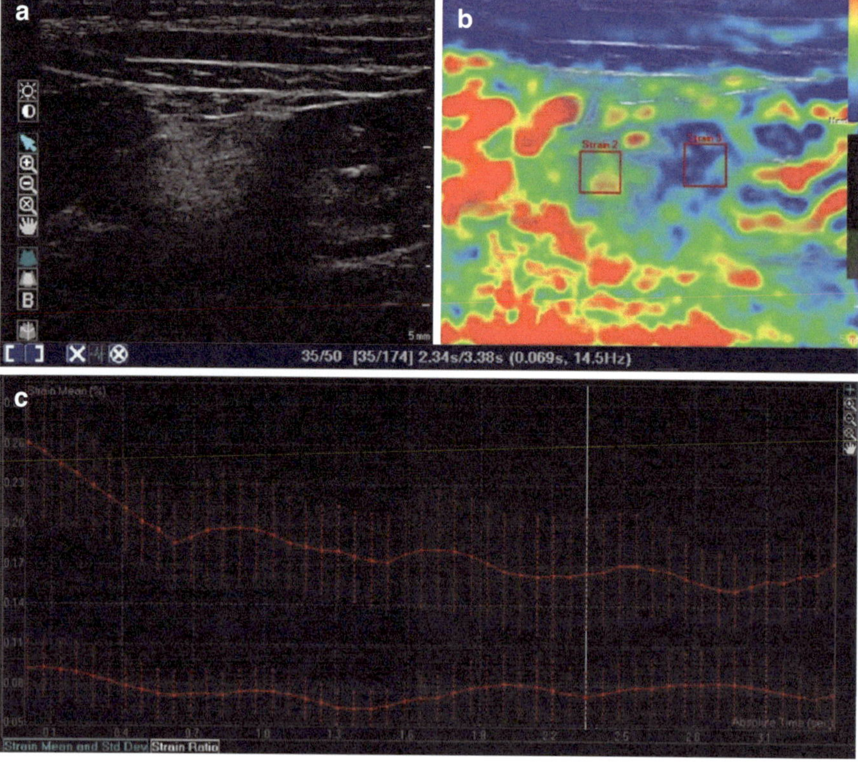

Fig. 21.1 Intestinal ultrasound image showing a thickened terminal ileum with a prevalently hypoechogenic pattern (**a**). Ultrasound elasticity image (UEI) at color scale with the selection of regions of interest in the mesenteric tissue [ROI 1] and in the bowel wall [ROI 2] to calculate tissue strain. The semiquantitative real-time assessment of wall stiffness shows a predominantly hard (blue) pattern (**b**). Quantitative strain values of ROI 1 [mesenteric tissue] and ROI 2 [ileal wall] plotted over time (**c**)

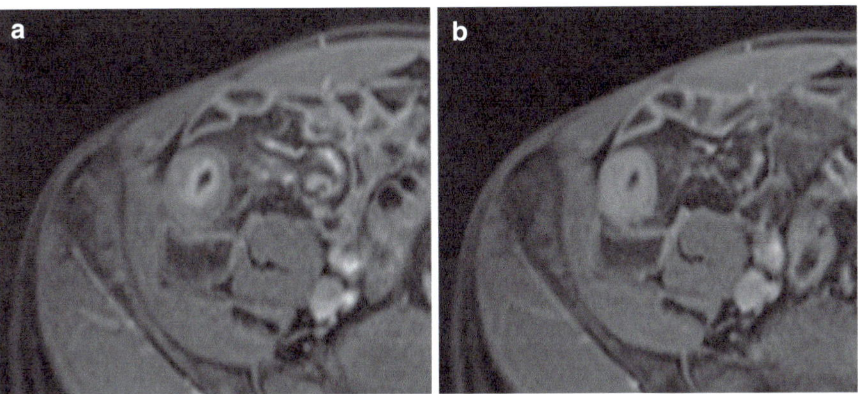

Fig. 21.2 Magnetic resonance (MR) enterography test showing a 9-cm segment of the distal ileum with wall thickening and contrast hyperenhancement. At delayed enhancement study the wall appeared stratified at the early phase (**a**) and homogeneous at the late phase (7 min) (**b**) with enhancement progression over time

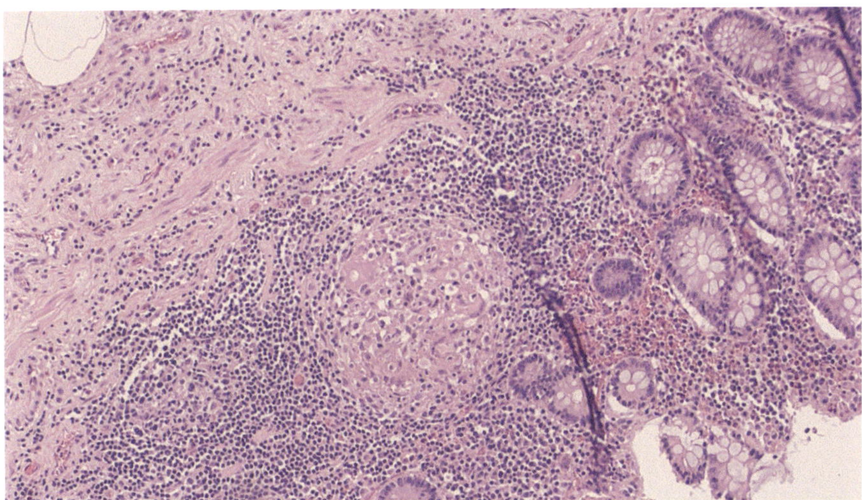

Fig. 21.3 Histopathology image of affected terminal ileum stained with hematoxylin/eosin (H&E) confirming the diagnosis of Crohn's disease with a typical finding of mucosal epithelioid cell granuloma

with ileo-colonic anastomosis; the postoperative course was regular. Histological examination confirmed the diagnosis of Crohn's disease with a typical finding of mucosal epithelioid cell granuloma (Fig. 21.3).

Azathioprine was reintroduced after surgery for prevention of postoperative disease recurrence. At ileo-colonoscopy 1 year after surgery, endoscopic remission (Rutgeerts i1) was observed. Clinical remission was maintained for nearly 2 years until 2018, when the patients started complaining of recurrent right flank pain and a slight increase in bowel movements. US with elastography was again performed to reveal a short (2–3 cm) thickened intestinal segment at the site of the anastomosis, with a soft (green) pattern, and a strain ratio of 0.9 at elastographic examination. Therefore, the treatment was enhanced with the starting of the patient on adalimumab (i.e., a 160/80 scheme of induction followed by 40 mg every other week) in June 2018, with the subsequent resolution of abdominal pain. To date, the patient still maintains clinical remission on adalinumab therapy Ileo-colonoscopy, perfomed in September 2020, evidenced endoscopic remission.

References

1. Fraquelli M, Branchi F, Cribiù FM, Orlando S, Casazza G, Magarotto A, et al. The role of ultrasound elasticity imaging in predicting ileal fibrosis in Crohn's disease patients. Inflamm Bowel Dis. 2015;21:2605–12.
2. Orlando S, Fraquelli M, Coletta M, Branchi F, Magarotto A, Conti CB, et al. Ultrasound elasticity imaging predicts therapeutic outcomes of patients with Crohn's disease treated with anti-tumour necrosis factor antibodies. J Crohns Colitis. 2018;12:63–70.
3. Rimola J, Planell N, Rodríguez S, Delgado S, Ordaas I, Ramirez-Morro A, et al. Characterization of inflammation and fibrosis in Crohn's disease lesions by magnetic resonance imaging. Am J Gastroenterol. 2015;110:432–40.

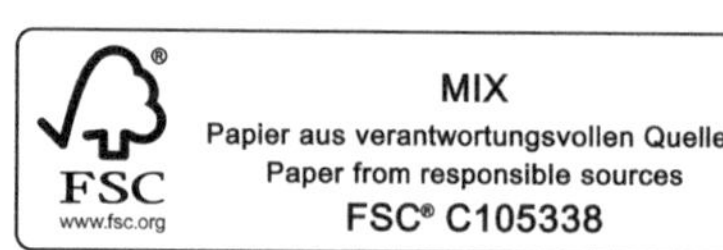

MIX
Papier aus verantwortungsvollen Quellen
Paper from responsible sources
FSC® C105338